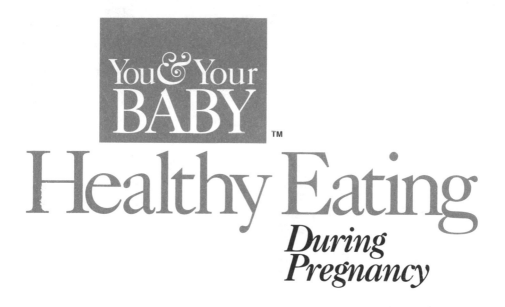

You & Your BABY™
Healthy Eating
During Pregnancy

D0711859

Dr. Laura Riley, OB/GYN
and Stacey Nelson, MS, RD, LDN

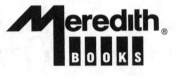

Meredith Books
1716 Locust Street
Des Moines, Iowa 50309-3023
meredithbooks.com

You & Your Baby™ is a trademark of Meredith Corporation.

First Edition.
Printed in the United States of America.
Library of Congress Control Number: 2006921322
ISBN-13: 978-0-696-23186-5
ISBN-10: 0-696-23186-7

Dr. Laura Riley

Life is a whirlwind for Dr. Laura Riley, author of *You & Your Baby: Pregnancy*, medical director of labor and delivery at Massachusetts General Hospital in Boston, and dedicated mom to daughters Natalie and Lauren. She is also assistant professor of obstetrics, gynecology, and reproductive biology at Harvard Medical School.

Dr. Riley has been committed to serving pregnant women for 15 years. At Boston City Hospital she focused on high-risk pregnant women, with an emphasis on HIV disease. In 1995 she joined Massachusetts General Hospital, where she currently practices, to focus on high-risk pregnancy with an emphasis on infectious disease complications of obstetrics. She has participated in numerous research projects. Her current project, sponsored by the National Institutes of Health, investigates epidural-related fever.

Dr. Riley is a consultant to the Centers for Disease Control (CDC). She has been on several major committees at the American College of Obstetricians and Gynecologists (ACOG); most recently she was chair of the Obstetric Practice Committee, which drafts guidelines for obstetric care in the United States. She has been quoted extensively in national publications, including the *Wall Street*

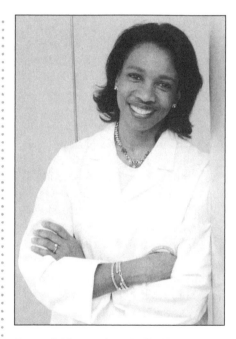

Journal, Newsweek, and *The New York Times*, and has appeared on NBC's *Today* and CBS's *The Early Show*. She has published numerous articles in peer-reviewed scientific journals.

Dr. Riley is a graduate of Harvard University. She received her medical degree at the University of Pittsburgh, completed an internship and residency in obstetrics and gynecology at the Magee-Womens Hospital of University of Pittsburgh, and completed subspecialty training in maternal fetal medicine at Brigham and Women's Hospital and in infectious disease at Boston University Medical Center.

Stacey Nelson

Stacey Nelson, M.S., R.D., LDN, is a senior clinical nutritionist with more than 17 years of clinical and community nutrition experience. She received a bachelor of science degree in nutrition sciences from the University of New Hampshire and a master of science degree in human nutrition and metabolism from Boston University. She completed her dietetic internship at the former New England Deaconess Hospital in Boston. Since 2000, she has been with the nutrition services department at Boston's Massachusetts General Hospital, where she also serves as the dietitian for the Vincent Obstetrics Service. Her areas of interest include perinatal nutrition, women's health, and adult weight management, in which she holds a Certificate of Training from the Commission on Dietetic Registration. She has been quoted in a variety of publications including *American Baby*

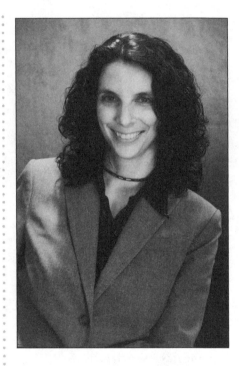

and *Babytalk* magazines, and she appears in the local media to comment on nutrition-related news and research.

acknowledgments

I thank Lauren, Natalie, Scott, my parents, and my aunts for their support in this project. While I worked on this book, they enjoyed an even healthier diet. I also appreciate the contributions of Dr. Michael Greene, Dr. David Nathan, and C. C. Martin who provided valuable editorial comments. Thank you to my pregnant patients and my obstetric colleagues who suggested many of the topics included in this book. Finally, I enthusiastically thank Stacey Nelson for providing great nutrition advice to my pregnant patients over the last 6 years and for taking the time and effort to write it all down. Stacey and I had the pleasure of working with a great team: Alice Lesch Kelly, a talented writer who helped us communicate the complicated science into a user-friendly book, and Stephanie Karpinske, our very patient editor and accomplished registered dietitian.

Laura Riley

There are many people to thank, but none as important as Laura Riley. Thank you, Laura, for the opportunity to write this book with you and for the information and support you provide each day at work. I'd also like to give thanks to Alice Lesch Kelly, without whom this book would not have been possible, and to our editor Stephanie Karpinske for her invaluable experience and guidance throughout this process. Great thanks to my family and friends, who were excited about this book when it was only a vague concept and became ever more excited as it took shape in the flesh. A special thank you to Lillian Sonnenberg, DSc, R.D., for her support and to all my fellow R.D.s at MGH Nutrition Services. And last but certainly not least, I'd like to thank all of my patients: It is because of their collective experiences and feedback that I knew the time for this particular book had come.

Stacey Nelson

6

Contents

contents

Here's where to go to find more information about the many topics this
book covers.

PART 2: Healthy Recipes for Before, During, and After Pregnancy

Check here for a handy index to recipes that make healthy eating both simple and
delicious for you and your whole family.

Get the calcium you need each day with these recipes. They offer a good variety of
high-calcium options beyond the traditional glass of milk.

Women need more iron during pregnancy, so make sure you get enough with
these many tasty dishes.

If you normally eat a diet low in fiber, now is the time to make a change. These
easy recipes will get you started.

Don't feel like eating much? Try one of these nutritious mini meals.

Instead of driving through a fast-food place to grab a bite to eat, try one of these
recipes for foods-to-go.

When time is short, it's tempting to head for the nearest restaurant, but
these dishes give you a fast and healthy homemade alternative.

The thought of a long kitchen cleanup keeps many people from cooking. These
one-dish dinners are designed to keep the aftermath to a minimum.

This section is meant to help you in those first weeks home with baby. Just make
these meals toward the end of your pregnancy, freeze them, and they'll be ready
when you need them.

Are you longing for dessert but still want to eat healthy? These treats are the
perfect answer.

From the Authors

Even before the amazing journey of pregnancy begins, most women are struggling to figure out the answer to the question: What is a healthy diet? Thousands of studies have been done, scores of guidelines from experts compiled, and data from every health and nutrition group imaginable offered. So much information is floating around out there that it is tempting to just throw up one's hands, eat whatever tastes good, and hope for the best. Pregnancy adds a whole new layer of complexity. Some health care providers may give you a detailed diet to follow, filled with warnings, "shoulds," and "shouldn'ts." Others may say, "Eat healthy" and "Don't gain too much weight"—and leave the details of how to do it to you.

Before I had children, I was in the latter group. I didn't know much about nutrition and therefore couldn't give my patients much guidance. Years of practice as an obstetrician and mother of two have forced me to learn the basics. I also realized that since I work among nutrition experts every day, I should tap into their wealth of knowledge.

In this book, I have teamed up with Stacey Nelson, a registered dietitian who has been helping pregnant women through this process for more than 12 years. We will give you the information necessary to determine what constitutes a healthy diet before you become pregnant and what the important differences are once you conceive and in the months after you deliver. Our book provides the most up-to-date information so that you can make informed, confident, and educated decisions. After all, the ultimate decision of what to eat or not eat rests with you! We hope the easy, personalized checklists and the numerous recipes and snack ideas will make this an informative, efficient, and fun journey for both pregnant and new moms. We're so excited to be a part of your pregnancy.

Laura Riley, M.D., OB/GYN

Stacey Nelson, M.S., R.D., LDN

a healthy
everyday diet

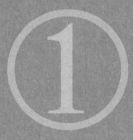

Eating a nutritious diet is one of the best ways to fight off disease and keep your body strong and healthy. But what exactly is a nutritious diet? Which foods should you choose and which should you avoid? Deciding what and how much to eat can be confusing, especially with so many fad diets out there. Don't worry—once you know the basics, putting together a smart eating plan is easier than it sounds. Essentially a healthy diet is one that includes plenty of vegetables, fruits, whole grains, and legumes, along with lean meats and low-fat dairy products. In this chapter, you'll learn all the important basics, including how to make good use of the U.S. government's new food pyramid.

A Healthy Everyday Diet

"You are what you eat," the old saying goes, and it's never been proved truer than it is today. Hardly a week goes by without news of a major research study that shows a connection between a healthy diet and a reduced risk of disease. But what is a healthy diet? The answer to that question has been evolving as scientists learn more about what nutrients various foods contribute and how those nutrients impact health. Before you learn what constitutes a healthy pregnancy diet, it's a good idea to brush up on the basics of good nutrition. This chapter tells you everything you need to know about healthy eating. The chapters that follow give specific guidelines, tips, advice, and information about a healthy pregnancy diet.

Dietary recommendations today are much different from what they were 50 years ago, 20 years ago, or even 10 years ago. In the 1990s, the U.S. Department of Agriculture developed a food pyramid that graphically described what kinds of food people should eat and in what amounts. In 2005, the Department of Agriculture revised the food pyramid and renamed it "MyPyramid." The new pyramid reflects the principles of the 2005 Dietary Guidelines for Americans, a set of recommendations the federal government issues every five years,

detailing the current scientific thinking on what constitutes a healthy diet.

The MyPyramid food guidance system helps you figure out what you should eat for optimal health. It also assists you in customizing your diet based on your size, age, gender, and level of physical activity.

Here's a look at some of the nutritional advice from MyPyramid, which represents the most up-to-date findings on healthy eating. Keep in mind that this chapter details the components of a healthy diet in general. Chapter 2 tackles what foods you should add or subtract to create a healthy diet during pregnancy.

If you'd like to find out more, or if you'd like to use some of the interactive online tools and diet trackers, go to www.mypyramid.gov and www.mypyramidtracker.gov.

MyPyramid Food Groups

MyPyramid divides foods into several groups. Within each group, it gives recommendations on which foods deliver the most nutritional power, as well as how much to eat.

Grain group

Grains are carbohydrate-rich foods made from wheat, rice, oats, cornmeal, barley, or other cereal grains. Grains are divided into two groups: whole grains and refined grains. Whole grains contain the entire kernel of the grain: the bran, germ, and endosperm. Refined grains are whole grains that have been processed. During processing, the bran and germ are removed. This gives the grains a finer texture, but it also removes most of the grain's nutrients. Because processed grains are stripped of their nutrients, many are enriched, which means certain nutrients (iron and vitamins from the B family) are added back into the products.

What grains contribute to the diet: Whole grains are rich in dietary fiber, several B vitamins (thiamin, riboflavin, niacin, and folate), and the minerals iron, magnesium, and selenium. Consuming whole grains helps reduce the risk of coronary heart disease, constipation, obesity, and some kinds of cancer. It also may help reduce blood cholesterol levels.

Daily recommendation for adults: 5–8 servings, depending on gender, age, and daily calorie level. At least half should be whole grain. (See "Healthy Eating Meal Plans," page 395.)

Selection tips: Choose breads, cereals, and pastas made with whole grains. Choose brown rice over white rice and whole wheat pasta over white pasta. Experiment cooking with unfamiliar grains such as bulgur, quinoa, and barley.

To incorporate grains into your diet: Substitute whole wheat flour for up to half of the white flour in home-baked muffins, cakes, or pancakes. (You may need to add extra leavening, such as baking powder or baking soda.) Add whole grain bread crumbs to meat loaf, stir whole wheat cereal into yogurt, and use rolled oats as a breading for fish.

Common whole grains
Amaranth
Brown rice
Buckwheat
Bulgur (cracked wheat)
Millet
Oatmeal
Popcorn
Quinoa
Sorghum
Triticale
Whole grain barley, rye, and cornmeal
Whole grain breakfast cereals
Whole wheat bread, crackers, pasta, rolls, tortillas
Wild rice

Common refined grains*
Cereals that aren't whole grain
Corn bread
Corn tortillas
Couscous
Crackers
Flour tortillas
Grits
Noodles
Pasta
Pita bread
Pretzels
White bread and rolls
White rice
*Some foods that you may think of as being refined, such as pasta, come in whole grain versions. Check the food label for the words "whole wheat" or "whole grain."

Whole Grain Foods and Serving Sizes	
Whole Grain Food	MyPyramid Serving Size
Bagel	½ small (2-ounce) bagel or 1 mini (1-ounce) bagel
Bread	1 slice
Bulgur	½ cup cooked
Cracker	5 whole wheat crackers or 2 rye crispbreads
English muffin	½ muffin
Oatmeal	½ cup cooked
Pancake	1 pancake (4½ inches in diameter)
Popcorn	3 cups popped
Ready-to-eat breakfast cereal	1 cup flakes or 1¼ cups puffed
Rice	½ cup cooked, or 1 ounce dry
Pasta	½ cup cooked, or 1 ounce dry
Tortilla	1 tortilla (6 inches in diameter)

Vegetable group

This group includes raw, cooked, fresh, frozen, and canned vegetables, as well as vegetable juice. Vegetables comprise five subgroups based on their nutrient content: orange, dark green, dried beans and peas, starchy, and other.

What vegetables contribute to the diet: Vegetables add a wide range of vitamins and minerals (especially vitamin A, folate, vitamin C, vitamin E, and potassium), as well as dietary fiber. Studies show that a diet rich in fruits and vegetables may reduce the risk of heart disease, stroke, type 2 diabetes, high blood pressure, and cancer (particularly cancer of the mouth, stomach, colon, and rectum).

Daily recommendation for adults: 2–3 cups, depending on gender, age, and daily calorie level (see "Healthy Eating Meal Plans," page 395).

Selection tips: Buy vegetables that are easy to prepare, including frozen vegetables, bags of prewashed and precut vegetables, and salad greens.

To incorporate vegetables into your diet: Add vegetables to pizzas, stews, soups, and pasta sauces. Serve raw veggies with low-fat dip. Shred carrots or zucchini into meat loaf, casseroles, muffins, and quick breads. Serve a vegetable main dish for dinner once a week. Cook and puree vegetables and use the puree to thicken stews, soups, and gravies.

Orange vegetables
Acorn squash
Butternut squash
Carrots
Hubbard squash
Pumpkin
Sweet potatoes

Dark green vegetables
Bok choy
Broccoli

Collard greens
Dark green leafy lettuce
Kale
Mesclun
Mustard greens
Romaine lettuce
Spinach
Turnip greens
Watercress

Dried beans and peas*
Black beans
Black-eyed peas
Garbanzo beans (chickpeas)
Kidney beans
Lentils
Mature lima beans
Navy beans
Pinto beans
Soybeans
Split peas
Tofu (bean curd made from soybeans)
White beans
*These foods are considered part of
   both the vegetable and the meat and
   beans group. See "Meat and beans
   group," page 15.

Starchy vegetables
Corn
Lima beans
Green peas
Potatoes

Other vegetables
Artichokes
Asparagus
Bean sprouts
Beets
Brussels sprouts
Cabbage
Cauliflower

Celery
Cucumbers
Eggplant
Green beans
Green or red sweet peppers
Iceberg lettuce
Mushrooms
Okra
Onions
Parsnips
Tomatoes
Turnips
Vegetable juice (such as tomato juice)
Wax beans
Zucchini

Fruit group
The fruit group consists of fruit that
is fresh, frozen, canned, raw, cooked,
or dried and may be whole, cut up, or
pureed. It also includes 100-percent
fruit juice.
   What fruit contributes to the diet:
Fruits offer a wide range of vitamins
and minerals (especially vitamin C,
potassium, and folate), as well as
dietary fiber. Studies show that a diet
rich in fruits and vegetables may
reduce the risk of heart disease, stroke,
type 2 diabetes, high blood pressure,
and cancer (especially cancer of the
mouth, stomach, colon, and rectum).
   Daily recommendation for adults:
1½–2 cups, depending on gender, age,
and daily calorie level (see "Healthy
Eating Meal Plans," page 395).
   Selection tips: Choose fresh, frozen,
dried, and canned fruits (canned in
water or natural juices, not heavy
syrup). Buy fresh fruit in season, when
it is at the height of flavor. For
convenience, buy precut fruits such as

pineapple chunks. Select juices that
are labeled 100-percent fruit juice.
   To incorporate fruit into your diet:
Top cereal with sliced fruit, mix berries
into yogurt, add fruit to salads and
main dishes, and serve baked apples
for dessert. Keep a bowl of fresh fruit
on the kitchen counter and a container
of fruit salad in the refrigerator for easy
snacking. Stock the fridge with
100-percent fruit juice, such as orange,
apple, grape, and grapefruit juices.

Common fruits
Apples
Apricots
Avocados
Bananas
Berries (strawberries, raspberries,
   blueberries)
Cherries
Grapefruit
Grapes
Kiwi fruits
Lemons
Limes
Mangoes
Melons (cantaloupe, honeydew,
   watermelon)
Nectarines
Oranges
Papayas

Peaches
Pears
Pineapple
Plums
Prunes
Raisins
Tangerines

Dairy group
This food group includes liquid milk
as well as foods that are made of milk,
such as yogurt and cheese. Note: Foods
such as cream and butter that are made
with milk but retain little or no calcium
are not included in this group.
   What dairy contributes to the diet:
Dairy offers calcium, potassium,
protein, and vitamin D. Milk products
help build and maintain bone mass,
reducing the risk of osteoporosis.
   Daily recommendation for adults:
3 servings.
   Selection tips: Full-fat dairy products
are usually high in artery-clogging
saturated fat, so whenever possible
choose milk, yogurt, and cheese that
are low in fat or fat-free. If you are
lactose-intolerant, choose lactose-free
dairy foods. If you don't like milk, buy
calcium-fortified juices, soy beverages,
or rice beverages and eat plenty of
calcium-rich nondairy foods such as

Fact or fiction? It's better to eat fruit than to drink fruit juice, even if it's
100-percent-pure fruit juice.
   Fact. Although whole fruit and fruit juice both contain vitamins and minerals, whole fruit
has far more fiber than juice does. Limit your juice intake to one fruit serving per day, even if
it is 100-percent fruit juice. And remember: Not all foods that have the word "fruit" in their
names are actually made with fruit. For example, fruit-flavored candies may be made with
no fruit or fruit juice at all. Always check the label.

canned fish (sardines, salmon with bones), calcium-fortified soy products, and leafy greens.

To incorporate dairy into your diet: Drink milk at meals, order milk-based coffee drinks such as café latte (made with fat-free milk), use milk instead of water when reconstituting condensed soups, use yogurt as a dip for fruit or a base for fruit smoothies, and make pudding with fat-free milk.

Common dairy foods
Chocolate milk
Fat-free milk (also called skim)
Frozen yogurt
Hard cheese (cheddar, mozzarella,
    Swiss, Parmesan)
Ice cream
Lactose-free or
    lactose-reduced milk
Low-fat milk (1% milk fat)
Process cheese (American)
Puddings made with milk
Reduced-fat milk (2% milk fat)
Soft cheese (ricotta, cottage cheese)
Strawberry milk
Whole milk (4% milk fat)
Yogurt (fat-free, low-fat, reduced-fat,
    or whole)

Meat and beans group
This group contains foods made from meat, poultry, fish, dried beans or peas, eggs, nuts, and seeds. Dried beans and peas are part of both this group and the vegetable group.

What foods from the meat and beans group contribute to the diet: Meat and beans are rich in protein, B vitamins (niacin, thiamin, riboflavin, and B_6), vitamin E, iron, zinc, and magnesium.

Beans and nuts provide dietary fiber. Nuts contain monounsaturated fatty acids and polyunsaturated fatty acids. Some fish, such as salmon and trout, are rich in omega-3 fatty acids; research suggests that eating these fish may reduce the risk of heart disease.

Daily recommendation for adults: 5–6½ 1-ounce-equivalent servings, depending on gender, age, and daily calorie level (see "Healthy Eating Meal Plans," page 395). A 1-ounce-equivalent serving is a serving that provides 1 ounce's worth of nutrients. For example, a 1-ounce-equivalent serving equals 1 ounce of cooked meat or fish, 1 egg, ½ ounce of nuts or seeds, 1 tablespoon of nut butter, ¼ cup of cooked beans or peas, ½ cup bean or lentil soup, ¼ cup (2 ounces) tofu, 2 tablespoons of hummus, or 1 ounce of tempeh (a fermented food made from soybeans).

Note: The mercury levels in some fish can be harmful to a fetus. (See "Mercury and fish," page 77.)

Selection tips: Meat and poultry contain saturated fat, so choose lean or low-fat meat or poultry, remove skin from poultry, and trim any visible fat. Fish, nuts, and seeds contain heart-healthy monounsaturated fats and make a good substitute for meat and poultry. If you're on a reduced-sodium diet, check labels for sodium content: Processed meats such as ham, sausage, frankfurters, and lunch meats have added sodium, and some fresh meats such as turkey and pork are basted with salty solutions.

To incorporate these foods into your diet: Serve fish several times a week,

top a salad with white-meat chicken,
make hamburgers and meat loaf with
ground white-meat poultry, sprinkle
nuts over salads or steamed vegetables,
add toasted nuts instead of meat to stir-
fries, serve veggie burgers and soy dogs
at cookouts, and add beans to soups,
salads, and chili.

**Common foods in the meat and
beans group**
Canned fish (anchovies, tuna, sardines)
Dried beans and peas (bean burgers,
    black beans, black-eyed peas,
    garbanzo beans/chickpeas, kidney
    beans, lentils, mature lima beans,
    navy beans, pinto beans, soybeans,
    split peas, tempeh, texturized
    vegetable protein, tofu, white beans)
Eggs
Finfish (catfish, cod, flounder,
    haddock, halibut, herring, mackerel,
    pollock, porgy, salmon, sea bass,
    snapper, swordfish, trout, tuna)
Meats (beef, bison, giblets, ham, lamb,
    liver, pork, rabbit, veal, venison)
Nuts and seeds (almonds, cashews,
    hazelnuts/filberts, mixed nuts,
    peanut butter, peanuts, pecans,
    pistachios, pumpkin seeds, sesame
    seeds, sunflower seeds, walnuts)
Poultry (chicken, duck, goose, turkey)
Shellfish (clams, crab, crayfish, lobster,
    mussels, octopus, oysters, scallops,
    shrimp, squid/calamari)

Oil group
Oils are fats that are liquid at room
temperature, such as vegetable oils
used in cooking. Oils come from
various plants as well as fish. Some
foods are high in oil.

Fats that are solid at room
temperature come from animal foods or
can be made from vegetable oils
through a process called hydrogenation.
Common solid fats include butter, beef
fat (suet or tallow), chicken fat, pork fat
(lard), stick margarine, and shortening.
These fats are high in saturated fat,
which can raise LDL (bad) cholesterol
levels in the blood.

A few plant oils, such as tropical
coconut and palm kernel oils, have
significant saturated fat, so for
nutritional purposes you can consider
them a solid fat.

The monounsaturated and polyunsaturated fat in vegetable oils is
believed to contribute to heart health.
However, oil is high in calories—
1 tablespoon contains about
120 calories—so don't go overboard.

What oils contribute to the diet: Oils
are the major source of vitamin E in
the American diet. Oils and oily foods
such as fish and nuts are rich in
monounsaturated and polyunsaturated
fats, which contain fatty acids that are
essential for good health. Most of the
fat in your diet should be monounsaturated or polyunsaturated, not saturated.

Daily recommendation for adults:
5–7 teaspoons, depending on gender,
age, and daily calorie level (see
"Healthy Eating Meal Plans," page
395). Keep in mind that 1 tablespoon
equals 3 teaspoons. In addition,
1 ounce of nuts or seeds or half of a
large avocado equals 3 teaspoons of oil.
Two tablespoons of nut butter equals
4 teaspoons of oil. Four olives equal
½ teaspoon of oil.

Selection tips: Choose oils that are

highest in polyunsaturated and monounsaturated fats and lowest in saturated fat. Select soft margarines that contain no trans fats. Limit butter and other animal fats.

To incorporate oils into your diet: Snack on nuts, replace meat sandwiches with nut butter sandwiches, cook with oil rather than butter, and bake or broil foods instead of frying.

Common foods in the oil group
Canola oil
Corn oil
Cottonseed oil
Foods that are made mainly with oil (certain salad dressings, mayonnaise, soft or liquid margarines with no trans fats)
Foods that are naturally high in oils (avocados, nuts, olives, some fish)
Olive oil
Safflower oil
Sesame oil
Soybean oil
Sunflower oil
Walnut oil

Discretionary calories
MyPyramid also contains a category of foods known as discretionary calories, which is 100 to 300 extra calories for treats such as butter, whole-fat dairy products, sauces, added sugars, honey, syrup, alcohol, sweetened yogurts, sweetened breakfast cereal, or fatty meats. As the name implies, use your discretion when incorporating calories from these sources.

Serving Sizes

Although MyPyramid gives daily recommendations in teaspoons, cups, and ounces, you may prefer to count servings using as a more "real world" approach. The following list translates your daily needs into easy-to-understand serving sizes; the Healthy Eating Meal Plans that start on page 395 are also organized by serving size.

Whole grains: 3 or more servings a day. (Total grains should be 5–8 servings a day.) One serving equals 1 slice of bread; 1 ounce of ready-to-eat cereal (about a cup of most cereals); or ½ cup of cooked cereal, rice, or pasta.

Vegetables: 3–5 servings a day. One serving equals 1 cup of raw vegetables, 1 cup of leafy vegetables such as spinach or lettuce, ½ cup cooked vegetables, or ½ cup vegetable juice.

Fruits: 2–4 servings a day. One serving equals 1 medium piece of fruit such as an apple, banana, or orange; ½ cup of chopped fresh, cooked, or canned fruit; ¼ cup dried fruit; or ¾ cup 100-percent fruit juice.

Dairy foods: 3 servings a day. One serving equals 1 cup of milk or yogurt, 1½ ounces of natural cheese such as cheddar or mozzarella, or 2 ounces of processed cheese such as American.

Protein: 2–3 servings a day. One serving equals 2–3 ounces of cooked meat, poultry, or fish (about the size of a deck of cards); 1 cup of cooked beans, 2 eggs; 2 ounces of hard cheese,; 2 tablespoons of peanut butter; or 1 ounce (about ¼ cup) of nuts.

Building Blocks of Food

Foods contain macronutrients (protein, fat, and carbohydrates) and micronutrients (vitamins and minerals). Knowing what role these food components play in your diet can help you use them to build a healthy eating plan.

Protein
Your body uses protein to build bones, muscles, cartilage, skin, and blood, as well as enzymes and hormones. Protein also helps control your body's fluid balance and is essential for a proper immune response.

Fat
Fat provides fatty acids that are necessary for a healthy brain and nervous system. Also, fat stores and transports fat-soluble vitamins A, D, E, and K. There are several kinds of fat.
- *Saturated fat* is found in animal products such as meat, butter, cream, and whole milk. It raises the levels of damaging LDL cholesterol in the blood, which can clog arteries and harm your cardiovascular system. Some vegetable oils, such as coconut oil, palm kernel oil, and palm oil, are saturated. Saturated fat is usually solid at room temperature.
- *Polyunsaturated and monounsaturated fats* are considered to be much more healthful than saturated fat because they raise levels of heart-healthy HDL cholesterol and lower levels of artery-clogging LDL cholesterol. They are found in nuts, olives, avocados, and vegetable oils. Two kinds of polyunsaturated fat are known as essential fatty acids because your body can't manufacture them and so must get them from foods. Linoleic acid, an omega-6 fatty acid, is an essential fatty acid found in soybean oil, corn oil, and safflower oil. (Linoleic acid is necessary because it is a precursor to hormone-like substances called prostaglandins; prostaglandins play a vital role in blood pressure and inflammation regulation, as well as in a variety of other body functions.) Alpha-linolenic acid is an omega-3 fatty acid found in fatty fish, omega-3-enriched eggs, walnuts, and flaxseed. Omega-3 fatty acids help build and maintain brain and eye tissue.

Your Daily Needs		
	% of Total Calories	Recommended Daily Allowance (in grams)
Protein	10–35%	46 g for nonpregnant women, 71 g for pregnant women
Fat	20–35%	
Omega-6 acid		12 g
Omega-3 acid		1.1 g
Carbohydrates	45–65%	130 g for nonpregnant women, 175 g for pregnant women
Fiber		25–40 g

You may have read news reports about EPA (eicosapentaenoic acid) and DHA (docosahexaenoic acid), two polyunsaturated omega-3 fatty acids that foster the healthy development of eye and nerve tissue. EPA and DHA are found in sardines, salmon, mackerel, and herring. These fats are now turning up in prenatal vitamins and infant formulas. Formula and supplement manufacturers believe these fatty acids help improve babies' vision and IQ. Although studies show that breastfed infants whose mothers' milk is rich in EPA and DHA have higher average IQs than babies fed with ordinary formula, no studies have established whether adding EPA and DHA to formula or supplements is as beneficial to babies as getting it from breast milk.

- *Trans fats* are found in hydrogenated fats, which are liquid oils that are made solid by the addition of an extra hydrogen molecule. Trans fats are found in stick margarine, shortening, and many commercially made bakery products. They are believed to be as dangerous to the heart as saturated fat.
- *Cholesterol.* Your body manufactures all the cholesterol it needs, but you

Smart Fiber Choices	
Instead of ...	... Try This
Apple juice (0 grams of fiber)	1 apple (3 grams)
White bread (1 gram)	Oat-bran pita (6 grams)
Saltines (1 gram)	Triscuits (3 grams)
Special K cereal (1 gram)	All Bran cereal (10 grams)
1½ tablespoons peanut butter (1 gram)	1 ounce of almonds (3.4 grams)

also get it from animal products such as meat, eggs, seafood, poultry, and dairy products. Limit intake to less than 300 milligrams a day.

You should limit your daily fat intake to no more than about 20–35 percent of total calories from fat, with a limit of 7–10 percent of total calories from saturated fats, 10–15 percent from monounsaturated fats, and 10 percent from polyunsaturated fats. Consume as few grams of trans fats as possible.

Carbohydrates

These are your body's primary fuel source. When your body needs energy, it uses carbohydrates far more easily than protein or fat. There are two kinds of carbohydrates: simple and complex.

6 high-fiber cereals

The following cereals have 6–14 grams of fiber per serving, which goes a long way toward meeting the recommended 25–40 grams of fiber per day.

- General Mills Fiber One
- Kellogg's All-Bran Original
- Kashi GOLEAN
- Shredded Wheat 'N Bran
- Multi-Bran Chex
- Kellogg's Raisin Bran

Fact or fiction? Fresh fruits and vegetables are always more nutritious than frozen or canned.

Fiction. A lot of people think fresh is always the best way to go, but frozen fruits and vegetables can be as nutritious as fresh—or even more nutritious if the fresh produce in your grocery store or refrigerator has been hanging around for a few days. Frozen produce is packed very soon after picking, which preserves its nutrients. It's also convenient and, in many cases, less expensive than fresh.

Canned food is another story. With the exception of beans and tomatoes, the produce that comes in cans is less nutritious than fresh because the nutrients leach out of the produce and into the water it's packed in. If you use the canning liquid, you'll save the nutrients, but you will also get too much sodium.

- *Simple carbohydrates* are found in table sugar, pancake syrup, jellies, jams, white bread, soda, candy, and cake. Simple carbohydrates require little processing by the body, so the sugar they contain is converted to glucose and dumped into the bloodstream quickly. This causes spikes in blood sugar levels.

- *Complex carbohydrates* are found in whole grain breads and cereals, vegetables, whole fruits, and beans. They are higher in fiber than simple (refined) carbohydrates. Because your body needs more time to break down complex carbohydrates, eating them helps keep the body's blood sugar levels stable. (For more information, see Chapter 7, "Blood Sugar Problems During Pregnancy," page 101.)

What's so special about dietary fiber?
Fiber is a kind of carbohydrate, but unlike other carbohydrates, your body cannot digest it. That's why it's sometimes referred to as "your body's broom." There are two types of fiber: insoluble and soluble. Because insoluble fiber goes through your digestive system without breaking down, it adds bulk to your stools. It also stimulates your intestines, which helps prevent constipation, hemorrhoids, irritable bowel syndrome, and diverticulosis, an intestinal disease. Soluble fiber may lower cholesterol and prevent heart disease, diabetes, and certain kinds of cancer.

Vitamins continued on page 21				
Vitamin	What it does	Recommended intake for adult women	Recommended intake during pregnancy (age 19 and older)	Sources
A	Keeps eyes and skin healthy. Protects against infections.	700 micrograms	770 micrograms	Carrots, sweet potatoes, spinach, vitamin A-fortified milk

Vitamins *continued from page 20*				
Vitamin	What it does	Recommended intake for adult women	Recommended intake during pregnancy (age 19 and older)	Sources
B vitamins (thiamin, riboflavin, niacin, B$_6$, folate, B$_{12}$)	Plays a key role in metabolism, helping your body release energy from protein, fat, and carbohydrates. Keeps the nervous system healthy and helps the body form red blood cells. Folate (folic acid) reduces the risk of neural tube defects in babies.	Thiamin: 1.1 milligrams Riboflavin: 1.1 milligrams Niacin: 14 milligrams B$_6$: 1.3 milligrams Folate: 400 micrograms B$_{12}$: 2.4 micrograms	Thiamin: 1.4 milligrams Riboflavin: 1.4 milligrams Niacin: 18 milligrams B$_6$: 1.9 milligrams Folate: 600 micrograms B$_{12}$: 2.6 micrograms	Whole grains, dairy products, meat, poultry, seafood, nuts, fish, spinach, dried beans and peas
C	Plays a part in the growth and repair of tissues, the absorption of iron, and teeth and gum health.	75 milligrams	85 milligrams	Citrus fruits, green sweet peppers, tomatoes, strawberries, broccoli
D	Maintains proper levels of calcium and phosphorus, thereby helping to build and maintain bone.	5 micrograms	5 micrograms	Milk and other fortified foods, salmon, and sunlight (your body can manufacture vitamin D in the presence of sunlight)
E	Protects cells from the damaging effects of oxidation.	15 milligrams	15 milligrams	Sunflower seeds, almonds, hazelnuts, wheat germ, peanut butter, corn oil, spinach, pecans
K	Aids in blood clotting and maintaining healthy blood, bones, and kidneys.	90 micrograms	90 micrograms	Spinach, broccoli, eggs, wheat bran, wheat germ, milk, strawberries

The daily recommendation for everyone is 25–40 grams of fiber a day. If you don't get much fiber and want to boost your intake, increase your fiber intake slowly to prevent bloating and intestinal gassiness. And as you eat more fiber, drink more water so you don't get constipated. It's always best to get nutrients from food, but if you can't consume 25 grams or more fiber a day, fiber supplements can help. Brands to try include Metamucil, FiberCon, and Benefiber.

Good sources of fiber include fruits, vegetables, whole grain breads and cereals, lentils, and beans. Whole foods are best: The more a food is processed, the less fiber it contains. For example, apple juice contains less fiber than applesauce, and applesauce contains less fiber than a raw apple.

Vitamins

Vitamins build and maintain healthy tissue, regulate your metabolism, and assist in many other body functions. Fat-soluble vitamins (A, D, E, and K) are stored in your body's fat and are used on an as-needed basis. Your body cannot store water-soluble vitamins (the B vitamins and vitamin C), so in order to have the amounts you need, you have to eat foods that contain them each day. All women of childbearing age should take a supplement containing 400 micrograms of folic acid.

Minerals

Minerals play a critical part in the healthy development and growth of bones, teeth, muscles, and blood. See the "Minerals" chart (page 23) for what minerals are important during pregnancy and why.

What's on a food label?

You can get just about all of the nutrition information you need about a food from its label, including the following:

- Serving size
- Number of servings in the container
- Calories per serving
- Amount of total fat, saturated fat, trans fat, calories from fat, cholesterol, and sodium per serving
- Grams of total carbohydrates, sugar, and dietary fiber per serving
- Grams of protein per serving
- Percentage of the daily value of vitamin A, vitamin C, calcium, and iron (these are required by the U.S. Food and Drug Administration)
- Percentage of the daily value of other vitamins and minerals with which the food is fortified or enriched
- Recommended daily values of fat, saturated fat, cholesterol, sodium, carbohydrates, and fiber based on both a 2,000-calorie diet and a 2,500-calorie diet
- Ingredients of the food

Minerals				
Mineral	What it does	Recommended intake for adult women	Recommended intake during pregnancy (age 19 and older)	Sources
Calcium	Builds bones and teeth, maintains bone mass, and is necessary for muscle and blood vessel expansion and contraction.	1,000 milligrams	1,000 milligrams	Dairy products, calcium-fortified orange juice, calcium-fortified soy products
Iron	Carries oxygen in the blood, promotes a healthy immune system, and is essential for cell growth regulation.	18 milligrams	27 milligrams	Beef, shrimp, tuna, chicken, pork, whole grains, blackstrap molasses, spinach, kidney beans
Magnesium	Builds bones, releases energy from muscles, and aids in the production of enzymes.	310 milligrams (age 19–30) 320 milligrams (age 31–50)	350 milligrams (age 19–30) 360 milligrams (age 31–50)	Spinach, peanut butter, pecans, black-eyed peas, lima beans, whole wheat bread
Potassium	Maintains healthy blood pressure. Necessary for muscle contractions. Regulates fluid/mineral balance.	4.7 grams	4.7 grams	Bananas, prunes, prune juice, dried peaches, sweet potatoes, white beans, tomato products, spinach, dairy products
Sodium	Helps your body hold on to water and maintain blood pressure. Contributes to muscle and nerve health.	1,500–2,300 milligrams	1,500–2,300 milligrams	Table salt, canned tomato products, canned soups, fast food, processed meats
Zinc	Helps the immune system function properly. Promotes cell reproduction and helps repair tissues.	8 milligrams	11 milligrams	Beef, wheat germ, crabmeat, wheat bran, sunflower seeds, black-eyed peas, almonds, milk, tofu

Food Labels and Nutrient Claims

The Food and Drug Administration closely regulates nutrient claims on food labels. Here are some of the claims you may see on labels, along with their FDA-mandated definition:

"Free." Contains no amount of, or only a very small amount of, one or more of these components: fat, saturated fat, cholesterol, sodium, sugars, and calories. For example, "calorie-free" means fewer than 5 calories per serving.

"Low." Can be eaten frequently without exceeding dietary guidelines for one or more of these components: fat, saturated fat, cholesterol, sodium, and calories
    Low fat: 3 grams or less per serving
    Low saturated fat: 1 gram or less per serving
    Low sodium: 140 milligrams or less per serving
    Very low sodium: 35 milligrams or less per serving
    Low cholesterol: 20 milligrams or less, and 2 grams or less of saturated fat per serving
    Low calorie: 40 or less per serving.

"Lean" and "extra lean." Can be used to describe the fat content of meat, poultry, seafood, and game meats
    Lean: less than 10 grams of fat, 4.5 grams or less of saturated fat, and less than 95 milligrams of cholesterol per serving and per 100 grams.
    Extra lean: less than 5 grams of fat, less than 2 grams of saturated fat, and less than 95 milligrams of cholesterol per serving and per 100 grams

"High." Can be used if the food contains 20 percent or more of the daily value for a particular nutrient in a serving

"Good source." Means that one serving of a food contains 10 to 19 percent of the daily value for a particular nutrient

"Reduced." Means that a nutritionally altered product contains at least 25 percent less of a nutrient or of calories than the regular product

"Less." Means that a food, whether altered or not, contains 25 percent less of a nutrient or of calories than another food. For example, pretzels that have 25 percent less fat than potato chips could carry a "less" claim.

"Light." Can mean either that a nutritionally altered product contains one-third fewer calories or half the fat of the reference food, or that the sodium content of a low-calorie, low-fat food has been reduced by 50 percent

"More." Means that a serving of food contains a nutrient that exceeds the daily value of the reference food by at least 10 percent

"Healthy." Means the food is low in fat and saturated fat and contains limited amounts of cholesterol and sodium, as well as at least 10 percent of the daily value of certain vitamins, minerals, protein, or fiber

The healthy way to read a food label

Pay attention to serving size and the number of servings per container. Before calculating nutritional information, ask yourself, "How many servings am I eating?" For example, a typical 19-ounce can of soup is two servings, not one.

Figure out if it's low-fat. Not everything you eat has to be low-fat, but it's nice to know what is and what isn't. What is considered low-fat? Foods that have 3 grams or less of fat per serving.

Look for starches that are whole grain. If it has at least 3 grams of fiber per serving, you can consider it a whole (or complex) grain.

Nutrition Facts:
Canned Green Beans

Serving Size ½ cup (121g)
Servings Per Container about 3½

Amount Per Serving

Calories 20	Calories from Fat 0

	% Daily Value*
Total Fat 0g	0%
Saturated Fat 0g	0%
Trans Fat 0g	0%
Cholesterol 0mg	0%
Sodium 10mg	0%
Total Carbohydrate 4g	1%
Dietary Fiber 2g	8%
Sugars 2g	
Protein 1g	

Vitamin A 6%	•	Vitamin C 4%
Calcium 2%	•	Iron 4%

* Percent Daily Values are based on a 2,000-calorie diet.

NOT A SODIUM-FREE FOOD
INGREDIENTS: GREEN BEANS, WATER

My Prepregnancy Diet

Use this page to assess how you ate before you were pregnant. It can show you what foods you eat a lot and what foods you should eat more of for a healthier diet both during pregnancy and after your baby is born.

Date _____

On most days, I eat the following:	S	M	T	W	Th	F	S
Number of servings of fruit							
Number of servings of vegetables							
Number of servings of protein							
Number of servings of refined grains							
Number of servings of whole grains							
Number of servings of dairy							
Number of servings of fat/oils							
Number of ounces of water							
Vitamin/mineral supplements I take:							
Amount of fiber in my diet:							

I could improve my diet by: _____

_____

_____

_____

_____

_____

_____

_____

_____

_____

your best
pregnancy diet

Now that you know the basics of healthy eating, it's time to learn how to eat healthfully during pregnancy. Different rules apply when you're expecting—you need more of many nutrients as well as additional calories. And there are foods you should avoid or eat only in moderation while you're pregnant. During the nine months your baby is growing inside you, eating the right foods is important. The foods you eat (or don't eat) can have a major impact on your baby's health, including her size, her risk of birth defects, and her health after birth. Smart choices can also reduce the possibility of gestational diabetes and other complications.

Your Best Pregnancy Diet

When making food choices during pregnancy, remember that whatever you eat, your baby eats too. That's not to say that the turkey sandwich you had at lunch actually crosses the placenta and makes its way into your baby's body. But the nutrients in it do. That's why it's important to eat a healthy diet during pregnancy. When you do, you give your baby the nutrients she needs to grow strong bones and muscles, well-functioning organs, and an intelligent mind.

A good pregnancy diet takes an everyday healthy diet, like the one described in Chapter 1, a step further. Because your body is supporting a growing baby, it requires more of some nutrients than it does when you're not pregnant. For example, when you're pregnant you need extra protein, iron, zinc, and folic acid. You also need extra calories, but not too many. The old adage says you're eating for two, but most women need only about 300 extra calories each day during pregnancy. Eating adequate amounts of certain kinds of fat is important during pregnancy as well. (Unfortunately, the fat you need more of is not the kind found in burgers and french fries.)

Certain foods and nutrients are best minimized during your pregnancy, including caffeine, trans fats, and simple carbohydrates. Some foods you should avoid completely. These include alcohol, raw meat, fish that might contain high levels of mercury, unpasteurized dairy products and juices, and other foods that may carry bacteria or pollutants that are dangerous to you and your baby. (See Chapter 5, "Foods That Can Harm," page 69.)

All this may sound complicated, but in practice it's not. If you keep junk food consumption to a minimum, watch your vitamin and mineral intake, and eat a diet that is rich in fruits, vegetables, whole grains, low-fat dairy products, and lean meats, you'll be going a long way toward building a strong, healthy baby.

Necessary Nutrients

It's always important to consume recommended amounts of vitamins and minerals, but it's even more crucial when you're pregnant. Don't worry, you don't have to carry a calculator around to figure out if you're getting what you need. Eating a healthy diet and taking a prenatal vitamin should cover it. However, it's still a good idea to know which vitamins, minerals, and other nutrients play a particularly important role during pregnancy—so important, in fact, that pregnant women are advised to boost their intake of these nutrients.

Choosing vitamin supplements

Food is the best source of most nutrients. However, during pregnancy, it's a good idea to take a daily multi-vitamin in case you fall short of any vitamins or minerals on any given day. Think of your daily prenatal vitamin as nutrition insurance—it's good to have even if you don't need it.

Typically multivitamins contain about 20 vitamins and minerals, including vitamins A, B_6, B_{12}, C, D, E, and K, folic acid, niacin, riboflavin (vitamin B_2), thiamin (vitamin B_1), iron, calcium, iodine, magnesium, zinc, and phosphorus. Most multivitamins contain at least 100 percent of the daily value (DV) for nearly all vitamins, but they usually don't contain 100 percent of the DV for most minerals.

Prenatal vitamins are available over the counter or by prescription. Either kind is fine. Keep these tips in mind when choosing a prenatal vitamin:

- Make sure your daily pill contains at least 400 micrograms of folic acid.
- Read the label to find out how to take it and store it safely.
- Stay away from herbal supplements and extracts and megadoses of vitamins, which may harm your baby. Few herbs have been thoroughly researched, and even fewer have been studied in pregnant women.
- Select a supplement with extra iron only if your doctor recommends it.
- If you have trouble getting enough calcium in your diet, add a daily calcium/vitamin D supplement. Most prenatal vitamins and multi-vitamins contain only small amounts of calcium. Select supplements that contain calcium carbonate, the kind of calcium your body uses best. (See "Choosing the best calcium supplement," page 91.)
- Look for the letters *USP* on vitamin labels. This shows that the vitamin meets the standards set by the

Is 'liquid energy' good for you?

Push your cart through the aisles of the grocery store and you're likely to notice shelves stocked with energy drinks with names such as Boost, Ensure, Resource, and Sustacal. Drinks like these have been used for years in hospital environments, and now they're being marketed as meal-replacement drinks, joining products such as Carnation Instant Breakfast and Slim-Fast shakes.

The truth is that these drinks don't make nutritional sense for the average person or the average pregnant woman. They are no match for a real meal, and some of them contain nearly as much sugar as a soda.

Grab one occasionally if you're in a bind and don't have time to eat a meal, but don't rely on them. For a fast meal, you're better off reaching for a container of cottage cheese, a couple of slices of whole wheat bread, and an apple. Or make your own energy drink—mix fat-free milk or yogurt in a blender with a soft fruit such as cantaloupe, peaches, strawberries, apricots, raspberries, or blueberries—and take it with you in a thermos.

U.S. Pharmacopeia, an organization that sets vitamin standards.

- Save money by buying store or generic brands; they are just as good as name brands.

Vital vitamin A

Vitamin A promotes good vision, cell and tissue growth, and embryo development. It also helps fight infection, and it works as a cancer-fighting antioxidant.

Vitamin A is a double-edged sword, though. Too much vitamin A can be dangerous to both you and your baby. In adults, excess vitamin A can cause bone and joint pain, liver damage, and nerve damage. In a developing fetus, too much vitamin A can cause birth defects such as cleft palate and faulty limb development.

Vitamin A is fat-soluble, which means your body stores whatever it doesn't use. Because your body holds on to the extra vitamin A, it is possible to get too much of it. At high doses, it can be harmful. The daily recommended maximum of vitamin A is 5,000 international units (IUs) or 1,500 micrograms. Only twice that amount has been associated with birth defects.

There are two forms of vitamin A: preformed and carotenoids.

Preformed vitamin A appears on labels as retinol or vitamin A palmitate or acetate. This is the form of the vitamin that's found in supplements and fortified foods, as well as animal foods such as liver, fish oil, milk, and eggs. Preformed means your body doesn't have to put the vitamin components together in order for them to do their job. It also means that in high amounts, they are more likely to do damage.

Carotenoids (such as beta-carotene), the other form of vitamin A, are found in many red, orange, yellow, and dark green leafy vegetables. Your body converts some carotenoids into vitamin A on an as-needed basis.

So go ahead and eat carrots, sweet potatoes, spinach, kale, mangoes, papayas, red peppers, milk, eggs, and other vitamin A-rich foods. It's highly unlikely that you'd get too much vitamin A from nonfortified food sources (with the exception of liver, which has far more vitamin A than any other food). But limit your intake of foods fortified with preformed vitamin A. Check the labels of fortified cereals and energy bars—if they contain palmitate or retinol, eat them only in moderation or choose another cereal or energy bar to avoid putting yourself over the recommended daily maximum of 5,000 IUs of vitamin A each day.

Folic acid fights birth defects

Folic acid is a B vitamin that helps prevent serious birth defects such as the neural tube defect spina bifida, congenital heart disease, and cleft lip. Since scientists discovered the power of folic acid and began advising women of childbearing age to take it, the number of babies born with neural tube defects in the United States has dropped significantly.

You may have heard folic acid referred to as folate. The two words aren't exactly interchangeable: Folate is the form of the B vitamin that's found in food, and folic acid is the synthetic form of the vitamin found in supplements and fortified foods. Surprisingly, your body actually absorbs folic acid better than folate.

Foods such as beans, asparagus, oranges, orange juice, peanuts, and leafy green vegetables contain folate, but it's nearly impossible for pregnant women to get the amount they need from food. That's why doctors prescribe daily multivitamin supplements that contain 400 micrograms of folic acid.

Folic acid supplementation is most effective when it's started a few months before conception because the neural tube begins to develop soon after conception and is closed by approximately day 56 after conception. Many women don't even know they're pregnant that early. According to the March of Dimes, if all women took 400 micrograms of folic acid every day throughout their childbearing years, as many as 70 percent of neural tube defects could be prevented.

Supplementing with folic acid is even more important if you take certain medications such as anti-convulsants or if you've already had a pregnancy affected by a neural tube defect. Doctors usually recommend that these women supplement with at least 1,000 micrograms of folic acid every day.

Crucial vitamin C

During pregnancy, vitamin C helps build red blood cells, blood vessels, gums, and collagen, a connective tissue that holds together bones, muscles, and other tissues. It also protects you from infection, helps wounds heal, and aids in the absorption of iron and folate.

You need about 85 milligrams of vitamin C a day during pregnancy, which is about 10 milligrams more than you needed when you weren't pregnant. Getting enough vitamin C is easy for most people: ¾ of a cup of orange juice provides about a day's worth of vitamin C. Other vitamin C-rich foods include guavas, red sweet peppers, papayas, oranges and other citrus fruits, broccoli, green sweet peppers, strawberries, and tomatoes.

Tofu for you

Calcium-fortified tofu, or soybean curd, has about as much calcium in a 5-ounce serving as plain yogurt. Because it takes on the flavor of other ingredients, it can replace meat in chili, stir-fries, casseroles, and pasta sauces. Tofu is a great base for smoothies and puddings, and it's even tasty when it's grilled like a slice of meat.

Tofu is sold in several forms: soft or silken (for dressings, smoothies, and shakes), medium-soft (for puddings and pie fillings), and firm or extra-firm for stir-frying, grilling, or using in casseroles, chili, or soups. Tofu is sold packed in water in the refrigerated section of the grocery store. Store in the refrigerator and use within a week. Follow package directions on storing: Tofu is best stored in water that is changed every day.

Critical calcium

Now that you're pregnant you need lots more calcium in your diet, right? Wrong. Contrary to what many people think, the recommended intake of calcium is the same for pregnant women as it is for nonpregnant women: 1,000 milligrams a day.

Of course, if you're like the vast majority of women, you don't get that much calcium. According to the March of Dimes, only 6 percent of U.S. women consume the recommended amount of calcium. On average, women of childbearing age in the United States get only 700 milligrams of calcium a day. If you don't get the calcium your body needs from foods, your body takes calcium from your bones in order to keep blood levels of calcium stable. Over time, not enough calcium can lead to osteoporosis.

Dairy foods are the best source of calcium. Eat three to four servings of dairy foods a day. Some fruits and vegetables contain calcium, but not enough to provide 1,000 milligrams a day. (For example, you would have to eat 10 cups of mustard greens or 20 oranges to tally 1,000 milligrams of calcium.) Also, the fiber in fruits and vegetables makes it harder for your body to absorb the calcium in those foods, so even if you could get 1,000 milligrams, your body wouldn't absorb it all. Choose fruits and vegetables that contain calcium, but don't count on produce alone to give you what you need.

Most milk contains added vitamin D because vitamin D helps your body absorb and use calcium.

If you can't stand the thought of drinking glass after glass of plain milk, see the alternatives in "Calculating Calcium" on the opposite page. Disguise your dairy by mixing milk or yogurt into fruit smoothies, sprinkling whole grain cereal and fresh berries into yogurt, eating pudding made with low-fat milk, or drinking decaffeinated café latte made with low-fat milk. And if you're lactose-intolerant, choose lactose-free milk or give yogurt a try—many people who are lactose-intolerant can handle yogurt.

What in the world is blackstrap molasses?

It's not surprising to see various fruits and vegetables listed as potent sources of various vitamins and minerals. But blackstrap molasses? Is it really that nutritious?

Yes. Blackstrap molasses, which is a by-product of the process of refining sugar cane into table sugar, contains the nutrients that are stripped away from the sugar cane plant. It is a rich source of calcium, iron, magnesium, potassium, selenium, copper, manganese, and vitamin B_6. For example, 1 tablespoon contains 170 milligrams of calcium (17 percent of your daily requirement) and 3.5 milligrams of iron (13 percent of what you need in a day).

If you like the robust, bittersweet taste of blackstrap molasses, stir it into baked beans, use it to baste chicken or turkey, mix with orange juice and fresh ginger as a sauce for vegetables, or add it to your favorite stir-fry.

Calculating Calcium	
Food	Milligrams of calcium per serving
1 cup fat-free plain yogurt	450
½ cup tofu processed with calcium	435
1 cup low-fat plain yogurt	415
1 cup fruit yogurt	315
1 cup fat-free milk	300
1 cup 2% milk	295
1 cup whole milk	290
1 cup low-fat (1% or 2% fat) chocolate milk	285
1 ounce Swiss cheese	270
1 cup calcium-fortified soymilk	250–300
¾ cup calcium-fortified orange juice	225
1 ounce cheddar cheese	205
3 ounces canned salmon with bones	205
1 ounce part-skim mozzarella cheese	185
1 tablespoon blackstrap molasses	170
½ cup pudding	150
½ cup frozen yogurt	105
½ cup turnip greens	100
½ cup ice cream	85
½ cup cottage cheese	75
½ cup mustard greens	50
½ cup broccoli	45
Source: American Dietetic Association	

Whatever you eat, be sure to spread your calcium intake throughout the day because your body can absorb only about 500 milligrams at a time.

Vitamin D: The calcium key

Vitamin D requirements do not change during pregnancy. However, pregnant women should make sure they're getting enough. Here's why: Vitamin D helps the body absorb bone-strengthening calcium and phosphorus. Without proper amounts of vitamin D, the calcium in your food may not make it to your bones.

Unfortunately many women don't get the vitamin D they need. Why? Researchers blame it on a lack of exposure to sunlight. In addition to being found in food, vitamin D is manufactured by the body when the skin is exposed to sun. Many people stay indoors when the weather is cold, and when it's warm, they slather on so much sunscreen the sun's rays can't get through. People who live in northern climates tend to be particularly low in vitamin D, which is stored in body fat.

You don't need a lot of sun to get the vitamin D you need: Vitamin D researchers recommend just 5 to 10 minutes a day of sunshine on your face and arms between the hours of 10 a.m. and 3 p.m. two or three days a week. That small amount of exposure—less than half an hour a week—will give your body the sunshine necessary to manufacture all the vitamin D it needs, but probably not enough to increase your risk of skin cancer. If you live north of Atlanta, the sun is too weak between November

Fact or fiction? If I don't get enough calcium in my diet, my baby will take what it needs from my bones.

Fact. If calcium intake is inadequate, your baby's body will use calcium stores in your bones. Your teeth are safe though. Your body won't grab calcium from your teeth if you don't get enough dietary calcium during pregnancy. And the old saying "You'll lose one tooth for every baby" is just a myth.

and February to make vitamin D, so during this time it's particularly important that you drink vitamin D–fortified milk and vitamin D–fortified orange juice. Of course, you should also be taking a prenatal vitamin.

Iron: An essential blood builder

Women need iron throughout their lives, but it's even more crucial during pregnancy. The amount of blood in your body increases by 50 percent during pregnancy, and iron is a major component of blood. Iron helps red blood cells transport oxygen through your bloodstream to cells in your body and your baby's body.

When you're pregnant you need 27 milligrams of iron a day. (That's up from the 18 milligrams you need when you're not pregnant.) During your first pregnancy appointment, your obstetrician will do a blood test that indirectly measures the iron in your blood. If your iron level is low and you are anemic, your doctor will recommend that you eat iron-rich foods or take extra iron in the form of a supplement. Take extra iron only if your doctor advises it.

Even if your iron levels are just fine, it's a good idea to eat iron-rich foods throughout your pregnancy. Iron-rich foods include lean red meats, dark-meat poultry, leafy green vegetables, oatmeal, blackstrap molasses, cooked beans, and dried fruits such as raisins, prunes, dates, apricots, and figs.

Dietary iron is absorbed better in an acidic environment, so wash down your prenatal vitamin with a glass of orange juice, tomato juice, white grape juice, or any other vitamin C–fortified juice.

Alert! The hidden danger of fortified foods

Having a cereal bar, energy bar, or smoothie that's fortified with 100 percent or more of the Recommended Daily Allowance (RDA) of many vitamins and minerals sounds like a healthy idea, but it may not be if you're pregnant. That's because consuming these fortified foods with other foods throughout the day could easily cause you to exceed the recommended daily maximum for certain vitamins and minerals—such as fat-soluble vitamins A, D, E, and K, as well as iron. Excess vitamin A can be dangerous for you and for your baby. So carefully monitor your intake of fortified foods and stay away from those super-fortified foods that claim to give you all the vitamins and minerals you need for the day.

Breakfast: It's your most important meal

Would you start a daylong car trip with an empty gas tank? Of course not. Unfortunately, that's pretty much what you do if you start your day on an empty stomach. Without the proper fuel in your tank, you'll feel worn out and have trouble concentrating.

A good breakfast prepares you for your day. Protein stimulates the brain's neurotransmitters, which carry messages within the brain. Complex carbohydrates release a slow, steady stream of energy and stave off a mid-morning blood sugar dip, which can lead to the headache, anxiety, and shakiness that interfere with concentration.

It's important, however, not to pack breakfast with too many carbohydrates. While some carbohydrates are needed to help the protein perk up the brain, too many can sedate the brain. Also, it's best to avoid simple carbohydrates such as sweet cereals, which give an immediate surge of energy that disappears quickly.

The best breakfast is one that is high in protein, low in fat, and moderately rich in complex carbohydrates. Some examples:

- Yogurt and cereal
- Scrambled eggs and whole wheat toast
- Whole grain cereal with milk and fresh fruit
- Peanut butter and banana on a whole wheat tortilla
- Whole grain waffles with fresh fruit and milk

Once a day, eat a meal that includes a high-iron food and a vitamin C–rich food such as strawberries, oranges, or tomatoes. Avoid milk and other high-calcium foods at that meal because calcium blocks iron absorption.

Finally, limit your intake of liver. Although it contains a lot of iron, it is also high in vitamin A. Too much vitamin A can cause birth defects. (See "Vital vitamin A," page 30.)

Sidestepping sodium

There's no doubt about it—Americans eat too much salt. But contrary to what you may think, you should not eliminate sodium from your diet during pregnancy. As your body manufactures more blood (during pregnancy, you have 50 percent more blood than prepregnancy), it needs sodium to help maintain normal blood pressure.

Instead, practice moderation with sodium. Excess sodium consumption can worsen hypertension (high blood pressure), but it does not cause pregnancy-induced hypertension, or preeclampsia. Start by reading labels and paying attention to how much sodium is in your favorite foods. Foods that are high in sodium include canned and dry soups, cured meats (ham, bacon, sausage), processed meats (hot dogs, deli meat), canned tomatoes, some kinds of peanut butter, some breakfast cereals, prepackaged frozen dinners, fast food, seasoned rice, snack foods (potato chips, pretzels, tortilla chips), gravy, and flavor enhancers such as taco seasoning, cooking sherry, chili

Fact or fiction? Whole milk is more nutritious than fat-free, or skim milk. **Fiction.** The only thing whole milk has that fat-free milk doesn't is fat. One cup of whole milk packs 8 grams of fat (including 5 grams of artery-clogging saturated fat) and 160 calories. The same amount of skim milk has no fat and only 100 calories. If you drink whole milk, switch to fat-free milk gradually, going from whole milk to reduced-fat 2% fat milk to 1% to skim. Try to drink skim milk even if you're underweight—if your doctor has recommended that you get extra calories, you're better off loading up on foods with heart-healthy unsaturated fats rather than whole milk.

sauce, meat tenderizer, soy sauce, steak sauce, and Worcestershire sauce.

During early pregnancy, some women find that the only foods they can stomach are salty foods such as crackers, pickles, pretzels, or potato chips. Such salt cravings may be your body's way of making sure you stay hydrated, because salty foods make you thirsty. If you had hypertension before becoming pregnant, keep your sodium intake on the lower side of the recommended range and consider seeing a registered dietitian for sodium recommendations that are tailored to your personal health profile.

The facts on fluoride

You need the same amount of mineral fluoride during pregnancy as you do when you're not pregnant. Most people get all the fluoride they need from their municipal drinking water. However, now is a good time to check your water to be sure it contains fluoride. (If you're not sure about the fluoride content of your tap water, contact your state's water board or local water supplier.) If you use well water or spring water, or if your municipality does not add fluoride to the water

supply, you may want to make some changes in your water-drinking habits.

Adequate intake of fluoride helps ensure that your baby has strong teeth—and that your teeth stay strong throughout your pregnancy too. Your baby's teeth begin forming long before birth, and without enough fluoride, they can be soft, mottled, or prone to decay. If the water you normally drink contains no fluoride, consider drinking a few servings a day of fluoridated tap water.

A safe and adequate intake of fluoride during pregnancy is 3 grams a day.

Protein: The cell builder

During the 1st trimester, a pregnant woman's daily protein requirement stays the same as it was before she conceived—about 46 grams. But in the 2nd and 3rd trimesters, as your baby gets bigger, it increases to approximately 71 grams a day. Your body uses protein to build cells, grow and repair tissues, expand blood volume, build and maintain the placenta, and manufacture hormones and enzymes.

For most women, getting enough protein is easy. Eat a bowl of cereal

Don't forget your teeth

It's recommended that pregnant women eat three small meals and two or three small snacks a day. Frequent small meals are better than infrequent large meals because small meals help keep blood sugar stable, minimize heartburn, and help prevent nausea.

But eating often throughout the day can take a toll on your teeth. Frequent snacking, especially on high-carbohydrate foods, invites tooth decay. The decay process begins with plaque, an invisible sticky layer of bacteria that forms on your teeth. These bacteria convert sugar and starch in the mouth to a kind of acid that eats away at tooth enamel. The longer the sugars stay in your mouth, the more damage the acids cause. Over time your teeth start to decay. That's why it's important to brush your teeth after each meal and snack, if possible, and to floss daily.

If you aren't sure how to brush and floss correctly, ask your dentist or dental hygienist to help you brush up on your tooth-care skills. If you are prone to gum disease, your dentist may recommend more-frequent professional cleanings while you're pregnant.

Don't have time to brush during the day? Veggies and cheese are smile-friendly snacks that can help remove plaque and boost tooth-building calcium phosphorus intake. Try carrots or celery sticks and a low-fat mozzarella string cheese or a slice of cheddar.

with milk for breakfast, a peanut butter sandwich at lunch with 1 cup of milk, 1 cup of yogurt as a snack, and a piece of grilled chicken with a side of beans at dinner, and you'll have all the protein you need for the day.

Lean meat is an excellent source of protein, but there are lots of other protein-rich foods to choose from, including fish, dairy foods, nuts and nut butters, eggs, dried peas, beans, tofu, hummus, and seeds.

When making your protein selections, opt for foods that are low in fat, particularly saturated fat. For example, select extra-lean cuts of beef and pork and white-meat chicken with the skin removed. Here are some delicious protein-rich foods, along with their protein content:

- 3½ ounces boneless, skinless chicken breast: 30 grams
- 4-ounce broiled hamburger patty made with extra-lean beef: 29 grams
- 4 ounces baked Atlantic salmon: 25 grams
- 8 ounces fat-free yogurt: 12 grams
- 8 ounces fat-free milk: 8 grams
- 2 tablespoons peanut butter: 8 grams
- ½ cup black beans: 7 grams
- 1 egg: 6 grams

Can you eat too much protein? There's no proof that it's dangerous, but there's no proof that it's a good idea either. Stick to a balanced diet with a reasonable amount of protein.

Brain-building fats

So many women have focused on cutting fat from their diets during the past decade that it's unbelievable to them to hear researchers recommend they put it back in. The researchers are not talking about all fats though—just

Fact or fiction? You need a lot of protein and carbohydrates in your diet, and just a small percentage of your total calories should come from fat.

Fact. Protein, carbohydrates, and fat all contribute to a healthy diet. But how much of each should you consume? A good guideline is to aim to get 50 percent of your calories from carbohydrates, 25 percent from protein, and 25 percent from fat. You don't have to meet this goal at every meal or even every day, but in general, it's a good guideline to follow.

heart-healthy monounsaturated and polyunsaturated fats.

Omega-3 fatty acids are important during pregnancy. They lower your risk for heart disease and boost your immune system. They also help your baby develop a healthy brain, nerves, and eyes.

Omega-3 fatty acids and omega-6 fatty acids are both essential fatty acids—which means that your body can't manufacture them, so you must get them from the foods you eat. Omega-6 fatty acids are found in soybean oil, corn oil, and safflower oil. Omega-3 fatty acids are found primarily in fatty fish such as tuna, salmon, sardines, and herring. Other kinds of fish and some vegetable oils have omega-3 fatty acids too, but in smaller amounts.

Since eating too much fish during pregnancy can be risky (see "Fish Facts," page 77), you can get omega-3 fatty acids from flaxseed. A safe and very rich source of alpha-linolenic acid (ALA or omega-3) is flaxseed oil. You can buy flaxseed as whole seeds, ground flaxseeds, and flaxseed flour. Keep in mind that flaxseed must be ground to help release the fatty acids; don't bother eating whole flaxseeds

because they simply pass through your body without any benefit except the fiber. Here are some ways to use flaxseed products:

- Replace some white flour in muffin and bread recipes with flaxseed flour.
- Stir ground flaxseed into muffin or quick-bread batter.
- Sprinkle ground flaxseed over cereal, oatmeal, salads, steamed vegetables, or yogurt.
- Look for pancake, waffle, and quick-bread mixes that contain flaxseed.

How much of these essential fatty acids do you need in pregnancy? Aim for the following:

- Omega-6: 13 grams a day
- Omega-3: 1.4 grams a day (For food sources, see "Omega-3-Rich Food," page 94.)

Carbohydrates: Important fuel

Carbohydrates are your body's main source of fuel. Although your body can burn protein and fat for energy, it's much more efficient to use carbs. (See "Carbohydrates," page 19, for an overview of simple and complex carbohydrates.)

Carbohydrates are an important part of your pregnancy diet and should be your main energy source—about half of the calories you eat should come from carbohydrates. Pregnant women need about 175 grams of carbohydrates a day, up from 130 grams a day when they're not pregnant. Aim to get as many of your carbohydrates from foods that are rich in complex carbohydrates, such as whole grain breads and cereals, beans, fruits, and vegetables.

Water: An essential nutrient

Water should be considered as vital a nutrient as carbohydrates, fats, protein, vitamins, and minerals—after all, 70 percent of the human body is made up of water. Pregnant women require a minimum of eight 8-ounce cups a day to help keep up with their increasing blood volume. The Institute of Medicine has set recommended fluid needs for pregnant women at approximately 2.3 liters a day (9–10 cups a day) and encourages breastfeeding women to drink 3.1 liters a day (approximately 13 cups a day).

When to Say "Less"

Cutting down on caffeine

When you drink a cup of coffee, your baby drinks it too. The caffeine you consume in coffee, tea, soft drinks, chocolate, and other foods crosses the placenta and enters your baby's system. Studies suggest a link between high caffeine consumption and miscarriage. Excessive amounts can affect the fetus's heart rate, but researchers are unsure whether caffeine harms a fetus, and if so, how much caffeine. Some studies link high caffeine intake to

low birthweight, sudden infant death syndrome, and infertility, but others find no relation.

To be safe, the American Dietetic Association recommends that pregnant women consume less than 300 mg of caffeine daily. As a general rule of thumb, 1 cup of regular coffee per day or 1–2 cups of tea per day is considered safe. Decaffeinated coffee and tea are fine. Add as much milk as you can to your drinks for a boost of calcium. And don't worry about treating yourself to an occasional dark chocolate bar—the caffeine content is fairly low. Use the "Caffeine Levels in Popular Beverages

Caffeine Levels in Popular Beverages and Foods	
Coffee (8-oz. cup)	
Brewed, drip method	96–288 mg
Brewed, percolator	64–272 mg
Instant	48–192 mg
Decaf, brewed	5 mg
Tea (8-oz. cup)	
Brewed, major U.S. brands	33–144 mg
Brewed, imported brands	40–176 mg
Instant	40–80 mg
Brewed iced tea (12-oz. glass)	67–76 mg
Bottled iced tea (12-oz. bottle)	6–50 mg
Other	
Cola (12-oz. can)	34–44 mg
Diet cola (12-oz. can)	36–45 mg
Root beer (12-oz. can)	0–22 mg
Mountain Dew (12-oz. can)	55 mg
Hot cocoa (12-oz. serving)	3–32 mg
Chocolate milk (8-oz. serving)	2–7 mg
Milk chocolate (1 oz.)	1–15 mg
Dark chocolate, semisweet (1 oz.)	5–35 mg
Baker's chocolate (1 oz.)	26 mg
Chocolate-flavored syrup (1 oz.)	4 mg
Red Bull Energy Drink (8.3-oz. can)	80 mg

Sources: FDA, American Beverage Association, National Soft Drink Association

and Foods" chart, page 39, to stay within the recommended limit.

Avoiding alcohol

It's difficult to order club soda when everyone else is drinking wine or beer, but it's the right choice. Pregnant women who drink alcohol risk having babies with fetal alcohol syndrome, the leading form of preventable mental retardation, as well as other physical and mental defects.

Nobody knows for sure how much alcohol it takes to harm a fetus or cause a miscarriage or a stillborn baby, and because each woman metabolizes alcohol differently, what may be acceptable for one woman would be too much for another. So what is the bottom line? Doctors know of no safe level of alcohol intake during pregnancy.

If you can't stop drinking, seek help immediately. Ask your obstetrician or health care provider for a referral to an alcohol treatment program or join an Alcoholics Anonymous support group (look in your phone book's white pages for contact information). For more information and referral to resources in your area, call 800-ALCOHOL (800-252-6465) or go to the U.S. Department of Health and Human Services' Substance Abuse Treatment Facility Locator at www.samhsa.gov and click on "Get help for substance abuse problems."

When to Say "Yes"

Small indulgences

Being pregnant doesn't mean you can't have a slice of cake on your birthday, pie at Thanksgiving, sugar cookies at Christmas, latkes at Hanukkah, or an ice cream cone on the Fourth of July. Those little indulgences are fine. In fact, they're a nice way to treat yourself to something out of the ordinary. However, little indulgences such as cake, candy, cookies, and chips should be just that—small amounts of special foods that you eat once in a while, not every day.

Because these treats tend to be high in fat, full of sugar, and devoid of most nutrients, they provide calories without adding any vitamins, minerals, or other important nutrients. Eating an occasional truffle can fit into a healthy eating plan, but a doughnut every morning and a candy bar every afternoon can add up to extra weight gain that won't do you or your baby any good. The excess pounds you gain during pregnancy will be ones you're trying to lose six months postpartum.

If you enjoy ice cream, have a small serving of your favorite kind. If you love chocolate, treat yourself once in a while to a small piece of high-quality Belgian chocolate. Savor it as you eat it, paying attention to how it smells, tastes, and feels in your mouth. How many times have you wolfed down a candy bar? If you eat slowly and mindfully, you'll enjoy a small portion more than you would a large portion that you eat quickly.

Foods that fight fatigue

The following food combos have a good balance of carbohydrate, fat, and protein—just what your body needs when your energy is low. These foods are rich in iron and vitamin C, which help the body's ability to absorb iron, especially from nonanimal sources.

- Chili with beef, ground chicken, or turkey, or a vegetarian variety with beans. The tomato base is rich in vitamin C, and the beans contain iron and fiber.
- Lasagna
- Spaghetti and meatballs
- Stir-fried chicken or beef with broccoli
- Grilled beef or chicken on a salad with tomatoes
- Black beans and cheese with rice and salsa
- Do-it-yourself trail mix. Blend a high-iron cereal (anything with 45 percent or more of the daily value) with nuts and dried fruit (try dried strawberries)
- Bean dip and salsa with baked chips or toasted pita wedges

Smart Shopping

Grocery store tips

Healthy eating starts in the grocery store. After all, you can't cook healthy food if you don't buy healthy food. Here are some tips on how best to shop for your healthy pregnancy diet:

Plan ahead. Use the recipes and menus in the back of this book for inspiration. As you plan, keep in mind how much time you'll have for meal preparation. When time is short, opt for a low-fat frozen dinner or soup or other convenience food. Round out the meal with fruit, vegetables, and milk.

Make a list. Write down the items you need so you don't have to rely on memory at the store. Then you'll be less likely to buy items you don't need.

Shop only once a week. Frequent shopping leads to impulse buys.

Eat before you go. You'll buy more if you have an empty stomach.

Shop the perimeter of the store. The healthiest foods (fruit, vegetables, fish, lean meats, low-fat dairy products) tend to be found on the outer aisles of the grocery store.

Choose the freshest produce. Fruits and vegetables taste best and last longer when they are firm, unbruised, and undamaged.

Buy locally grown produce in season. A fruit or vegetable retains more nutrients and flavor when it's transported across town rather than across the world.

Shop at several stores. If you have time, go to an ordinary grocery store or discount store for staples, a whole foods store or farmer's market for produce, and ethnic markets for specialty foods, spices, and flavorings.

Pick frozen and canned too. Frozen fruits and vegetables are as nutritious as fresh, so stock up. Canned is OK too, but avoid canned foods with high sodium content, fruits packed in heavy syrup, and vegetables packed in oil. Choose water-packed when possible.

Select the leanest meats. Avoid "prime" meats because they are loaded with saturated fat. The leanest grade is "select," followed by "choice." The leanest cuts of beef include:

- Beef: eye of round, top round, sirloin, and lean or extra-lean ground beef
- Pork: tenderloin, sirloin, and top loin
- Veal: shoulder, ground veal, cutlets, and sirloin
- Lamb: leg-shank
- Poultry: white meat or thigh meat without skin, and ground breast meat
- Lunch meats: 95- to 99-percent fat-free. (Reheat until steaming; see "Listeria," page 70.)

Use your nose when buying fish. The flesh of fish should spring back when pressed, its surface should glisten, and it should not smell fishy. Be sure that any seafood you buy has been refrigerated properly; don't buy cooked seafood if it is displayed in the same food case as raw fish because the raw fish can contaminate it with bacteria.

Pack your cart (and grocery bags) with food safety in mind. Keep raw meat, poultry, seafood, and eggs separate from ready-to-eat foods. Place raw foods inside plastic bags to contain juices that could harbor bacteria.

Get nutty about nut butters. Try other nut butters besides peanut butter, such as almond or cashew butter. Choose unsalted varieties when possible.

Take your time in the produce aisle. Browse around to find what's fresh, what's new, and what's on sale. Add a new fruit or vegetable to your cart every week.

Educate yourself on how to read food labels. They help you compare foods and find the healthiest choices.

Read bread labels carefully. Choose breads that list "100-percent whole wheat" or "100-percent whole grain" as the first ingredient on the label. Those labeled simply "wheat" breads—even if they are brown in color—may not contain whole grains. True whole grain bread contains at least 3 grams of fiber per serving.

Go right home, especially when it's hot outside. Get perishables into the refrigerator quickly to avoid or slow bacterial growth.

Healthy brown-bag meals

A good lunch contains moderate amounts of protein and complex carbohydrates and is low in saturated fat. That means passing up greasy cheeseburgers and other fast foods that leave you feeling lethargic in the afternoon.

The best way to ensure a healthy lunch is to pack it yourself. Here are some ideas for what to tuck into your lunch bag (along with a piece of fruit and some fat-free milk):

- Salmon salad sandwich
- Salad of greens, white-meat chicken, barley, and beans
- Mildly spiced chili with beans
- Minestrone or chicken noodle soup and a green salad
- Low-fat cheese and tomato on whole wheat bread or tortilla
- Peanut butter and jelly on whole wheat bread

weight gain
during pregnancy

*Gaining the right amount of weight—
not too much, not too little—is very
important when you're pregnant. The
energy and nutrients in the food you
eat help your baby grow and develop.
Knowing how much to gain can be
tricky. Many factors come into play,
including your prepregnancy weight
and your activity level. The amount
you gain during each trimester is an
issue. In this chapter you'll learn all
the ins and outs of pregnancy weight
gain: tips for underweight women,
tips for overweight women, and most
important, how to achieve the slow,
steady weight gain that is best for
your baby's health.*

Weight Gain During Pregnancy

If you added the local pizza delivery's phone number to your speed dial the minute after you found out you were pregnant, watch out. Pregnancy does not give you license to eat anything you want. A healthy pregnancy requires smart weight gain, for both your baby's health and yours.

One of the first questions most women ask their obstetricians is "How much weight should I gain during my pregnancy?" Although the answer varies according to your prepregnancy weight, one thing holds true for women of all sizes: If you gain too much or too little weight, or if you gain too slowly or too quickly, your risk of complications may rise.

If you don't gain enough weight, you increase the risk of having a small baby or a baby who is born prematurely. Small and premature babies are more likely than normal-size babies to have health problems at birth and chronic health problems throughout their lives. Ironically, low-birthweight babies are more likely than normal-weight babies to become obese later in life. Scientists believe this happens because an underweight baby's body learns to be super-efficient at storing fat and continues to store fat aggressively throughout life.

If you gain too much weight, you increase the risk of several complica-

tions for both yourself and your baby. Keep these potential problems in mind:

- You may have a very large baby. Big babies are more difficult to deliver, and the bigger your baby, the more likely you are to need a cesarean delivery, a forceps delivery, or a vacuum-assisted delivery.
- Excess weight is associated with an increased rate of neural tube defects, miscarriage, and stillbirth.
- Studies show that big babies are likely to grow up into overweight children. They're also more likely to develop type 2 diabetes.
- Gaining excess weight during pregnancy increases your risk of gestational diabetes and preeclampsia, as well as back and knee pain, hemorrhoids, and varicose veins.
- Putting on too much weight makes it tougher to get back to your prepregnancy weight after your baby is born. Research shows that women who gain more than the recommended weight during pregnancy and who fail to lose this weight within six months of giving birth are at much higher risk of being obese as long as a decade later.

How Much Is Enough?

The right gain for you

Studies show that as many as one-third of pregnant women say they receive no advice on pregnancy weight gain from their health care provider. If your doctor doesn't talk to you about this topic, be sure to bring it up yourself. Although guidelines detail the recommended weight gains, your obstetrician should be the one to determine exactly how much you should gain based on your health history and your body mass index (BMI). BMI compares your weight to your height in order to determine whether you're at a healthy weight.

The chart below outlines the general guidelines for pregnancy weight gain for a single baby. (Recommendations differ for multiples. See "Twins, triplets, and beyond," page 48.) Tell your doctor if you lost or gained a large amount of weight shortly before

Weight Gain Recommendation

Prepregnancy BMI	Recommended weight gain
Underweight (BMI less than 18.5)	28–40 pounds
Normal weight (BMI 18.5–24.9)	25–35 pounds
Overweight (BMI 25–29.9)	15–25 pounds
Obese (BMI greater than 30)	At least 15 pounds

Body Mass Index

BMI	19	20	21	22	23	24	25	26	27	28	29	30	31	32	33	34	35
Height (inches)	Body Weight (pounds)																
58	91	96	100	105	110	115	119	124	129	134	138	143	148	153	158	162	167
59	94	99	104	109	114	119	124	128	133	138	143	148	153	158	163	168	173
60	97	102	107	112	118	123	128	133	138	143	148	153	158	163	168	174	179
61	100	106	111	116	122	127	132	137	143	148	153	158	164	169	174	180	185
62	104	109	115	120	126	131	136	142	147	153	158	164	169	175	180	186	191
63	107	113	118	124	130	135	141	146	152	158	163	169	175	180	186	191	197
64	110	116	122	128	134	140	145	151	157	163	169	174	180	186	192	197	204
65	114	120	126	132	138	144	150	156	162	168	174	180	186	192	198	204	210
66	118	124	130	136	142	148	155	161	167	173	179	186	192	198	204	210	216
67	121	127	134	140	146	153	159	166	172	178	185	191	198	204	211	217	223
68	125	131	138	144	151	158	164	171	177	184	190	197	203	210	216	223	230
69	128	135	142	149	155	162	169	176	182	189	196	203	209	216	223	230	236
70	132	139	146	153	160	167	174	181	188	195	202	209	216	222	229	236	243
71	136	143	150	157	165	172	179	186	193	200	208	215	222	229	236	243	250
72	140	147	154	162	169	177	184	191	199	206	213	221	228	235	242	250	258

conceiving because it may impact your weight-gain goals.

Weight gain and activity levels

BMI calculations do not take into account whether your body weight comes primarily from muscle or fat. Muscle is denser than fat, so if you're a normal-weight woman who is very muscular, you could have a BMI in the overweight range. Be sure your doctor knows the shape you're in when making weight-gain suggestions. Better yet, roll up your sleeve and show off your biceps.

Slow and steady

What matters is not just what you gain but how you gain. The best way to gain weight during pregnancy is slowly and steadily. Here's a good guideline for normal-weight mothers:

- During the 1st trimester, gain a total of 1 to 4 pounds.
- During the 2nd and 3rd trimesters, gain about 1 pound a week.

Why is slow and steady weight gain best? Fast weight gain, particularly in the 1st trimester, benefits neither you nor your baby—it basically just makes you fat. Gaining too slowly can be a problem, especially in the 3rd trimester when your baby's body and brain are undergoing rapid growth. If you don't gain enough during the 3rd trimester, your baby may not grow properly.

Overall, women who gain slowly and steadily, especially during the first 20 weeks, are more likely to have full-term pregnancies and to give birth to healthy-weight babies. Take these eat-smart tips to heart to keep your weight gain slow and steady:

Limit white foods (white bread, white rice, white crackers, white pasta). They can cause blood sugar spikes that leave you feeling hungry shortly after eating.

Limit fast food. If you must eat fast food, choose healthier options, such as a salad with grilled chicken and low-fat dressing, chili on a baked potato, or a grilled chicken sandwich topped with vegetables, not mayonnaise. Also choose milk instead of soda.

Watch your fruit juice intake. Even if you're drinking 100-percent fruit juice, the calories still add up quickly.

Stay away from sugary soda. It can add hundreds of calories to your diet each day. Get your bubble fix from seltzer instead.

Eat bulky, filling foods such as salads, raw vegetables, and popcorn.

Head for the low-fat or fat-free dairy products instead of full-fat options.

Fact or fiction? If you're obese, there's a good chance your baby will be too.

Fact. A child's risk of becoming obese actually begins before birth. Studies show that children with obese mothers are much more likely to become obese than children with normal-weight mothers. Overweight and obese children have a higher risk of type 2 diabetes and heart disease. It can be hard to stick to a healthy eating plan during pregnancy, particularly if you're hungry all the time, but it's worth the effort.

Don't restrict fat intake too much.
Your baby's developing eyes and brain
need the fatty acids from the foods you
eat. Choose healthy fats such as
vegetable oils and nuts.

Eat lots of high-fiber foods such
as nuts, whole grains, fruits, and
vegetables. They fill you up and help
you feel full longer.

Fill up on beans. They are nutritional
powerhouses, and because they have so
much fiber they make you feel full.
Canned beans are fine; there's no need
to go through the time-consuming
process of soaking and cooking dried
beans. Rinse canned beans before
using to remove excess sodium. Mix
beans into salads, soups, or stews;
spread hummus (made from chickpeas
and sesame paste) instead of
mayonnaise on sandwiches, and serve
low-fat bean dip with fresh vegetables.

Drink plenty of water, aiming for 9 or
10 cups a day.

Eat wet foods. Foods that contain
liquid—soups, stews, and smoothies,
for example—make you feel fuller than
dry foods with the same number of
calories. For example, a 100-calorie
bowl of soup will leave you feeling
fuller than a 100-calorie bag of chips.

Get moving. Swim, walk, do yoga, or
take a pregnancy exercise class. (Be
sure to check with your health care
provider before exercising.)

Eat before you reach the point of
feeling ravenous. You're more likely to
overeat when you're hungry. Eat three
small meals and two or three small
snacks each day.

Special Weight Concerns

What if you're overweight?

If your prepregnancy BMI is greater
than 25, you may be tempted to try to
avoid weight gain during pregnancy.
It's understandable, but it's not a good
idea. Even an obese woman needs to
put on 15 pounds so that her baby can
get the nutrition and calories it needs
to grow.

Here's a good guideline for
overweight mothers:

- During the 1st trimester, gain a total
of 1 to 4 pounds.
- During the 2nd and 3rd trimesters,
gain about ½ pound per week.

It's never a good idea to go on a
weight-loss diet during pregnancy. If
you do, you may not get enough of the
iron, folic acid, and other important
nutrients your baby needs to grow.
Also, weight loss forces your body to
mobilize its fat stores for energy,
causing ketones to build up in your

Where Does the Weight Go?

Here's a look at how a 29-pound weight gain
during pregnancy is distributed in your body:

Blood	3 pounds
Breasts	2 pounds
Uterus	2 pounds
Baby	7.5 pounds
Placenta	1.5 pounds
Amniotic fluid	2 pounds
Fat, protein, and other nutrient stores	7 pounds
Retained water	4 pounds

Source: March of Dimes

blood. Over time, this may be harmful to the developing fetus.

What if you're underweight?

If you start your pregnancy with a BMI under 18.5, you need to gain 28 to 40 pounds. Underweight women should start gaining weight as early in their pregnancy as possible because gaining even a couple of extra pounds in the 1st trimester is associated with lower rates of premature delivery.

Here are good guidelines for underweight mothers:

- During the 1st trimester, gain 5 pounds.
- During the 2nd and 3rd trimesters, gain 1 to 1½ pounds a week.

Putting on extra pounds when you're underweight isn't simply a matter of loading up the grocery cart with fattening foods. Instead, follow these tips to gain weight the healthiest way for you and your baby:

- Add healthy fat (vegetable oil, nuts and nut butters, olives, avocado) to your diet rather than saturated fat (ice cream, cheese, butter).
- Choose snacks that are high in protein and calories but low in volume so you don't fill up as quickly. Try nuts and dried fruits.
- Add nonfat dry milk, soy protein powder, whey protein powder, or silken tofu to smoothies.
- Snack on energy bars that are not overly enriched with vitamins and minerals. A good choice is a Luna bar. (See "Alert! The hidden danger of fortified foods," page 34.)
- Add protein to your carbohydrates. For example, add slivered almonds

to your breakfast cereal, low-fat cheese to your crackers, and black bean dip to your bread.

- Eat frequently throughout the day, having a protein-rich snack or meal every 2 to 3 hours.
- If you are very active, ramp down your intensity a bit so that you burn fewer calories.
- Eat plenty of fruits and vegetables but boost calories with added protein and healthy fats. Spread soy butter on apple slices, dip vegetables in olive oil-and-vinegar dressing, and pair fresh berries with yogurt.

If you're still not gaining enough weight, try to figure out why. Are you full from drinking too much water? Eating too much fiber? Exercising too much? Skipping meals because you are stressed or anxious? Keeping a food record for a few days can help pinpoint your intake pattern. (See "Keeping a food diary," page 53.) Once you have a handle on why you're not gaining, try to make changes in your diet or behavior. If that doesn't help, talk with your health care provider and see a registered dietitian.

Twins, triplets, and beyond

You'll need to gain extra weight if you're carrying multiple babies. Your doctor will make the call regarding how much weight to gain based on your prepregnancy weight, your activity level, and your health history.

Twins: Early weight gain is associated with the best outcome in twin pregnancies. In general, women should gain 24 pounds during the first 24 weeks of pregnancy and an additional 10 to 20 pounds (about 1 to 1½ pounds per week) during the following weeks. The total weight gain target for normal-weight women carrying twins is 35 to 45 pounds.

Triplets: As with twins, early weight gain is recommended. Aim to gain 36 pounds by week 24 and an additional 15 pounds (approximately 1 to 1½ pounds per week) during the following weeks. The total weight gain target for normal-weight women carrying triplets is at least 50 pounds.

Quadruplets or more: Talk with your doctor and a registered dietitian for specific guidelines.

In addition to needing more calories, a woman carrying multiples requires extra vitamins and minerals. Although precise requirements for vitamins and minerals in multiple pregnancies is unknown, the Institute of Medicine recommends that women bearing more than one fetus take supplements that provide additional zinc, copper, calcium, vitamin B$_6$, folic acid, vitamin C, vitamin D, and iron.

As for increased calorie intake, plan on adding 500 calories a day for twins and 650 calories a day for triplets. Eat an extra serving of dairy, as well as extra protein, fruits and vegetables, and heart-healthy fats such as olive oil-based salad dressings, nuts and nut butters, olives, and avocados.

Your New Calorie Counts

Added pregnancy calories

If the first thing newly pregnant women ask their health care providers about is weight gain, the second is usually about food: "How much more can I eat?" For those of us who love ice cream sundaes and potato chips, the answer, unfortunately, is "Not much." Most women need to add only about 300 calories to their daily tally by the 2nd trimester. (Most normal-weight pregnant women carrying one baby need to consumer a total of 2,500 to 2,700 calories a day.)

That number can vary based on how much you exercise. If you are very active, you may need to eat more during pregnancy than a sedentary woman. Although you should gain the recommended amount of weight, you may need to take in more than the suggested 300 extra calories a day. In order to gain a pound or so a week, you may need to eat 400 or even 500 extra calories a day.

Likewise, if you're sedentary, 300 extra calories a day may be too much. You may gain enough on just 100 extra calories each day. Because it's difficult to get all of the nutrients you need each day with just 100 extra calories' worth of food, you should increase your activity level a bit so you can eat 200 or even 300 extra calories. You should also be extra mindful about limiting your intake of empty calories.

How should you spend your extra 300 calories? Keep in mind that you need not just extra calories but extra nutrients as well. During pregnancy, you require more of certain nutrients than before you became pregnant, including protein, vitamin A, vitamin C, B vitamins (including thiamin, riboflavin, niacin, folate, and B$_{12}$), iron, magnesium, selenium, and zinc. (For more on recommended vitamin and mineral intake during pregnancy, see Chapter 2.) And although calcium and fiber recommendations are the same before and during pregnancy, many women don't get enough normally, so it's important to make sure you're getting enough during pregnancy.

Three hundred calories isn't much, so spend them wisely on nutritious foods such as fruits, vegetables, lean protein, and whole grains. Here are some healthful choices that add up to approximately 300 calories:

- 1 piece whole wheat toast spread with 2 tablespoons nut butter
- 1 cup raisin bran cereal with ½ cup fat-free milk and a small apple
- 3 ounces roasted lean chicken breast and ½ cup cooked squash
- 1 flour tortilla (7-inch), ½ cup refried beans, ½ cup cooked broccoli, and ½ cup cooked red sweet pepper
- 1 cup fat-free fruit yogurt and a medium orange
- 1 baked potato with skin, topped with 1 ounce low-fat cheese and ½ cup each of broccoli and cauliflower
- 2 cups fresh spinach topped with ¼ cup fresh mushrooms, ½ ounce shredded Swiss cheese, and a sliced hard-cooked egg, sprinkled with 1 tablespoon olive oil and 1 tablespoon balsamic vinegar
- 2 slices whole wheat bread, 2 ounces lean turkey, lettuce, and tomato
- 1 cup beef and bean chili sprinkled with ½ ounce cheddar cheese

Your calorie calculator

Calorie needs differ based on factors such as your height, prepregnancy weight, activity level, and metabolism. Your doctor or registered dietitian should make the final determination on how many calories you should eat each day, but in general, you can use the following formula to figure out your daily calorie intake target:

Multiply your prepregnancy weight (in pounds) by 13 if you're sedentary, 15 if you're moderately active, and 17 if you're highly active. Then add 300. The sum is the number of calories you need each day during pregnancy.

For example, if you weighed 150 pounds before pregnancy and are moderately active, you need approximately 2,550 calories per day. (The calculation looks like this: 150×15=2,250; 2,250+300=2,550.)

Once you know how many calories you need each day, you can use the calorie-specific meal plans in this book (see "Healthy Eating Meal Plans," page 395) to build a more personalized healthy pregnancy diet.

Note: This is a rough estimate of daily calorie needs based on your starting BMI. You may find that you need more or fewer calories to promote a healthy rate of weight gain. Let your weight gain be your guide to see if you may need to change to a higher- or lower-calorie checklist.

Sugar and pregnancy

Sugar in all its forms—white sugar, brown sugar, honey, corn syrup, pancake syrup, jelly, hard candy, and molasses—contributes flavor and calories to the diet, but not much else. (The exception to this rule is blackstrap molasses. See page 32.) In addition to increasing your risk of cavities and gum disease, sugar promotes weight gain, boosts triglyceride levels in the blood, and causes blood sugar levels to skyrocket.

The most sinister kind of sugar may be high-fructose corn syrup, a sweetener added to soda, sweetened drinks, and many processed foods. Although it is a sugar, high-fructose corn syrup may not act like a sugar in your body. The theory is that it is digested, absorbed, and metabolized differently from ordinary sugar and does not have the same effect on blood sugar, insulin, or the hormones that regulate appetite. As a result, high-fructose corn syrup may not be as satisfying as regular sugar, and that could lead you to eat more and more of it. In addition, evidence suggests that high-fructose corn syrup encourages the liver to produce excessive amounts of heart-damaging triglycerides.

Many researchers believe the use of high-fructose corn syrup in processed foods is a major contributor to obesity. The consumption of high-fructose corn syrup in the United States has increased by more than 1,000 percent since 1970, mirroring the rapid increase in American obesity. Without the research to back it up, however, this is just a theory.

Limit sugar, especially high-fructose corn syrup. If you crave sweets, have a piece of fruit. Fruit contains natural sugar, which triggers a jump in blood sugar, but it also contains fiber, which helps slow down the blood sugar roller coaster. If you have to have sugar, pair it with protein. For example, eat chocolate pudding made with milk, or applesauce with almonds.

Your Pregnancy Appetite

Your up-and-down appetite

During pregnancy, your appetite is all over the place: One minute you're craving a cheeseburger and fries; the next minute you're sure you can't eat anything more than a cracker. It's normal for your appetite to fluctuate.

Most women find that in the 1st trimester, they have less interest than usual in eating. Foods you ordinarily love may make you nauseous. You may even have food aversions. For example, the smell of barbecuing meat may send you to the bathroom. Don't force yourself to eat something you don't want. No matter how healthy a food is, it's not going to help you if you force it down and then have it come back up. Besides, pregnant women who purposely eat a food that repulses them often find that they lose their taste for that food after pregnancy—sometimes years after.

Stick to mild-flavored foods that don't have much of an odor. Pungent food can set you off faster than you can say "Limburger cheese." (For more help on relieving nausea, see Chapter 4, "Managing Morning Sickness and Other Eating Problems," page 59.)

I'm hungry all the time!

You may find that pregnancy gives you a ferocious appetite, particularly in the 3rd trimester. If you find that you're starving all the time, go ahead and eat—but eat smart. Eat a small meal or snack every 3 hours to prevent yourself from getting too hungry.

When your stomach growls, consider it a golden opportunity to give your body healthy foods. You're likely to crave carbohydrates—starchy foods are very appealing, particularly in the 1st trimester. Try not to give in to too many all-carbohydrate snacks though. Adding some protein can keep your blood sugar level even. So sneak some in by eating a few almonds with your apple, a few slices of hard-cooked egg with your crackers, or some ricotta cheese with your pasta.

Finally, drink lots of water and fill up on high-fiber, high-fluid foods that will leave you feeling satisfied without adding too many excess calories.

Managing Weight Gain

When it's too much, too fast

If you find yourself gaining too much weight, sit down and try to figure out why. Are you eating loads of junk food? Do you reward yourself with food? Are you grabbing food whenever you feel tired or stressed? Are you filling up on sweets instead of facing a difficult or nerve-wracking situation? A food diary may help you uncover the whys. (See "Keeping a food diary," opposite.)

Once you understand why you're overeating, you can work on changing your behavior. If you eat when you're stressed, for example, try calming down with stress-management techniques such as deep breathing, mindful walking, yoga, warm showers, or a pregnancy massage. If you want to treat yourself to something special, buy that CD you've had your eye on or go to the movies with a friend. And if you're facing problems that seem insurmountable, ask for help. Talk with a trusted friend or family member or seek counseling with a trained therapist. Out-of-control eating will only make things worse.

Perhaps you're eating too much without even realizing it. In America's

Burn, Baby, Burn

Get moving! Here are the approximate number of calories burned during various activities.

Activity	Calories burned by a 150-pound person in 30 minutes*
Leisurely walking (2 miles per hour)	85
Brisk walking (4 miles per hour)	170
Gardening	135
Raking leaves	145
Dancing	190
Leisurely bicycling (10 miles per hour)	205
Swimming laps, medium intensity	240
Jogging (5 miles per hour)	275

*If you weigh more than 150 pounds, you'll burn more calories; if you weigh less, you'll burn fewer.

Source: U.S. Surgeon General

crazy 24–7 schedules, many rush through meals at their desks, in cars, and while they multitask. It's time to stop squeezing meals into your busy day and take time to eat mindfully and really enjoy your food. Allow plenty of time for your meal, serve food on attractive dishes, shut off the television, push aside the newspaper, and let the answering machine pick up your calls. Focus on really tasting your food rather than rushing through it. People who eat more slowly usually eat less than those who speed through their meals.

Take a look at what you're drinking. You may be eating all the right foods, but if you're enjoying those healthy foods with four or five glasses a day of sugary soda, fruit juice (even if it's 100-percent fruit), or sweetened lemonade or iced tea, you're probably getting a lot more calories than you need. Some women find that their weight gain problems disappear when they replace sweet drinks with unsweetened drinks or water.

And don't forget to think about how much you're moving. If your doctor has given you the OK for exercise, go for it. Take a walk, sign up for a prenatal exercise class, work out with a pregnancy exercise video, do prenatal yoga, go for a swim. You may think you're too tired to exercise, but you'll probably discover that exercise energizes you and relieves fatigue. (For more fitness information, see Chapter 9, "Keeping Fit During Pregnancy," page 133.)

Keeping a food diary

A food diary is an excellent way to keep track of what you eat and to determine whether you're getting the nutrients and calories you need. It also helps you become more aware of why you eat, which is particularly important if you are gaining too much weight. In a food diary, you write down what, when, where, how much, and why you eat meals and snacks throughout the day. If you want, you can write down how you feel emotionally as you eat each meal and snack.

Keeping a food diary for a week can tell you a lot about your eating habits. It will show you when and where you

Expanding Portion Sizes		
	Average portion size and calorie count 20 years ago	**Average portion size and calorie count today**
Bagel	3 inches in diameter, 140 calories	6 inches in diameter, 350 calories
Cheeseburger	Small patty, 333 calories	Large patty, 590 calories
Spaghetti and meatballs	1 cup spaghetti, 3 small meatballs, 500 calories	2 cups spaghetti, 3 large meatballs, 1,020 calories
Soda	6.5 ounces, 85 calories	20 ounces, 250 calories
Blueberry muffin	1.5 ounces, 210 calories	5 ounces, 500 calories

Source: U.S. Department of Health and Human Services

Controlling Portions

As you plan your healthy diet, think about portion control. Average portion sizes in America have ballooned over the past 20 years or so, and what you consider to be one portion may actually be two or three.

The best way to know if you're eating proper portion sizes is to measure them once or twice with a measuring cup, measuring spoons, or scale. When you're out at a restaurant or having dinner at someone's house, or you don't have time to measure, use these handy portion guidelines to determine the size of one serving:

Serving	... compares in size to
Grains	
1 cup of cereal flakes	fist
1 pancake	compact disk
½ cup cooked rice, pasta, or potato	baseball
1 slice of bread	cassette tape
1 piece of corn bread	bar of soap
Vegetables and fruit	
1 cup of salad greens	baseball
1 baked potato	fist
1 medium fruit	baseball
½ cup fresh fruit	half a baseball
½ cup chopped vegetables	lightbulb
¼ cup raisins	large egg
Dairy and cheese	
1½ ounces	4 stacked dice or 2 cheese slices
½ cup ice cream	half a baseball
Meat and alternatives	
3 ounces meat, fish, or poultry	deck of cards
3 ounces grilled or baked fish	checkbook
2 tablespoons peanut butter	ping-pong ball
Fats	
1 teaspoon margarine or spread	1 die

tend to overeat, what foods you eat too much of, and what kinds of emotions trigger poor eating. Then, after you have a good understanding of your eating habits, you can work to improve your diet.

Use a notebook for your food diary or the Healthy Eating Meal Plans (page 395). Feel free to keep a small notebook if you need more room for documenting your emotions and other information.

Eating in restaurants

Portion control is particularly difficult when you're eating away from home. It's easier if you keep these tips in mind:

Eat small. Order an appetizer as your main course or split an entrée with your dining companion.

Start with a salad. A salad with low-fat dressing can fill you up and help you get the vegetables you need for the day. Choose a garden salad and ask the waiter to leave off croutons, meat, bacon bits, and other fatty toppings.

Go to the bar. Take advantage of grocery store and restaurant salad bars, but choose wisely. Avoid creamy dressings, fried noodles, shredded cheese, and croutons. Instead, select lots of greens and vegetables and sprinkle with low-fat dressing, nonfat dressing, or oil and vinegar.

Take half home. When your waiter brings your meal, ask for a take-out container and immediately pack half to take home. That way you won't be tempted to eat more than half.

Order healthier fare. Choose broiled meat and fish instead of fried, baked potatoes instead of french fries, and vegetable-based soups instead of creamy chowders.

Read between the lines. Look for menu items that are baked, braised, blackened, broiled, grilled, poached, roasted, steamed, or stir-fried. Foods prepared in these ways are often lower in fat and calories than those that are fried or sauteed.

Get the bread out. Out of sight, that is. Ask the waiter to take away the breadbasket. Bread and butter add calories and fat, raise blood sugar, and fill you up before you even order your meal. If you're starving when you sit down, ask the waiter to bring you a glass of tomato juice or side salad right away.

Order the smallest size. In a world full of super sizes, smaller is better. You might even be able to order child-size drinks, french fries, and desserts.

Ask the waiter to hold the sauce or dressing. Or have it on the side and dip your food into it rather than pouring it all over everything.

Drink smart. Choose water, unsweetened iced tea, seltzer, or fat-free milk instead of sweet, calorie-laden drinks.

Forget the "value meals." Sure, it may be economical to buy an extra-large order of fries, but all that food is no good for your health no matter how much you save. Buy the smallest size even if it's not a bargain. Or buy the larger size and share it with a friend (or several friends). If you're alone, drop what you don't want to eat into the trash.

Eat smart in fast-food joints. It's not as hard as it seems to eat well in fast-food restaurants. Choose salad with low-fat dressing, a single hamburger with no mayonnaise, a baked potato, a grilled chicken sandwich without sauce, or a small cup of chili.

Dieting during pregnancy

One word you need to know about dieting during pregnancy is *Don't*. Although it's very important not to overeat during pregnancy, it's even more important that you stay away from weight-loss deprivation diets.

No matter what your weight, you should never go on a calorie-reducing diet while you're expecting. If you do, your baby may suffer. Your baby needs the vitamins, minerals, and energy that your diet provides. Starve yourself and you're starving your baby too.

Low-carbohydrate diets are particularly dangerous during pregnancy. Carbohydrates are the ideal fuel source for you and your baby because they're more efficient at delivering energy than protein or fat. If you don't eat enough carbohydrates, your body will have to burn fat for energy. Sounds great, right? Wrong. When the body burns fat, substances called ketones are released into the blood. Ketones can harm your baby—even a moderate amount of ketones in your blood is dangerous. That doesn't mean you should go wild with carbohydrates. A moderate carbohydrate intake is best for you and your baby.

Reducing dietary fat isn't a great idea either. Your baby's developing brain and eyes need the fatty acids in the foods you eat. Again, moderation makes the most sense. Be sure to include healthy fats in your diet but don't go overboard.

Perhaps you were dieting before you became pregnant. If so, now's the time to adjust your diet by adding calories, carbohydrates, fat, or whatever you may have drastically cut back. If you've been on a low-carbohydrate diet, add carbohydrates gradually so that your blood sugar levels don't suddenly skyrocket. Focus primarily on whole grains, legumes, and whole fruits because they don't cause blood sugar to spike the way processed carbohydrates and fruit juices do.

If you've been on a meal-replacement diet, you probably don't have to give up the prepackaged foods that have helped you lose weight, provided they aren't too high in sodium. You do, however, need to round them out with other foods. Make a prepackaged meal more nutritious by adding a salad, fruit, milk, some bread, or some vegetables.

Although it is best for both you and your baby to give up a deprivation diet, you can increase your calorie count healthfully. If you're not sure how to do it, see a registered dietitian for advice.

Eating disorders and pregnancy

Approximately 5 percent of American women have a history of eating disorders such as anorexia nervosa and bulimia nervosa. Women with eating disorders often have trouble getting pregnant because dieting, excessive exercise, and low body weight affect their endocrine system, which regulates pregnancy hormones.

If they do manage to get pregnant, women with eating disorders are at an increased risk of miscarriage, premature birth, stillbirth, preeclampsia, gestational diabetes, cesarean delivery, having a baby with low birthweight and birth defects such as blindness and mental retardation, developing postpartum depression, and suffering from weak and fragile teeth and bones, according to Anorexia Nervosa and Related Eating Disorders, Inc. (ANRED), a nonprofit education organization.

Babies born to women with eating disorders may develop a range of physical, social, intellectual, mental, and emotional developmental difficulties.

Pregnancy can worsen an eating disorder. If you had an eating disorder in the past, pregnancy may cause it to recur even if you have recovered fully from it.

How do you know if you have an eating disorder? Check the following list of warning signs, and if some of them describe your behavior, get help as soon as possible. Your doctor should be able to refer you to a counselor who specializes in eating disorders.

The warning signs of eating disorders include:

- Skipping meals
- Taking tiny portions
- Not wanting to eat in front of others
- Chewing food and spitting it out before swallowing
- Eating only a small selection of foods
- Eating only low-calorie or low-fat foods
- Drinking large amounts of diet soda
- Eating very little or no fat
- Being obsessed with food and reading food labels
- Secretly gorging on large amounts of food
- Forcing yourself to vomit after eating
- Using laxatives, diet pills, water pills, or "natural" products from health food stores to promote weight loss
- Being obsessed with your body's appearance
- Feeling that you can never be thin enough to satisfy yourself
- Feeling self-hatred
- Compulsive exercise
- Believing that if you are thinner, your life will be much better
- Having trouble concentrating

continued on page 58

continued from page 57

If you think you have an eating disorder, seek professional help from a registered dietitian, therapist, or psychologist specializing in eating disorders and consider joining a support group. Even slight undernutrition during pregnancy can increase your risk of going into labor and delivering your baby early, which means a low birthweight. Although more research needs to be done on eating disorders during pregnancy, evidence suggests people with eating disorders are more likely to have been born prematurely and with low birthweight.

If you can control your disordered eating habits and follow a healthy pregnancy diet, your risk of pregnancy complications plummets. The sooner you start eating a normal diet, the greater the chance that you'll have a healthy pregnancy and give birth to a healthy baby.

During pregnancy, try your best to gain the recommended amount of weight, eat a healthy pregnancy diet, and avoid purging and using laxatives or diuretics. Be sure to tell your doctor about your eating disorder history.

managing
morning sickness
and other eating problems

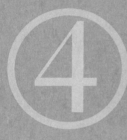

It's annoying but true: Nausea and vomiting are a very real part of most women's pregnancies. Some lucky women sail through pregnancy with only an occasional upset stomach. Others are so sick their bodies have to receive fluids and nutrients intravenously. Most women are in the middle. The nausea and vomiting they experience goes away by the 2nd trimester. What can you do if you're feeling sick to your stomach? This chapter shares tips that include staying hydrated; eating smaller, more frequent meals; and avoiding certain foods. And remember, no matter how crummy you feel, mild morning sickness won't hurt your baby.

Managing Eating Problems

Cute maternity clothes and gift-filled baby showers will play a starring role in your pregnancy. Unfortunately for most women, so will nausea and vomiting and other eating problems. About three-quarters of pregnant women experience some kind of nausea and vomiting, also known as morning sickness even though it occurs throughout the day, not just in the morning. About 50 percent of women experience both nausea and vomiting, 25 percent suffer nausea only, and a lucky 25 percent are unaffected.

Morning Sickness

Who is affected?

Morning sickness usually starts within the first 9 weeks of pregnancy and ends by around 13 weeks. Some women simply feel nauseous; others gag, vomit, retch, or experience dry heaves. In the vast majority of cases, morning sickness is nothing more than an annoyance. (A small number of women suffer from debilitating nausea and vomiting—a condition known as hyperemesis gravidarum—that is so severe it can threaten their baby's health. See "Severe Nausea," page 62.)

Nobody knows exactly why pregnant women feel nauseated, but fluctuating hormone levels are the likely culprit.

Some people believe that nausea and vomiting, as well as food aversions, are an evolutionary adaptation that developed to protect women and their babies from potentially dangerous foods. Most health care providers, however, consider that a myth.

Another myth is that morning sickness is hereditary. The evidence doesn't bear this out. Morning sickness patterns vary not only between mother and daughter but also between pregnancies. You may have a fair amount of nausea and vomiting with one baby and hardly any with the next. (This is true only of mild morning sickness; hyperemesis gravidarum does appear to have a genetic component.)

Although morning sickness has not been linked to any kind of vitamin deficiency, studies show that women who begin taking a prenatal vitamin before pregnancy are less likely to suffer from nausea and vomiting than those who start taking the vitamins after they become pregnant.

Prevention and coping tips

No matter how lousy it makes you feel, mild morning sickness poses no risk to you or your baby, provided you don't become dehydrated. Even when you can't eat, try to drink water. If you can't stomach water, add a lemon wedge or try diluted fruit juice, ice chips, unsweetened seltzer, frozen 100-percent-fruit-juice bars, or decaffeinated tea or coffee. Try different temperatures—some women who can't keep cold water down do fine with warm water. Take small, frequent sips rather than gulping down large amounts all at once.

Here are some tips on how to prevent and cope with mild nausea and vomiting. Not all of them work for every woman, so experiment to see what might help you:

- Get up slowly in the morning. Hurrying out of bed can trigger a bout of nausea.
- Keep a few crackers on your nightstand. Eat them before getting out of bed.
- Avoid strong odors. As much as possible, stay away from perfume, body lotion, cooking foods, soiled diapers, restrooms, barbecue fires, smelly fish, pungent raw foods (such as garlic), and pet odors. Just the thought of such strong odors can bother you. Even fragrances that you enjoyed before pregnancy can make you feel sick now. Don't toss your perfumes in the trash though; you'll enjoy their scents again later in your pregnancy or after your baby is born.
- Avoid spicy or fatty foods. They can upset your stomach.
- Stay out of the kitchen. Ask someone else to do the cooking or rely on raw produce and foods that don't require cooking. As much as possible, take advantage of the times when you feel good by preparing future meals to have on hand when you don't feel so great. For ideas, see the "Make-

Ahead Meals" recipe section, starting on page 347.
- Keep fresh air flowing. Open the windows or run air-conditioners or fans in your house, at work, and in the car.
- Eat three small meals and two to three small snacks a day. Avoid large meals. For ideas, check out the "Light Mini Meals" recipe section, starting on page 251
- Don't drink with food. It may fill you up too much. Instead, take small sips with your food—just enough to moisten it—but wait 15 or 20 minutes after a meal to drink the majority of your beverage.
- Take your prenatal vitamin at night or with food. The iron in the vitamin may upset your stomach, and sometimes food can settle it. If you take the vitamin before bed, you may sleep through the worst of the nausea. Although vitamin manufacturers recommend taking prenatal supplements in the morning without food, it's better to take them at night and keep them down than to take them in the morning and have them come right back up. If you haven't started taking a prenatal vitamin yet, begin as soon as possible.
- Keep blood sugar levels stable. Peaks and valleys in blood sugar can trigger nausea. Don't let yourself get too hungry because that causes blood sugar levels to plummet. As much as possible, avoid all-carbohydrate snacks and meals. Just a little protein with your carbohydrates—a smear of peanut butter on your bread, a bit of cheese on your crackers, a touch of

cottage cheese with your apple—can help keep blood sugar from surging and crashing.

- Switch to chewable vitamins. A children's chewable multivitamin may sit better in your stomach than a big pill you swallow whole. As long as the chewable vitamins contain 400 micrograms of folic acid, they're as good as adult vitamins.
- Ask your doctor about vitamin B_6 supplements. Some women find that 10–25 milligrams three or four times a day keeps nausea at bay.
- Ask your doctor about antihistamines. The American College of Obstetricians and Gynecologists recommends treatment with vitamin B_6 alone or three or four daily doses of 10 milligrams of vitamin B_6 plus 10–12.5 milligrams of doxylamine, an antihistamine that is considered safe during pregnancy. Researchers don't know why an antihistamine might help with nausea and vomiting, but studies show that it sometimes does.
- Talk with your doctor about taking ginger capsules. Some women find that ginger reduces nausea.
- Don't worry too much about what you're eating. Good nutrition is important, but at this point, if all you can keep down is white bread, go ahead and eat it. What matters most in the 1st trimester is adequate energy intake. You'll have time to catch up on your healthy eating when you start feeling less nauseous.
- Avoid eating very hot with very cold foods. For example, don't have a meal that combines a hot soup with a cold glass of milk.

- Eat cool foods. They have less odor than warm foods. Try cold cooked meats, cold cheese, and hard-cooked eggs that have been chilled in the refrigerator.
- Try tart, sour, or salty snacks. (See "Snacks that help relieve nausea," opposite page.)
- Wear Sea-Bands. These acupressure wristbands—designed for ocean travel—help some women with morning sickness too. The knitted, elasticized bands contain plastic studs that apply constant gentle pressure to an acupressure point on each wrist, which may aid in reducing nausea. According to Eastern medical tradition, pressure on this point frees up blocked chi, or life energy. It may sound implausible, but some pregnant women swear by their Sea-Bands. You can buy them at natural-food stores and most pharmacies. They are washable and reusable.

Severe Nausea

Hyperemesis gravidarum

When nausea and vomiting are so bad that you can't keep any food or fluids down, take it seriously. It may be hyperemesis gravidarum. Although it is a rare condition—it affects fewer than 2 percent of pregnancies—it is a medical problem that requires treatment. Babies born to women with hyperemesis are more likely to be underweight than babies whose mothers did not have hyperemesis.

Unlike morning sickness, which

Snacks that help relieve nausea

Sometimes sour and salty foods can help with that queasy feeling. Here are some tasty snacks that are worth a try:

- Granny Smith apple with cheddar cheese or nuts
- Almonds and dried cherries or cranberries
- Celery sticks with chive cottage cheese or hummus
- Pickle spear with a slice of cheese
- Pretzel nuggets with peanut butter or cheese
- Gingersnaps and a cup of milk
- Lemon yogurt

Try to eat every three to four hours, even if you feel nauseous. Some women find that keeping something in their stomach staves off feelings of nausea. Try also to stay hydrated. Don't gulp down a huge glass of water because it's likely to make you feel queasy. Instead, have a glass or bottle of water by your side and sip it slowly throughout the day. If cold water bothers you, try warm water or tea. If you choose tea, keep track of caffeine and limit yourself to 300 milligrams a day (see "Caffeine Levels in Popular Beverages and Foods," page 39). You may enjoy weak tea almost as much as you enjoy strong tea; the less time you leave a tea bag in hot water, the less caffeine your tea will contain.

usually lasts 3 months, hyperemesis may continue throughout pregnancy. Although the condition itself is rare, it's the most common cause of hospital admission during early pregnancy and is second only to preterm labor as the most common reason for hospitalization during pregnancy.

One of the dangers of hyperemesis is dehydration, which can stress the body, increase pulse rate, and decrease blood pressure. If not properly treated, hyperemesis can also cause vitamin deficiencies, particularly of water-soluble vitamins that the body is not able to store.

While it's important to know the risks of hyperemesis, keep in mind that in the vast majority of women, hyperemesis either goes away on its own or can be successfully treated, and most women with hyperemesis give birth to perfectly healthy babies. In fact, women who experience nausea and vomiting during pregnancy—even when it advances to hyperemesis— have a lower rate of miscarriages than women who have no such symptoms.

Risk factors. Although health care providers don't know what causes hyperemesis, some women are more likely to develop it, including those carrying more than one fetus, those carrying a female baby, daughters and sisters of women who have had it, those who are sensitive to motion, those who have a history of migraines, and those who had hyperemesis during a previous pregnancy.

Signs of hyperemesis. Call the doctor if you experience any of the following:
- Constant vomiting, to the point that

you can't keep food or even liquids
down for 24 hours
● Vomiting immediately after eating or
drinking anything
● Vomiting blood
● Severe headaches
● Loss of need to urinate or dark-
colored urine
● Weight loss
● Pounding or racing of your heart
  If you are vomiting excessively—
even if you think it may be the result
of a stomach bug—call your health care
provider. When there is a risk of
dehydration or malnourishment, it's
better to be safe than sorry. If your
vomiting starts for the first time when
you are in the 2nd or 3rd trimester,
your doctor may want to rule out other
possible causes of vomiting.
  With hyperemesis, the sooner you
seek treatment the better because
hyperemesis becomes more difficult to
treat as symptoms progress. Vomiting
and dehydration cause fatigue, which
triggers more vomiting, which makes
you more fatigued—it's a downward
spiral. Treatment in the early stages
may prevent more serious complications and hospitalization.
  Treatment. Intravenous (IV) fluids
are given to pregnant women who
become dehydrated from excessive
vomiting. If you need IV fluids, your
doctor will probably advise you to go to
your local hospital, where you will be
hooked up to an IV and given a dilute
salt solution. The IV solution may
contain electrolytes and an antiemetic
(nausea) drug. You'll stay at the
hospital until you are properly
hydrated, are no longer vomiting

excessively, and can manage sipping
fluids at home.
  If vomiting continues and you are
losing weight, your health care provider
will probably admit you to the hospital,
where there are a number of safe
treatments available.
  In addition to an intravenous saline
solution, vitamins and antiemetics will
be administered. Some women
improve with antiemetics given as
rectal suppositories rather than pills.
Your provider may treat you with
vitamin B$_6$ alone or in combination
with doxylamine.
  If you are still unable to hold down
fluids, there are other options that are
safe for you and your baby. In extreme
cases, several days of IV may be
needed; a feeding tube with high-
calorie nutrition is also helpful for
many women. Studies show that even
adding steroids to the IV fluid can do
the trick.
  The key is to keep a positive
attitude. Most women who have
hyperemesis gravidarum will recover
within days; it rarely takes weeks.
Even though you may feel horrible,
your baby is growing happily. Don't
blame yourself if you have
hyperemesis—it's something that
happens, not something you bring on.
  Additional testing. Generally in the
course of all of this upheaval, you will
have an ultrasound to see how many
babies are present. In cases of
hyperemesis, additional studies are
done to see if there are other explana-
tions to account for extreme symptoms,
such as hyperthyroidism.
  Remember, even as you recover,

reintroduce a bland diet in small portions. You still may benefit from Sea-Bands, so don't give those up just yet. (For more information on Sea-Bands, see "Prevention and coping tips," starting on page 60.)

Mouth Issues

When good foods taste bad

Some pregnant women develop an unpleasant metallic taste in their mouth. Even plain water takes on a disagreeable taste that may trigger vomiting. Still others find sweet-tasting food to be unusually offensive. This is called dysgeusia. Here are some tips on how to cope with taste changes:

To mask a bitter or metallic taste, make a beeline for sour and tart foods. Sour and tart tastes are especially helpful with meats, so marinate meat in vinegar, low-sodium soy sauce, and citrus juices. Sour and tart tastes will also stimulate salivation, which helps wash away the annoying metallic taste; they also combat "dry mouth." Try adding lemons to your water, drinking lemonade, and sucking on sour citrus drops. Use plasticware instead of silverware to combat that metallic aftertaste too.

To tame overly sweet tastes, avoid concentrated sweets. Add a tiny pinch of salt to canned/jarred fruits or other sweet dishes.

Pay attention to what foods taste best and work with them! If salty appeals, stick to peanut butter, cheese, and cottage cheese for proteins. Add some pickles or olives to other dishes.

Rinse your mouth frequently between meals. Brush teeth and tongue with a small soft brush. Try a rinse of ½ teaspoon baking soda mixed with ½ teaspoon salt and 1 cup warm water. Keep mouth moist throughout the day with frequent sips of fluid, sugar-free candies, and artificial saliva products if necessary.

Excessive salivation

No, you're not imagining it—pregnancy can cause you to salivate more than usual, particularly during your 1st trimester. As with many of the other minor annoyances of pregnancy, nobody is sure what causes this, but hormones may be the culprit.

Excessive salivation, which is also called ptyalism, is more common in women with hyperemesis. It also occurs more often in women with heartburn because heartburn causes an increase in stomach acid, which in turn triggers salivation.

Although excess salivation is bothersome, it won't hurt you or your baby, and it will probably go away by the end of your 1st trimester. Nausea can make it worse, so by taking steps to prevent nausea (such as eating smaller meals and avoiding foods that trigger nausea), you may help curb excess salivation as well.

Ironically, drinking plenty of water can help because it washes saliva out of your mouth and into your stomach, where it is less bothersome. You can also spit saliva out into a cup or sink. Some women find that brushing their teeth frequently (with a soft brush that won't be too rough on tender gums) and sucking on hard candies (choose sugarless to prevent tooth decay) help make the saliva less unpleasant to swallow, although neither will decrease saliva production.

Cravings and Aversions

When you hate foods you love

You adore broccoli. Before you conceived, you ate it all the time. Now the thought of it turns you green. It's not unusual to no longer like the foods you used to love. You may be repulsed by the smell, texture, taste, or appearance of certain foods. Even seeing a picture of them in a magazine or a commercial for them on television may make you queasy.

Foods that trigger aversions include meats, fish, poultry, and eggs; pungent foods such as mushrooms, coffee, garlic, and strong cheese; highly spiced foods; and fatty or fried foods. Food aversions may come and go—a food that disgusts you today you may love again tomorrow—or they can last throughout pregnancy.

If a food repulses you, avoid it and look for other, more palatable foods that provide similar nutrients.

Constant cravings

Pizza, pasta, pie. What are you craving? Some of the items pregnant women crave most are chocolate, pickles, chips, and ice cream. If you're feeling nauseated and having trouble keeping food down, it's fine to eat what you crave—at least you'll get something in your stomach. If you're feeling fine, though, try to stick to a healthy diet and eat only small amounts of the sweets and other low-nutrient, high-fat foods you are craving.

Pica and nonfood cravings

What if you want to eat soap or burnt matches? This craving for nonfood substances is called pica. Common cravings include dirt, clay, sand, stones, paper, laundry starch, soap, ashes, chalk, paint, burnt matches, or talcum powder, as well as unusually large amounts of foods ordinarily eaten only in very small quantities, such as baking powder and cornstarch.

Eating nonfood items can be incredibly dangerous because of the potentially toxic impurities they contain. For example, soil and clay can contain lead, which can cause miscarriage, preterm delivery, low birthweight, and developmental delays in babies. Soil and clay can also contain parasites such as the one that causes

Fact or fiction? If you find yourself craving a certain food, your body must need the nutrients in that food.

Fiction. There's no evidence that cravings correspond to vitamin or mineral deficiencies. If you crave a hamburger, for example, it's probably because you like hamburgers, not because you need extra iron.

toxoplasmosis. Nonfoods can cause severe constipation, perforations of the gastrointestinal tract, and intestinal blockages. Finally, some nonfood substances bind to the nutrients in your body, robbing you and your baby of their value.

Some women crave ice and chip it off the inside of their freezer. This can be hazardous because that ice can harbor dangerous levels of bacteria.

Although the cause of pica is unknown—and no clear evidence shows a nutrient deficiency to be the culprit—deficiencies in iron, calcium, zinc, and certain other vitamins have been associated with it. Tell your doctor if you're craving nonfoods; she may test your blood to see if your iron or other nutrient stores are low.

Eating clay and other nonfoods has been traditional in some cultures for centuries. Scientists are looking into whether any nonfoods supply nutrients that a pregnant woman needs or whether nonfoods such as clay bind to and carry away toxins in your body. However, until their research is completed, avoid all nonfood items. To satisfy your cravings, look for foods with similar taste or texture. For example, if you crave the chalky taste of clay, see if an over-the-counter antacid such as Tums satisfies your craving. (Consume antacids in moderation, though.)

Should you see a dietitian?

If you have a nutrition-related health concern or have nutrition questions that your doctor can't answer, consider seeing a registered dietitian. Most health insurance companies cover visits with a dietitian, particularly if your pregnancy is considered nutritionally high-risk, meaning you have diabetes, hypertension, or other diet-related heath concerns. Call your insurance company before scheduling an appointment because some require you to get a referral from your primary care physician or obstetric provider.

Look for a dietitian with the letters R.D. after his or her name. R.D. stands for "registered dietitian," and it means that the dietitian is certified by the American Dietetic Association (ADA). In order to get certification, a dietitian must earn a bachelor's degree with food and nutrition sciences course work; complete an accredited six- to 12-month practice program at a health care facility, community agency, or food service corporation; and pass a national examination administered by the Commission on Dietetic Registration. After certification, R.D.s must complete continuing professional education requirements to maintain their registration. Many R.D.s hold additional certifications in specialized areas of practice, such as pediatric nutrition, diabetes education, or prenatal nutrition.

Don't be fooled by people who call themselves "nutritionists." They are not registered dietitians, and they may not have the education and training that an R.D. has. In fact, many so-called nutritionists are in business primarily to sell unproven dietary supplements or herbal products.

continued on page 68

continued from page 67
It's a good idea to visit an R.D. if you:

- Are underweight
- Are overweight
- Are pregnant with more than one baby
- Have been advised by your doctor to go on bed rest or to make a major cut in your activity level
- Gained or lost a large amount of weight shortly before your pregnancy
- Have severe morning sickness
- Don't eat any foods from certain food groups
- Have phenylketonuria (PKU)
- Started your pregnancy with preexisting chronic health problems such as diabetes, high blood pressure, heart disease, gastrointestinal reflux, high cholesterol, HIV, kidney or liver disease, or irritable bowel syndrome
- Have a history of eating disorders
- Had gastric bypass surgery before getting pregnant
- Have a history of substance abuse or alcohol abuse
- Have given birth to a baby with a neural tube defect
- Are a teenager
- Are unsure what to eat, how many calories to consume, or how much weight to gain
- Need motivation to eat well
- Have unusual food cravings (for example, cornstarch or baking soda) or are craving nonfood substances such as clay or dirt (see page 66)
- Are interested in receiving individualized nutrition counseling
- Are a vegan (a vegetarian who eats no animal products)
- Would like advice about planning healthy meals or making smart choices in restaurants

Ask your doctor to refer you to an R.D. or get a recommendation from the American Dietetic Association (www.eatright.org or 800-366-1655).

foods that
can harm

The food supply in the United States is among the safest in the world. Despite that, some 76 million Americans get sick each year as a result of foodborne illness, and 5,000 of them die. Pregnant women are particularly vulnerable to foodborne illness. However, you can prevent most food-safety problems by making proper food choices and by handling and storing food correctly. In this chapter, you'll learn about smart food handling and why it's so important to you and your baby.

Foods That Can Harm

Pregnant women are particularly vulnerable to foodborne illness. When you're pregnant, your immune system may not fight off harmful bacteria as well as it does when you're not expecting. Harmful bacteria that make their way into your body can cross the placenta and infect your baby, whose developing immune system is no match for them. Pregnant women who contract foodborne illnesses are at risk for serious health problems and miscarriage, and their babies are at increased risk of being born early and having birth defects.

In general, foodborne illnesses cause symptoms such as stomach cramps, vomiting, diarrhea, fever, headache, and body aches, although sometimes you can be infected and feel fine.

Harmful Bacteria

You will most likely be able to prevent potential problems from foodborne illnesses by following smart and simple food-handling and storing rules. You should also be aware of some of the most common food pathogens, which include the following:

Listeria

These bacteria can be found in refrigerated ready-to-eat foods (such as dairy products, packaged lunch meats, deli meats, poultry, and seafood), unpasteurized milk, and milk products made from unpasteurized milk (such as raw-milk goat cheese).

Listeriosis, the infection caused by listeria, can be devastating to your baby. A fetus with listeriosis has a higher risk of miscarriage, premature birth, or stillbirth and newborns can develop mental retardation, blindness, seizures, and paralysis. Listeriosis occurs 20 times more often in pregnant women than in nonpregnant adults, possibly because the immune system is weakened during pregnancy.

The symptoms of listeriosis may include fever, muscle aches, chills, and sometimes nausea or diarrhea. It can develop into a blood infection or meningitis, an infection of the membranes in the brain. Symptoms of meningitis include severe headache and a stiff neck.

If you suspect you have listeriosis, contact your doctor immediately. Antibiotics can prevent the bacteria from infecting your baby if administered early enough. At any rate, it's always a good idea to tell your doctor about any flu-like symptoms.

To protect yourself from listeriosis, follow these U.S. Food and Drug Administration guidelines:

- Do not eat hot dogs or luncheon

meats, including deli meats such as ham, turkey, and bologna, unless they are heated until steaming hot.

- Do not consume unpasteurized milk or any foods made from it. Stay away from soft cheeses such as feta, Brie, Camembert, Roquefort, blue-veined, queso blanco, queso fresco, or Panela (unless they have been made with pasteurized milk; check the label). Hard cheeses, process cheeses, cream cheese, and cottage cheese are safe, as is any cheese that has been thoroughly heated.

- Do not eat refrigerated pâtés or meat spreads because listeria thrive at refrigerator temperatures. Canned and shelf-stable versions are safe for pregnant women to eat.

- Avoid refrigerated smoked seafood unless it has been cooked (for example, in a casserole). At the grocery store or deli counter, refrigerated smoked seafood, such as salmon, trout, whitefish, cod, tuna, and mackerel, is most often labeled "nova-style," "lox," "kippered," "smoked," or "jerky"; avoid all of these. Canned and shelf-stable versions can be eaten safely.

Toxoplasma

Toxoplasma is a parasite that is found on unwashed fruits and vegetables; in raw or undercooked meats, poultry, and eggs; and in water, dust, and soil. It can cause toxoplasmosis, an illness that can cause hearing loss, mental retardation, and blindness in newborn babies who were infected by it while in their mother's uterus.

To keep you and your baby safe from toxoplasmosis, fully cook meat, poultry, and eggs (see "Safe Cooking Temperatures," page 77) and avoid foods made with raw or partially cooked eggs, such as cookie batter, eggnog, hollandaise sauce, and some Caesar salad dressings. Also, wash fresh fruits and vegetables thoroughly with tap water before eating. If there is a firm surface, such as on apples or potatoes, scrub the produce with a brush. Do not use detergent or soap, however, because unsafe residue may remain on the produce.

Toxoplasma can also turn up in cat-litter boxes and outdoor places where cat feces may be found, such as gardens and sandboxes. If you must clean the litter box, use gloves and wash your hands thoroughly with warm water and soap afterwards. Also, be sure to wear gloves when gardening or handling sand in a sandbox.

Most nonpregnant people who are exposed to the toxoplasma parasite experience a mild infection and then develop a protective resistance to it. However, if a woman who has not been previously exposed to the parasite first acquires an infection a few months before or during pregnancy, she may pass it to her unborn baby.

Toxoplasmosis may cause no symptoms or it may cause only mild flu-like symptoms. However, if you get toxoplasmosis there is about a 40 percent chance that you'll pass it on to your baby. Antibiotics may help reduce the severity of symptoms in your baby after birth, but the best thing for your baby is to prevent toxoplasmosis in the first place.

Salmonella

These bacteria, which can cause an illness called salmonellosis if they are ingested, are spread through direct or indirect contact with the intestinal contents or waste of animals and humans. Pregnant women are at no higher risk than other people of getting salmonellosis, but if they do contract it, it can be dangerous. Rarely, salmonella bacteria are passed to the fetus, where they can cause miscarriage, stillbirth, or premature labor.

Foods that commonly carry salmonella bacteria include unpasteurized milk products; raw or undercooked meat, eggs, and poultry; raw sprouts (alfalfa, clover, radish, broccoli); and cream-based dessert fillings made with raw eggs or dairy.

Symptoms of salmonellosis include headache, diarrhea, abdominal pain, nausea, chills, fever, and vomiting within 12 to 36 hours of ingestion.

To be safe, avoid the foods that may carry salmonella and follow safe food-handling rules.

Vibrio parahaemolyticus

These bacteria live in brackish salt water along the coasts of the United States and Canada. They are present in higher concentrations during the summer and can contaminate fish and shellfish, especially oysters. The bacteria can cause a gastrointestinal illness in humans called vibrio infection. Infection leads to diarrhea, vomiting, abdominal cramping, fever, and chills. Vibrio infection during pregnancy has not been well studied, so researchers aren't sure what kind of risk it may pose to an unborn baby. To protect yourself, completely cook all shellfish, particularly oysters. Infection with vibrio bacteria is treated with antibiotics that are believed to be safe during pregnancy.

Clostridium botulinum

In rare cases these bacteria, which can be found in moist, low-acid foods, can produce a toxin that causes botulism, a disease that leads to muscle paralysis. Never eat food from containers that show the telltale signs of clostridium botulinum contamination: leaking, bulging, or badly dented cans; cracked jars; jars with loose or bulging lids; cans with a foul odor; or any container that spurts liquid when opened. Don't even taste suspicious food because a tiny amount can be deadly to both mother and baby.

Fact or fiction? Rinsing meat with water before cooking removes bacteria and makes the meat safer to eat.

Fiction. The latest guidelines from the U.S. Department of Agriculture advise against washing raw poultry, beef, pork, lamb, or veal before cooking because doing so makes it more likely that harmful bacteria will be spread around the kitchen. Don't worry: Thorough cooking will destroy bacteria on the surface of the meat, so washing is unnecessary. (See "Safe Cooking Temperatures," page 77.)

Four ways to fight foodborne illness

Here are four simple ways to lower your risk of catching a foodborne illness:

Concentrate on cleanliness. Wash your hands with warm water and soap before and after handling food, after using the bathroom or changing a diaper, and after handling pets. Wash cutting boards, dishes, utensils, and countertops with hot water and soap and replace cutting boards when they become worn. Rinse raw fruits and vegetables thoroughly under running water before eating.

Separate raw foods from cooked foods. Keep raw meat, poultry, and seafood away from ready-to-eat foods. Use two cutting boards: one for raw foods and another for foods that won't be cooked. Do not place cooked food on an unwashed plate that held raw meat, poultry, or seafood because bacteria from the raw food could contaminate the cooked food.

Cook thoroughly. Cook foods completely and use a food thermometer to check for doneness. (See "Safe Cooking Temperatures," page 77.)

Keep it cool. Set your refrigerator at 40 degrees F or below and set the freezer at 0 degrees F or below. Use an appliance thermometer to make sure your refrigerator and freezer are at the proper temperatures. Refrigerate or freeze perishable foods promptly and use them before they spoil. (See "Safe Storage Times for Refrigerated Foods," page 75.) Unfortunately, you can't rely on your senses to tell you if a food is unsafe. Dangerous bacteria generally do not affect the taste, smell, or appearance of a food. If you inadvertently forget to refrigerate a food that should be chilled, throw it away if it's been out more than 2 hours (or 1 hour if the air temperature is warmer than 90 degrees).

Store canned goods and other non-perishables in a cool, dry place. Don't keep them above the stove, under the sink, in a damp garage or basement, or in any place that is exposed to high or low temperatures.

Be cautious when eating home-canned meats, vegetables, and jams. Improperly preserved food can become contaminated by bacteria or toxins. For guidelines on safe canning, visit the University of Georgia's National Center for Home Food Preservation website at www.uga.edu/nchfp.

Proper Food Handling

Meat safety

Raw meat and poultry can carry all kinds of toxins. The best way to protect yourself is to keep raw meat and its juices away from countertops and other foods and to wash your hands and your work surfaces carefully after handling raw meat.

In the grocery store, never buy meat or poultry in packaging that is torn or leaky. Place raw meat packages into plastic bags to contain any juices.

As meat ages, bacteria multiply. Check expiration dates and don't buy meat that is past its date. Once you get home from the grocery store, refrigerate or freeze meat immediately. Throw away meat or poultry that smells bad, is sticky or tacky to the touch, or is slimy. Spoiled meat may fade or darken in color, but don't judge a meat by color alone because some color changes are normal for fresh meat and poultry.

If you normally thaw frozen meat on the countertop or in hot water, now is a good time to learn a safer way to do it. Frozen meat left to thaw at room temperature is a prime breeding ground for bacteria. As soon as a food becomes warmer than 40 degrees F, any bacteria it harbored before freezing can begin to multiply.

Here are three safe ways to thaw frozen meat:

- In the refrigerator. This requires planning because it takes time. A pound of ground beef or boneless chicken breasts requires a full day to thaw in the refrigerator, and a large item like a frozen turkey needs 24 hours in the refrigerator for every 5 pounds of weight. After thawing in the refrigerator, poultry and ground meat should be cooked within one or two days. Red meat will last three to five days.

- In cold water. This is faster than thawing in the refrigerator but can be a mess. Place the meat in a leak-proof package or plastic bag. Submerge it in cold water, changing the water every 30 minutes. Using this method, a pound of meat or poultry will defrost in about an hour. Whole turkeys will take about 30 minutes per pound to thaw.

- In the microwave. This is a quick way to thaw meat, but it also requires immediate cooking after defrosting because some areas of the meat can become warm and may even start to cook in the microwave.

No matter how you defrost meat, be sure to keep raw meat juices away from ready-to-eat foods and off countertops because they could contain bacteria. If meat juices leak onto a countertop or table, wash the surface well with hot, soapy water.

If you marinate your meat, do so in a covered dish in the refrigerator and never on the counter. Meat and poultry can be marinated for several hours or days. If you intend to use some of the

---

Fact or fiction? If the meat you are thawing releases water, that means it's going bad and you shouldn't eat it.

Fiction. It's normal for defrosting meat to release water, and it's safe to eat. You'll probably be surprised to learn that meat contains a lot of water—in fact, meats and poultry are more than half water. So when frozen meat and poultry are thawed, the water seeps out of the meat. This change can affect the taste and texture of the meat—it may be drier than fresh meat when cooked—but does not make it unsafe. Flash-frozen meats will produce less water, and taste better, than home-frozen meats when they are defrosted.

Safe Storage Times for Refrigerated Foods

Food	Refrigeration time
Eggs (in shell)	3 weeks
Hard-cooked eggs	1 week
Liquid pasteurized eggs and egg substitutes	Unopened: 10 days Opened: 3 days
Cooked egg dishes	3–4 days
Commercially made mayonnaise	2 months
Salads made with egg, chicken, tuna, ham, or pasta	3–5 days
Frozen dinners	Keep frozen until ready to heat
Prestuffed pork, lamb chops, and chicken breasts	1 day
Store-cooked dinners and entrées	3–4 days
Raw ground beef, turkey, veal, pork, and lamb	1–2 days
Raw stew meat	1–2 days
Canned ham	Unopened: 6–9 months Opened: 3–5 days
Fully cooked whole ham, vacuum-sealed at plant, undated and unopened	2 weeks
Fully cooked whole ham, vacuum-sealed at plant, dated and unopened	Go by the "use by" date on package
Fully cooked whole ham	7 days
Fully cooked half ham	3–5 days
Fully cooked ham slices	3–4 days
Corned beef in pouch with pickling juices	5–7 days
Hot dogs	Unopened package: 2 weeks Opened package: 1 week
Luncheon meats	Unopened package: 2 weeks Opened package: 3–5 days
Bacon	7 days
Raw sausage	1–2 days
Smoked breakfast sausage links and patties	7 days
Summer sausage labeled "keep refrigerated"	Unopened: 3 months Opened: 3 weeks
Pepperoni	2–3 weeks
Leftover cooked meat, poultry, and fish (pieces or in casseroles)	3–4 days

Source: U.S. Department of Agriculture

continued on page 76

Safe Storage Times for Refrigerated Foods *(continued from page 75)*	
Gravy and broth	1–2 days
Cooked meat and fish patties and nuggets, including chicken nuggets	1–2 days
Soups and stews	3–4 days
Fresh steak, chops, and roasts	3–5 days
Variety meats (tongue, liver, heart, kidneys, chitterlings)	1–2 days
Fresh poultry (chicken, turkey, giblets)	1–2 days
Fried or baked chicken leftovers	3–4 days
Leftover poultry covered with gravy	1–2 days
Fresh fish and shellfish	1–2 days
Pizza (cooked)	3–4 days
Stuffing (cooked)	3–4 days

marinade as a sauce on the cooked food, reserve a portion of it before putting the raw meat into it. Or reuse the marinade in which the raw meat sat, but pour it into a saucepan and bring it to a full boil to destroy any bacteria in it.

The safe way to cook

Cooking kills harmful bacteria that may be present in meat, poultry, seafood, and eggs. If you don't cook these foods thoroughly, however, bacteria can survive and make you sick. Experienced cooks often decide whether meat, chicken, or fish is completely cooked by looking at it or piercing a piece of it to check the color of the juices. However, looks can deceive, particularly with ground meat, which can look fully cooked before it actually is.

The most reliable way to determine whether meats are cooked thoroughly is to use a food thermometer, which measures the internal temperature of the meat. Turkeys and chickens are sometimes sold with pop-up thermometers. These are reliable if they've been placed into the meat properly, but it's a good idea to use a second meat thermometer in other parts of the bird to be sure it's fully cooked.

The chart, opposite, shows internal temperatures to which various meats should be cooked to ensure safety.

Brown-bag lunch safety

Packing a meat sandwich into a paper bag, taking it to work, and letting it sit in your desk drawer for three hours is a foodborne illness waiting to happen. Instead, be sure to keep it chilled. You can prepare your lunch the night before and keep it in the refrigerator overnight. Then, in the morning, take it to work and store it in a refrigerator at work. If none is available, pack it in an insulated lunch box or bag with a small ice pack or frozen juice box.

Fact or fiction? You shouldn't put hot food directly into the refrigerator.

Fiction. Hot food can be placed directly into a refrigerator—it's safer than leaving it on the counter to cool. However, a large pot of soup, stew, or spaghetti sauce should be divided into small portions and put in shallow containers before refrigerating. The food can cool to a safe temperature more quickly when in small containers.

Another option is to make your sandwich the night before and freeze it. Take it to work, and by the time you're ready to eat it, it should be thawed. (Don't freeze sandwiches containing mayonnaise, lettuce, or tomatoes because they don't defrost well.) Foods that don't require refrigeration include fresh fruits, vegetables, unopened canned meat and fish, chips, breads, crackers, peanut butter, jelly, mustard, and pickles.

If you prefer a hot lunch, ladle soup, stew, or chili into a preheated thermos. (To preheat, fill the thermos with boiling water and let it stand for a few minutes. Empty it, then ladle in the

Safe Cooking Temperatures

Type of food	Final doneness temperature
Poultry	170 degrees F for white meat, 180 degrees F for dark meat
Stuffing inside poultry	165 degrees F
Beef, medium to well	160–170 degrees F
Pork	160–170 degrees F
Ground meat and poultry	160–170 degrees F
Combination dishes such as casseroles	165 degrees F

Source: FDA

hot food.) Keep the thermos tightly closed until lunchtime to keep the food hot (140 degrees F or higher).

Fish Facts

Mercury and fish

Fish and shellfish are an important part of your diet whether you're pregnant or not. Fish and shellfish provide high-quality protein. Most are low in artery-clogging saturated fat and rich in heart-healthy monounsaturated fats and omega-3 fatty acids.

Unfortunately, some kinds of fish contain high levels of mercury, (also known as methylmercury), which can harm your baby.

Mercury is a by-product of industrial pollution. Factories and coal-burning power plants pump it into the air, and it falls from the air into waterways, where bacteria in the water convert it into methylmercury, the type of mercury that is harmful to people. Children born to women who eat large quantities of mercury-laden fish during pregnancy are at risk for nervous system damage, developmental delays, and reduced brain function.

Nearly all fish contain traces of mercury, but large fish that live long tend to have the highest levels of mercury because they've had more time to accumulate it in their fatty tissues while feeding in polluted waters. The U.S. Food and Drug Administration recommends pregnant women avoid eating the following large, long-lived fish: swordfish, king mackerel, shark, and tilefish. (Nursing mothers, women who plan to become pregnant, and young children should avoid them as well.)

Levels of mercury in other fish can vary. For that reason, you can safely eat up to 12 ounces (two or three meals) of other fish and shellfish a week. Good choices include shrimp, canned light tuna (see "Tuna tales," below), salmon, pollock, and catfish. Generally, frozen and fast-food fish sticks and fish sandwiches are made from fish that are low in mercury. To reduce your chances of mercury exposure, however, do not eat the same kind of fish or shellfish more than once a week.

Check local advisories about the safety of fish caught by family and friends in local waters. Local fish and shellfish may have significantly higher or lower mercury levels, depending on how much mercury is found in those waters. Your community health department can be a source of information about this. If no advice is available, you can safely eat up to 6 ounces (one meal) per week of fish you catch from local waters—but don't eat any other fish during that week.

If you accidentally eat more than the recommended amount of fish in one week, don't worry. Just be sure to cut back on fish for the next week or two.

For further information about the safety of locally caught fish and shellfish and to find a list of state, local, or tribal health departments, visit the Environmental Protection Agency's Fish Advisory website at www.epa.gov/ost/fish.

For information about the risks of mercury in fish and shellfish, call the U.S. Food and Drug Administration's food safety hotline at 888-SAFEFOOD (888-723-3366) or visit its food safety website at www.cfsan.fda.gov.

Say "no" to raw fish

No matter how much you'd love to aim your chopsticks at a platter of sushi, it's

Tuna tales

Tuna salad is a brown-bag lunch staple. Is it safe to eat during pregnancy? Yes, but in moderation, says the FDA.

Tuna steaks and canned albacore (white) tuna generally contain higher levels of mercury than canned light tuna, so choose canned light tuna whenever possible. Because albacore tuna and tuna steaks contain higher levels of mercury, eat no more than 6 ounces (one can) per week. If you're not crazy about the taste of light tuna, mix it with low-fat mayonnaise and dress it up with fresh herbs such as dill or parsley or with chopped onions, celery, carrots, or other vegetables. Even better, try boneless, skinless canned salmon. It has less mercury than tuna and a lot of omega-3 fatty acids.

How do you know if fish is fresh?

Fish spoils quickly, so it's important to know how to spot safe fish at the grocery store. Here are some things to look for:

- Fish should smell fresh and mild, not "fishy" or ammonia-like.
- Whole fish should have eyes that are clear and bulge only a little. Only a few fish, such as walleye, have naturally cloudy eyes.
- Whole fish and fillets should have firm and shiny flesh. Dull flesh is a sign of age.
- Fresh whole fish should have bright red gills that are free of slime.
- There should be no darkening around the edges of fish.
- There should be no brown or yellowish discoloration on the fish.
- Press the fish's flesh with your finger. If it doesn't spring back, it isn't fresh.

best to steer clear of raw or under-cooked fish or shellfish while you're pregnant. Raw fish is more likely to contain parasites, viruses, or bacteria that can make you sick. Shellfish such as oysters and clams are particularly risky because they may be polluted by raw sewage and can contain harmful pathogens that can cause severe gastrointestinal illness. Also, since shellfish pump water through their bodies, they can become sources of concentrated contaminants such as viruses. Once a virus is on or in shellfish, it can live even after the shellfish has been fished out of the water.

Nut Allergies

The truth about peanuts

Nuts and nut butters are ideal pregnancy foods. They contain fiber, protein, vitamin E, folate, and heart-healthy monounsaturated fat. Eating nuts and nut butters can help lower cholesterol and stabilize blood sugar.

They've also been shown to help with weight control because they have a strong satiety value, meaning they keep hunger at bay longer than many other foods, particularly those that are high in carbohydrates.

But many pregnant women wonder: Will eating peanuts during pregnancy increase the risk of my child having a peanut allergy? There has been much debate about this topic, and the results of previous research have been mixed. But a large study in 2004 at the University of Manitoba, Canada, showed that food avoidance does not prevent allergy. The study followed certain "high risk" children until the age of 2; these children had at least one relative with either asthma or another allergic disease.

The results were surprising. At 2 years of age, the children who had the higher rates of certain food allergies (particularly egg and milk) had mothers who *avoided* those foods during their 3rd trimester of pregnancy and during lactation. There was no difference in the rate of nut allergies between the children of mothers who ate nuts during pregnancy and the children of women who didn't.

In summary, the researchers concluded that pregnant or breastfeeding women who avoid certain foods, including nuts and peanuts, do not prevent the development of allergy to those foods in their children—and they may in fact increase the odds.

That being said, each woman must do what makes her comfortable. Talk to your doctor if you have questions, but feel free to work those nuts, seeds, and nut butters into your repertoire. As always, variety and moderation are key.

Herbs and Remedies

All kinds of claims are made about the power of herbal supplements, herbal teas, and other so-called natural plant-based remedies. Some believe that red raspberry, wild yam, and homeopathic treatments can relieve the nausea and vomiting associated with morning sickness. Stay away from these products. Some of them are quite powerful, and most haven't been studied carefully to determine whether they are safe, particularly for pregnant women and their babies. The U.S. Food and Drug Administration does not regulate natural products as stringently as it does prescription medications, so their quality, purity, and potency can vary from brand to brand—even from bottle to bottle within the same brand.

Even though they're "natural,"

herbal remedies can be dangerous when overconsumed. Large amounts of some herbal teas, including red raspberry leaf and peppermint, are thought to cause uterine contractions and may increase the risk of miscarriage or preterm labor, according to the March of Dimes.

The March of Dimes recommends pregnant women abstain from using botanicals in therapeutic doses and in particular advises against using peppermint, red raspberry leaf, black or blue cohosh, ephedra, dong quai, feverfew, juniper, pennyroyal, Saint-John's-wort, rosemary, and thuja. It is safe, however, to use botanicals in small amounts in cooking.

Because so little is known about the action of botanicals and other natural products, the American Academy of Pediatrics recommends pregnant women limit their consumption of herbal teas made from filtered tea bags to two 8-ounce servings a day.

It's fine to use fresh or dried herbs in cooking—they add wonderful flavor, especially to foods that are low in fat. But talk with your doctor before using any medicinal herbs, herbal supplements, homeopathic remedies, or other natural products.

Food Additives

Artificial sweeteners

Artificial sweeteners are everywhere these days. You'll find them in low-calorie foods such as diet cola and sugarless gum; in foods such as yogurt, cookies, and candy; and even in some milks, breads, and pastas. These chemicals are generally believed to be safe during pregnancy, although in large amounts some can cause side effects (see the chart below). They can be a great tool for women with type 2 diabetes or gestational diabetes who are advised to limit their intake of simple carbohydrates and sugars.

The only artificial sweetener that you may want to avoid during

Common Artificial Sweeteners			
Sweetener	**Description**	**Other names**	**Safety warnings**
Sugar alcohols (sorbitol, mannitol, xylitol, erythritol, tagatose, polyclycitol, polyclucitol, isomalt, lactitol, maltitol)	Made by adding hydrogen atoms to sugars; they contain up to about half the calories of sugar.	None	Eating more than 50 grams of sorbitol or 20 grams of mannitol can cause a laxative effect of bloating, diarrhea, and gas.
Saccharin	Discovered in 1879; it was used during the two world wars to sweeten foods when there were sugar shortages.	Sweet'N Low, Sugar Twin	In large quantities, causes bladder cancer in lab animals. However, having fewer than six servings a day is believed to be safe for humans.
Aspartame	Made from amino acids; approved by the FDA in the early 1980s.	NutraSweet, Equal	People with phenylketonuria (PKU) cannot metabolize aspartame. Some people say aspartame gives them headaches.
Acesulfame-K	First approved by the FDA in 1988; sometimes combined with aspartame in soft drinks.	Sunett, Sweet One	None known
Sucralose	Discovered in 1976; approved by the FDA in 1998.	Splenda	None known
Neotame	Has a chemical structure similar to aspartame; received FDA approval in 2002.	None	None known. Although it's similar to aspartame, people with PKU are not sensitive to it.

Source: U.S. Food and Drug Administration

pregnancy is saccharin, which can cross the placenta and may remain in fetal tissues. Although there is no evidence that saccharin is harmful to the fetus, both the American Diabetes Association and the American Dietetic Association recommend that it be used in moderation during pregnancy. And just to be cautious, consume all artificial sweeteners in moderation—stick to no more than two to four servings a day.

You may feel like you have to be a scientist to figure out whether a food contains artificial sweeteners because they have so many different names. The "Common Artificial Sweeteners" chart, page 81, can help you determine what's in the foods you eat.

MSG

Some pregnant women find that the salty food additive MSG (mono-sodium glutamate), which is often used in Asian restaurants, gives them headaches or worsens bloating. However, MSG is believed to be safe, even for pregnant women. If you're uncomfortable eating it, check labels (it's found in many prepackaged foods, including soups, frozen dinners, and sauces) and request that it not be used in food you order in a restaurant.

Cured meats

Hot dogs, ham, bacon, salami, sausage, prosciutto, and other cured meats contain food additives known as nitrites, nitrates, and nitrosamines. Studies of whether these food additives are harmful to a developing fetus have yielded mixed results. For example,

Pesticides and Produce

According to the Environmental Working Group, a nonprofit research organization, the following fresh fruits and vegetables are consistently **the most contaminated with pesticides:**

Apples
Celery
Cherries
Grapes
Nectarines
Peaches
Pears
Potatoes
Red raspberries
Spinach
Strawberries
Sweet peppers

These fresh fruits and vegetables consistently have **the lowest levels of pesticides:**

Asparagus
Avocados
Bananas
Broccoli
Cauliflower
Corn
Kiwi fruits
Mangoes
Onions
Papaya
Pineapple
Sweet peas

one study shows that prenatal exposure to nitrosamine may be associated with an increased risk of type 1 diabetes. But although researchers suspected a link between these food additives and brain tumors in children, studies have failed to prove that a link exists. Because of the uncertainty of the effect of cured meats on your baby, eat these foods in moderation; they're full of fat and salt, so you shouldn't be eating much of them anyway. Or choose noncured varieties. And remember to reheat the meats until steaming.

Fact or fiction? Conventionally grown produce and conventionally raised animal products are dangerous and should be replaced with organic foods.

Fiction. Organic foods are financially out of reach for most people, and there is no solid evidence that people who eat organic foods are healthier than those who don't. That said, if you feel more comfortable buying organic foods and it's in your budget, go for it. If you can't afford an all-organic diet, switch to organic animal products (meat, milk, eggs) that have not been treated with hormones or antibiotics and choose organic when you buy any of the 12 fruits and veggies that, according to the Environmental Working Group, have been shown to contain the most pesticide residue (see chart, opposite). Whether you choose organic produce, conventionally grown produce, or some of each, what matters most is that you consume the recommended number of servings of fruits and vegetables every day. And whether you choose conventional or organic, be sure to wash all produce carefully before eating.

Other Dangers

Lead

Lead is a highly toxic metal that occurs naturally in the earth but is spread by human activity. For many years, lead was used in water pipes, gasoline, and paint. The federal government banned its use in the 1970s. Lead poses health risks for everyone, but the danger is greatest for unborn babies and young children. Exposure to high levels of lead during pregnancy contributes to miscarriage, preterm delivery, low birthweight, and developmental delays in the infant.

Lead is particularly damaging to the body's central nervous system and red blood cells, which carry oxygen in the blood. Even low levels of lead can affect a child's cognitive development and IQ. Children with high lead levels are more inattentive, hyperactive, and disorganized, and they are less able to follow instructions.

Your home's water pipes. Lead is found in some drinking water. If your city or town uses old lead pipes, or if you have lead pipes in your home, it can leach into the water. Lead is still used in some metal water taps, interior water pipes, and pipes connecting a house to the main water pipe in the street. Lead in tap water usually comes from the corrosion of older fixtures or from the solder that connects pipes. When water sits in leaded pipes for several hours, lead can leach into the water supply.

The only way to know whether your tap water contains lead is to test it because you can't see, taste, or smell lead in drinking water. Ask your water provider whether your water system has lead in it or check with your local health department. For homes served by public water systems, your local water authority's data on lead may be available on the Internet. If your water provider does not post this information, call and ask.

Most water systems test for lead as a regular part of water monitoring. However, these tests measure lead only in the water system, not in your house. If you'd like to find out more about having your water tested, contact the Environmental Protection Agency's Safe Drinking Water Hotline at 800-426-4791.

If you have lead pipes, run the tap water for 2 minutes every morning before using it for drinking or cooking. Do not use hot tap water for mixing formula, drinking, or cooking. (It is safe to bathe in because lead is not absorbed through the skin.) Some home water filters remove lead, but others don't, so if you use a home water filter, read the manual to find out if it removes lead.

You can also reduce the risks of lead by eating a healthy diet. Foods that are high in calcium and iron, such as meat, beans, spinach, and low-fat dairy products, reduce the amount of lead absorbed by the body.

Traditional folk medicines. Lead has also been found in some traditional folk medicines used by East Indian, Indian, Middle Eastern, West Asian, and Hispanic cultures. The lead is sometimes added because it's thought to be useful in treating some ailments. Other times, it is accidentally added during grinding, coloring, or other methods of preparation. Lead has been found in powders and tablets given for arthritis, infertility, upset stomach, menstrual cramps, colic, and other illnesses, as well as in traditional beauty products. The following remedies contain significant amounts of lead, according to the Centers for Disease Control, and should be avoided:

- Greta and Azarcon (also known as alarcon, coral, luiga, maria luisa, or rueda). These are traditional Hispanic remedies taken for an upset stomach (*empacho*), constipation, diarrhea, and vomiting. They are also used on teething babies. These finely ground orange-colored powders have a lead content as high as 90 percent.
- Ghasard. This brown powder is an Indian folk remedy.
- Ba-baw-san. This Chinese herbal remedy is used to treat colic pain or to pacify young children.

Additional sources of lead. Lead crystal glassware and some ceramic dishes contain lead. To be cautious, avoid lead crystal glassware. Recently manufactured ceramic dishes probably don't contain lead paint. If you're not sure because you bought the plates on an overseas vacation or at a shop that sells handmade pottery, it's best to minimize their use while you're pregnant. Put them on display so you can enjoy their beauty, but eat from dishes that you know are lead-free.

vegetarianism
during pregnancy

Is it safe for pregnant women to eat a vegetarian diet? The answer is yes. You and your baby can get all of the nutrients you both need from a plant-based diet. Doing so requires smart planning, however, because several nutrients such as B_{12} are crucial during pregnancy and are found primarily in animal foods such as fish, meat, and eggs. Vegetarians, particularly those who don't eat animal products at all, have to make sure they get enough protein. And, like meat eaters, vegetarians need to get extra calories so that they gain adequate weight during pregnancy. This chapter helps you put together a vegetarian eating plan that is healthy for you and your baby.

Vegetarianism During Pregnancy

Like most people, you probably grew up eating meat. Beef, pork, lamb, and chicken took center stage on the dinner plate, barely leaving room for starches and vegetables. Today more and more people are deciding that they no longer want to give meat a starring role in their diets. Instead, they build a diet around plant foods such as grains, fruits, vegetables, legumes, nuts, seeds, and soy foods. Some include eggs, milk, or fish; others shun animal products completely.

People embrace vegetarianism for many different reasons: to be healthier; to take a stand for the rights of animals; because they don't like the taste of meat; to help the environment; to avoid the hormones, antibiotics, and pesticide residues found in animals; because of religious beliefs; to protect themselves from animal-borne diseases such as mad cow disease; because they believe that humans are meant to eat plant food and not animal food; or to save money.

As many as 10 percent of American adults are vegetarian. However, many more—estimates range as high as 40 percent—are "flexitarians," meaning they avoid meat sometimes and incorporate some vegetarian meals into their diets (see "How to be a 'flexitarian,'" page 89). People of all ages are adopting vegetarian diets.

Types of Vegetarians

Vegetarian lingo 101

There are several kinds of vegetarians:

Lacto-ovo vegetarians do not eat meat, fish, or poultry. They do eat dairy and egg products.

Ovo vegetarians do not eat meat, fish, poultry, or dairy products. They do eat egg products.

Lacto vegetarians do not eat meat, fish, poultry, or eggs. They do eat dairy products.

Semi-vegetarians do not eat red meat. They do eat fish, poultry, eggs, dairy products, and plant foods.

Vegans do not eat any animal products including meat, fish, poultry, eggs, dairy, and honey. In addition, most vegans do not use any nonfood animal products including silk, leather, fur, and wool.

Is It Safe for Baby?

Pregnancy concerns

A properly planned vegetarian diet can meet all of a person's nutritional needs. But is a vegetarian diet safe during pregnancy? The answer is absolutely yes: Babies born to well-nourished vegetarian moms are as healthy as babies born to well-nourished meat-eating moms. A vegetarian diet can be absolutely fine for you and your baby provided you get all of the calories and nutrients you need.

Before you run to the kitchen and toss out all of the meat, though, consider that it can be more difficult to plan a nutritious diet if you don't eat meat. It's even tougher if you shun all animal products. That's not to say that it can't be done. But it requires extra planning, particularly when it comes to certain nutrients, such as protein, calcium, vitamin D, vitamin B_{12}, zinc, riboflavin, iron, and omega-3 fatty acids. Also, if you're a vegan, you must take steps to ensure that you are getting enough calories each day.

Remember that there is such a thing as a poor vegetarian diet. Think about it: If your breakfast is a refined-flour bagel with cream cheese and coffee, your lunch is pizza with a side of greasy french fries and a sugary soda, and your dinner is packaged macaroni and cheese followed by a hot-fudge sundae for dessert, you're not eating any meat. But you're not getting many nutrients either. Plenty of junk foods qualify for a vegetarian diet, including potato chips, french fries, soda, white bread, candy, cake, and sugary fruit juices. The fact that you don't eat meat doesn't automatically make your diet a healthy one. You have to make nutritious substitutions in place of the meat and add plenty of fruits, vegetables, whole grains, and legumes to your diet. A poorly planned vegetarian diet can be far less nutritious than a well-planned diet that includes meat products.

You can make your vegetarian diet even healthier by keeping your intake of sweets and high-fat foods in check (unless you are eating healthy oils to gain weight), choosing whole grains rather than refined grains, eating a wide variety of foods, and, if you choose to eat dairy products, picking low-fat varieties.

Most pregnant women should take prenatal vitamins, but it's even more important for vegetarians to do so. A prenatal vitamin provides a little extra insurance that you'll get enough vitamins and minerals, particularly those that are found primarily in animal foods.

Lessons for meat eaters

On average, vegetarians tend to be healthier than meat eaters. Vegetarians have lower rates of obesity, heart disease, high blood pressure, diabetes, and some forms of cancer. (Researchers aren't sure whether vegetarians are healthier because they don't eat meat or because they tend to take better care of themselves in other ways, such as by exercising and not smoking.) Vegetarians tend to eat more fiber, vitamins, minerals, and cancer-fighting antioxidants and fewer artery-clogging fats and cholesterol.

You can receive some of the nutritional benefits of vegetarianism without shunning animal foods completely. Here are 12 lessons that meat eaters can learn from vegetarians:

- Soy is a nutritious, flexible food that can be a delicious meat and dairy replacer. It comes in a variety of forms. (See "Soy sense," page 95.)

- A world of grains that most meat eaters have never heard of, let alone cooked, is out there. Push aside the white rice and try bulgur, quinoa, pearl barley, and brown rice. Serve them with meals or toss them into salads for chewiness and a nutty taste. They're an excellent source of fiber, iron, and B vitamins.

- Nuts are for more than cocktail parties. They contain heart-healthy oils as well as fiber and vitamins. Go beyond peanuts, though, and try cashews, almonds, pecans, hazelnuts, macadamias, and pistachios. Or try soy nuts, which technically aren't nuts but dry-roasted soybeans. They have the same good-for-you oils as true nuts do. Experiment with nut butters too.

- Soup doesn't have to come from a can—and it doesn't have to contain chicken and noodles. Soup is a great way to combine vegetables, legumes, and grains in a healthy, hearty meal. You can whip up your own vegetable soup by simmering chopped vegetables (carrots, onions, garlic, celery, cabbage, green beans, chopped tomatoes, or whatever you have on hand) in a saucepan with canned vegetable broth and canned tomato sauce (choose low-salt varieties). When the vegetables are tender, add some canned beans, cooked grains, or pasta and you'll have a fabulous main-dish soup in less than half an hour.

- Vegetables can be the star of the meal. Who needs a hunk of beef when a spicy vegetable stir-fry or a vegetarian lasagna is on the menu?

- Olive oil is better than butter. Switching from butter to olive oil or trans fat-free olive oil margarine is good for your heart.

- Vegetarians eat a lot of vegetables that you walk right past in the grocery store. Go beyond peas, corn, and carrots and boost your vegetable intake with turnips, celeriac, salsify, jicama, all kinds of squash, tomatillos, rhubarb, parsnips, and rutabagas. You can expand your fruit horizons with passion fruit, guava, kumquats, pawpaw, lychees, star fruit, and plantains. Plan on trying at least one new fruit or vegetable each week.

- Veggie burgers taste good. Years ago they were nothing special, but today's veggie burgers are delicious. Grill them and serve them on whole wheat buns with sliced red onion, romaine lettuce, ketchup, and sliced tomatoes on the side.

- You don't need iceberg lettuce for a salad. Your salads will be much more nutritious (and tasty) with greens such as spinach, romaine, chicory, arugula, watercress, dandelion, radicchio, and mizuna.

- There's more to leafy green vegetables than spinach. Add variety and nutrients with greens such as bok choy, turnip greens, collard greens, and kale.

- Beans are nutritional powerhouses. Add them to soups, salads, chili, and stew or eat them plain.

- Pumpkin seeds aren't just for Halloween. Pumpkin seeds—along with sesame seeds, sunflower seeds, and flaxseeds—are a rich source of

How to be a 'flexitarian'

A flexitarian is a flexible vegetarian, someone who augments a vegetarian diet with some animal foods. Flexitarians can be vegans who occasionally eat meat, fish, eggs, or milk, or they can be carnivores who've heard so much about the health benefits of vegetarianism that they incorporate vegetarian foods into their diet while continuing to eat some animal products. They can be lacto-ovo vegetarians who decide to add some fish to their diet, or ovo vegetarians who sometimes consume dairy products, or lacto vegetarians who occasionally scramble up some eggs for breakfast. Or they can be carnivores who eat only chicken and fish but cut beef, pork, and other meats from their diet. In other words, flexitarians don't follow one rigid set of diet guidelines. Instead, they make up the rules as they go along.

Pregnant vegetarians who take a flexitarian approach may stick with a mainly plant-based diet, adding occasional animal foods that provide nutrients such as calcium, iron, and vitamin B$_{12}$—those that are hard to get from plant foods. Or they may eat some animal foods during pregnancy and go back to nonmeat vegetarianism after their babies are born. The way you structure your flexitarian diet is completely up to you.

nutrients. Toast them for the best flavor. Munch on them for snacks or add them to salads and trail mix.

Your Body's Needs

Calories

Getting adequate calories and gaining the recommended amount of weight are vital during pregnancy. Since vegetarians tend to be leaner than meat eaters, vegetarian women have to be especially aware of their calorie intake and weight gain while they're expecting. If you don't gain enough weight, you're at increased risk for having a small baby or a baby who is born prematurely.

Vegetarians who include dairy and eggs in their diet usually have no trouble getting the calories they need. However, vegans may have to work harder to boost their calorie intake by an average of 300 calories a day (and more if they start their pregnancy underweight). If you're an underweight vegan, consider adding dairy or eggs to your diet, even if it's just for a few months. If all animal foods are unacceptable, boost your calorie intake with high-calorie plant foods. See the chart at left for high-calorie vegan-friendly foods.

High-Calorie Vegan Foods

- Nuts and nut butters
- Seeds
- Granola
- Vegetable oils such as olive, safflower, canola, and peanut oil
- High-fat vegetables such as avocado
- Meat substitutes (known as meat analogs) such as vegetarian hot dogs, cheeses, burgers, and lunch meats (choose full-fat rather than reduced-fat versions)

Protein

As mentioned in Chapter 1, your body uses protein to help build cells and bones; increase blood volume; build your placenta; grow and repair muscles, cartilage, skin, and blood; and manufacture enzymes and hormones. Protein also helps control your body's fluid balance.

During your 1st trimester, your daily protein requirement stays the same as it was before you conceived—about 46 grams. But as your baby gets bigger in the 2nd and 3rd trimesters, your body needs more protein, and your daily requirement increases to approximately 71 grams a day.

You don't have to eat meat, dairy, or eggs to get the protein you need. Plant proteins alone can provide all of the amino acids (the building blocks of protein) that your body needs.

For meat-eating women, getting enough protein is easy. In fact, most American women eat more protein than they need. Women who don't eat meat can also get all of the protein they need with smart food choices. For example, if you eat a high-protein cereal with soymilk for breakfast (choose a cereal with at least 9 grams of protein), a peanut butter sandwich on whole wheat bread at lunch, and vegetarian chili with beans at dinner, you'll have all the protein you need for the day.

Contrary to what people believed years ago, you do not have to combine certain kinds of protein foods within a given meal in order to get "complete" proteins with all of the essential amino acids. As long as you eat a variety of foods each day that provide a mix of proteins, you will get the amino acids you and your baby need.

Many vegetarians replace animal protein with soy protein. That's a good choice because soy protein has been shown to be as high in quality as animal protein.

Plant Sources of Protein

- Soy foods
- Dried beans
- Lentils
- Sea vegetables such as spirulina, kelp, dulse, and alaria
- Nuts and nut butters
- Seeds
- Meat substitutes (known as meat analogs) such as vegetarian hot dogs, burgers, cheese, and lunch meats
- Soy-based protein powder
- Whole grain bread

Calcium

You may think that it's impossible to get enough calcium if you don't eat dairy products. The fact is, calcium is available in many nondairy sources. Calcium-fortified soy foods are a particularly good source.

If you don't eat meat, you may not need as much calcium as meat eaters. Studies show that vegetarians absorb and retain more calcium from foods than do nonvegetarians. That may be because diets high in certain amino acids (such as those in eggs, meat, poultry, and dairy) may increase loss of calcium from bone.

Use the "Healthy Eating Meal Plans" (page 395) to track your

Choosing the best calcium supplement

Synthetic calcium supplements are better for you than natural calcium supplements. Here's why: Natural sources of calcium, including oyster shells, shark cartilage, and bonemeal, may contain lead and other heavy metals and toxins that can be unsafe for your baby and you. If you use calcium supplements, choose the synthetic version, made from calcium carbonate (which is absorbed best when taken with food) or calcium citrate (which can be taken with or without food).

calcium-rich food intake. Aim for 1,000 milligrams of calcium a day. If you don't eat dairy foods and find you can't get enough calcium from plant foods, talk with your doctor about taking a daily calcium supplement. (Check out the tasty "High-Calcium Recipes," page 193.) And remember, spread your calcium intake throughout the day because your body can absorb no more than 500 milligrams at a time.

Plant Sources of Calcium

- Calcium-fortified soy products and fruit juices
- Calcium-fortified cereals
- Broccoli
- Dark green leafy vegetables (collard greens, bok choy, kale, turnip greens)
- Blackstrap molasses

Vitamin D

Vitamin D helps your body absorb calcium. Because it is found primarily in milk, people who don't drink milk may miss out on vitamin D. (For more information, see "Vitamin D: The calcium key," page 33.) Your body can also manufacture vitamin D when you are exposed to sunlight. Those who live in northern climates or have darker skin are more likely to lack this essential vitamin.

To get the vitamin D you need, seek out vitamin D-rich foods such as fortified soymilk, rice milk, and cereals. Or spend 5 to 15 minutes a day exposing your face, hands, and forearms to the sun without wearing sunscreen. (The darker your skin, the more sun exposure you need to manufacture adequate amounts of vitamin D.) Vitamin D supplements, which can be taken alone or combined with calcium, are another option.

Vitamin B_{12}

This important B vitamin helps build and maintain healthy nerve cells and red blood cells, which carry oxygen from your lungs to the cells in your body. Vitamin B_{12} is also a building block of DNA, the genetic material in all cells.

Vitamin B_{12} is naturally found only in animal foods, including meat, fish, poultry, eggs, milk, and dairy products. It is also found in fortified foods such as fortified breakfast cereal and fortified soy products. Some brands of nutritional yeast also contain B_{12}, but be sure to check labels carefully for B_{12} content.

You don't need much vitamin B_{12}—the daily requirement is just 2.6 micrograms during pregnancy. (Nonpregnant women should get 2.4 micrograms daily. Breastfeeding mothers need 2.8 micrograms daily.) If you eat animal products, you can get a day's worth of B_{12} easily; eat just 3 ounces of beef or 2 ounces of rainbow trout and you're all set. If you're a vegetarian who eats eggs or dairy, you most likely get plenty of B_{12}. But if you're a vegan and don't eat any animal food at all, you need help getting the B_{12} you need.

Your choices are to take a B_{12} supplement (after discussing it with your doctor) or to eat fortified foods. Soy companies are starting to fortify some of their products with B_{12} because they recognize that vegans, who tend to eat a lot of soy, need B_{12} fortification.

Getting enough B_{12} is also important after pregnancy, particularly if you are breastfeeding. In adults, vitamin deficiencies ordinarily take a long time to appear, but in babies they can develop within a few months. Vitamin B_{12} deficiency in infants can result in irreversible nerve damage. If you follow a strict vegan diet, be sure to talk with your baby's pediatrician about vitamin B_{12} supplementation for you (while breastfeeding) and your baby.

Sources of Vitamin B_{12}	
Food (serving sizes are after cooking)	Micrograms per serving
Clams, 3 ounces	84.1
Fortified breakfast cereals (100% fortified), ¾ cup (pregnant women should avoid eating too many fortified foods; see page 34)	6.0
Sockeye salmon, 3 ounces	4.9
Farmed rainbow trout, 3 ounces	4.2
Top sirloin of beef, 3 ounces	2.4
Fortified nondairy milk, ½ cup	0.4–1.6
Nutritional yeast (such as Red Star Vegetarian Support Formula), 1 tablespoon	1.5
Fortified breakfast cereals (25% fortified), ¾ cup	1.5
Plain nonfat yogurt with 13 grams protein per cup, 1 cup	1.4
Haddock, 3 ounces	1.2
Milk, 1 cup	0.9
Ham, 3 ounces	0.6
1 whole egg	0.6
American pasteurized cheese food, 1 ounce	0.3
White-meat chicken (½ breast)	0.3

Don't forget riboflavin

Some studies have shown that vegetarians get less riboflavin than nonvegetarians, although riboflavin deficiencies usually don't occur. If you are a vegetarian, you can boost your riboflavin intake by making sure to include some of these riboflavin-rich foods: asparagus, bananas, beans, broccoli, figs, kale, lentils, peas, seeds, sesame tahini, sweet potatoes, tofu, tempeh, wheat germ, and enriched bread. Riboflavin helps your baby grow. Some researchers believe that riboflavin may protect against preeclampsia: Women who are deficient in riboflavin are at an elevated risk for developing this dangerous condition.

Iron

Iron carries oxygen in your blood. If your blood is low in iron, you may be diagnosed with iron-deficiency anemia. If you are starting your pregnancy low in iron, your doctor will recommend an iron-rich diet and/or a supplement. The best way to prevent anemia is to eat foods that are rich in iron.

Anemia can cause fatigue, a sense of malaise, and sensitivity to cold. If you are anemic during pregnancy, you may not fight infections as well as you do when not pregnant. More important, when you lose blood at delivery—even the normal amount—you may be too weak to take care of your baby.

Vegetarians have a greater risk of iron deficiency than meat eaters because the richest sources of iron are red meat, liver, egg yolk, and other animal products. However, if you plan your diet carefully, you can get enough iron from plants. For example, a cup of legumes has about as much iron as 3 ounces of meat.

Food contains two kinds of iron: heme iron and nonheme iron. Heme iron, which is found in meat, poultry, and fish, is more easily absorbed by the body. The iron in dairy products, eggs, and plant foods is largely nonheme.

Because the body can't absorb iron from plants as easily as it can absorb iron from animal foods, it's important for vegetarians to take steps to increase absorption of iron in the foods they eat. One way to do that is to consume a vitamin C–rich food with a high-iron food since vitamin C enhances iron absorption. An example of this would be drinking orange juice with your iron-fortified cereal or adding sweet peppers to a bean burger. Some foods block iron absorption, so you should avoid them when you're eating a high-iron food. These include high-calcium

Plant Sources of Iron

- Legumes (kidney beans, black-eyed peas, lentils)
- Dried fruits (apricots, prunes, raisins)
- Dark green leafy vegetables (spinach, turnip greens, chard, beet greens)
- Bulgur
- Prune juice
- Blackstrap molasses
- Nuts
- Seeds
- Fortified breads and cereals
- Whole grains

foods, tea (including herbal tea), coffee, cocoa, and high-fiber foods.

For a selection of delicious iron-rich meals, go to Chapter 15, "High-Iron Recipes," starting on page 207.

Zinc

Zinc plays a part in many biochemical reactions in your body and helps your immune system function well. Vegetarians are at high risk of zinc deficiency, not only because meats contain more zinc than plant foods but because animal protein increases zinc absorption from foods. Getting enough zinc is important because this mineral helps your body and your baby's body grow and develop normally. If you are a vegan, consider eating some shellfish, which is an excellent source of zinc. Or talk with your doctor about supplementing with extra zinc.

Plant Sources of Zinc

- Soy foods
- Meat analogs
- Whole grains
- Wheat germ
- Legumes (white beans, kidney beans, chickpeas)
- Nuts and nut butters
- Pumpkin seeds

Omega-3 fatty acids

Fish and eggs are the primary sources of omega-3 fatty acids (linolenic acid), which help build and maintain healthy eye tissue. Keep in mind that during pregnancy, the recommended intake of omega-3 fatty acids increases; you should get 1.4 grams of linolenic acid

a day. If you don't eat fish or eggs, you can increase your omega-3 fatty acid intake by adding flaxseed to your diet. (See "Brain-building fats," page 37, for more on foods made from flaxseed.)

Omega-3-Rich Foods

- Canola oil, 1 tablespoon: 1.3 g–1.6 g
- Flaxseed, ground, 1 tablespoon: 1.9 g–2.2 g
- Tofu, ½ cup: 0.7 g
- Walnuts, ¼ cup: 2.7 g

Source: USDA Nutrient Database, 200

Meal Solutions

Planning a menu

If your meals usually consist of a meat, starch, and vegetable, making vegetarian meals may seem daunting. But it's easier than you think. Here are a few tips:

- Look for ways to transform your favorite meals into vegetarian versions. Many dishes that contain meat, poultry, or fish can be made vegetarian simply by leaving out the meat or replacing it with a nonmeat alternative. For example, substitute meat with soy crumbles (a soy product that looks like ground meat) in pasta sauce, in lasagna, or on pizza; take the meat out of tacos or burritos and add beans instead; or make stir-fries with tofu instead of meat.
- Experiment with meat substitutes such as veggie burgers, soy crumbles, and soy-based hot dogs.
- Build meals around low-fat protein sources, such as beans, nut butters,

The Vegetarian Food Guide	
Grains At least half should be whole grains	5–8 servings per day
Vegetables	3–5 servings (2–3 cups) per day
Fruits	2–4 servings (1½–2 cups) per day
Dairy or dairy substitutes Milk, cheese, or yogurt—either cow's milk or soymilk	3–4 servings per day
Protein Beans, nuts, nut butters, seeds, eggs, and meat substitutes	2–3 servings per day (one protein serving equals 1 cup cooked beans, 2 eggs or 3–4 egg whites, ½ cup tofu or tempeh, or 2 tablespoons peanut butter or nuts/seeds). All of these are equivalent to a 2–3-ounce portion of protein.
Oils Choose heart-healthy liquid vegetable oils such as olive, canola, and peanut	5–7 teaspoons per day
Discretionary calories Sugar, alcohol, butter, whole-milk dairy products	100–300 calories per day

soy cheese, tempeh, and tofu. (Or if you eat dairy and eggs, add yogurt, low-fat cheese, and eggs to the list of high-protein meal options.)

● Check out ethnic cookbooks (Chinese, Mexican, Thai, Indian) for meat-free recipe ideas.

● Round out your meals with a glass of calcium-fortified soymilk.

Eating in restaurants

Avoiding meat doesn't mean you have to avoid restaurants. Asian and Indian restaurants offer the greatest variety of vegetarian dishes, but most restaurants have some nonmeat dishes on the menu. Some even offer soy options. With a little creativity, you can even put together a vegetarian meal in a steak house.

Many restaurants will modify meals for vegetarians by omitting meat from stir-fries, substituting meatless sauces, or adding vegetables, legumes, or pasta to your plate to replace the meat.

Soy sense

Many vegetarians make soy foods a centerpiece of their diet. Soy foods are a rich source of protein and serve as a helpful replacement for meat, poultry, fish, and even dairy products. Like meat protein, soy protein is "complete." That means soybeans contain all the amino acids that are essential to human nutrition and that must be supplied by food because your body cannot manufacture them.

People in Asia and elsewhere in the world have used soy for centuries, but Americans only recently began to incorporate it into their diets. Consumption of soy foods has risen steadily during recent years, not just because vegetarians buy them but because nonvegetarians have started recognizing their value too. Scientific evidence suggests that soy lowers levels of LDL ("bad") cholesterol in the blood, reduces risk of heart disease, helps maintain bone density, and may help ward off some kinds of cancer, including prostate and colon.

Soy foods contain phytoestrogens, plant-based chemicals that mimic the action of the hormone estrogen in your body. However, because estrogen has been implicated in some kinds of breast cancer, the jury is still out on whether women who have had estrogen-positive breast cancer or a family history of breast cancer should avoid soy. Some studies show a protective effect; others show the opposite. If you have breast cancer in your family, talk with your doctor about what part soy can play in your diet.

Most grocery stores carry soy foods. If your store doesn't, try Asian markets or health food stores. Choose whole food rather than soy supplements, which have not been adequately tested. The following are some of the most common whole food sources of soy protein:

Tofu is made from pureed cooked soybeans processed into a custardlike cake. It has a neutral flavor and can be stir-fried, mixed into smoothies, or blended to a cream-cheese-like texture for use in dips or as a cheese substitute. It comes in firm, soft, and silken textures.

Soymilk is a soy beverage that is usually used in place of milk. Soymilk is produced by grinding dehulled soybeans and mixing them with water to form a milklike liquid. It can be consumed as a beverage or used in recipes as a substitute for cow's milk. Soymilk, sometimes fortified with calcium, is available plain or in flavors such as vanilla, chocolate, and coffee.

Soy nut butter tastes similar to peanut butter and is great in sandwiches and on crackers.

Soy dairy products, including cheese, yogurt, ice cream, and whipped toppings, are made with soymilk.

Soy flour is created by grinding roasted soybeans into a fine powder. The flour adds protein to baked goods, and because it also adds moisture, it can be used as an egg substitute in these products. Soy flour is also found in cereals, frozen desserts, and pancake mixes.

Textured soy protein is made from defatted soy flour, which is compressed and dehydrated. It can be used as a meat substitute or as filler in dishes such as meat loaf.

Tempeh is made from whole cooked soybeans formed into a chewy cake and used as a meat substitute.

Miso is a fermented soybean paste used for seasoning and in soup stock.

Meat analog products, such as soy sausages, soy burgers, soy hot dogs, and soy cold cuts, as well as soy yogurts and cheese, are used as substitutes for their animal-based counterparts.

Edamame are large soybeans that are harvested when the beans are still green and sweet tasting. They are usually boiled for 15–20 minutes and served as a snack or a main vegetable dish. They are high in protein and fiber and contain no cholesterol. Edamame are sold shelled or still in the pod.

Roasted soy nuts are whole soybeans that have been soaked in water and then baked until browned. High in protein, soy nuts are similar to peanuts in taste and texture.

Hydrolyzed vegetable protein (HVP) is a flavor enhancer that can be used in soups, broths, sauces, gravies, canned and frozen vegetables, meats, and poultry. It is a protein obtained from any vegetable, including soybeans. A chemical process breaks down the protein into amino acids.

If you've never used soy foods before, they can be intimidating. Don't worry, though. It's fairly easy to incorporate these foods into your diet. Here are some suggestions:

- Pour soymilk on cereal or in coffee.
- For breakfast, use soymilk and/or soy flour as an ingredient in homemade muffins, quick breads, pancakes, and waffles.
- Spread soy cream cheese on a bagel.
- Stir chopped fresh fruit into soy yogurt.
- Make delicious sandwiches with soy deli meats, soy nut butter, or soy cheese.
- Top pizzas with soy cheese, soy sausage, or soy crumbles, which are similar to ground beef.
- Grill soy hot dogs, burgers, and marinated tempeh.
- Cube and stir-fry tofu or tempeh and add to a salad.
- Snack on roasted soy nuts.
- Blend soymilk or silken tofu into smoothies.
- Use miso as a base for vegetable soups.

After Baby Is Born

Can vegetarians breastfeed?

It takes some extra planning and careful attention to your nutrient intake, but yes, you can continue to follow a vegetarian diet while nursing your baby. Forget the myth that you have to drink milk to make milk. If you're getting protein and calcium from nondairy sources, there's no need to drink cow's milk. Here are some things you'll need to be sure to get plenty of while you nurse:

Calories. Breastfeeding mothers need about 500 calories more than their usual intake (that's about 200 more than during pregnancy). To get those extra calories, you'll need to increase your consumption of protein and healthy fats because it would take a lot of fruits and vegetables to add up to 500 calories.

Increase your calorie input with soy, nuts, legumes, and, if you eat them, eggs and dairy products. Also, choose foods with healthy fats such as vegetable oils, avocados, and olives for calorie-dense additions to your diet.

Protein. You'll need about the same amount of protein you needed during pregnancy. An extra serving of milk, soy, or peanut butter will cover you. (For more on eating nuts while breastfeeding, see "The truth about peanuts," page 79.)

Calcium. Babies need calcium for their growing bones, and you need it to protect against bone loss. During breastfeeding, your calcium requirement stays at 1,000 milligrams a day. If you can't get it from foods, take a supplement.

Vitamin D. Vitamin D recommendations also stay the same. Eat vitamin D-fortified foods if you live in a northern climate or don't get 5 to 15 minutes of sun a day. At the grocery store, choose products such as soymilk and orange juice that are fortified with calcium and vitamin D since vitamin D helps your body absorb calcium. Ask your pediatrician if you should give your infant vitamin D supplements. (For more information see "Supplements: Does your baby need them?" page 168.)

Vitamin B$_{12}$. You need even more B$_{12}$ when you're breastfeeding than you did during pregnancy, so be sure you're getting enough. If you're not, discuss supplements with your baby's pediatrician or a registered dietitian.

Iron. Although your iron needs decrease after your baby is born from 27 milligrams to 9 milligrams, you should still make sure you have enough iron in your diet.

Zinc. Your zinc need does go up a bit while breastfeeding. If you don't eat meat or fish, you'll need to continue to track your zinc intake to make sure you're getting enough. If you took a zinc supplement during pregnancy, talk with your doctor about whether to continue it while breastfeeding. The answer will probably be yes.

DHA. This omega-3 fatty acid helps a baby's eyes and brain develop. It is found mainly in fish, so if you don't eat fish, you should take other steps to ensure that your baby is getting enough DHA. Babies can make DHA

from another fatty acid called linolenic acid, which is in your breast milk if you eat enough foods that contain it. While nursing, be sure to include these linolenic acid-rich foods in your diet: flaxseed oil, ground flaxseed, canola oil, and soy oil. (See "Omega-3-Rich Foods," page 94.)

Prenatal vitamin. Whether or not you eat meat and other animal foods, continue to take your prenatal vitamin while breastfeeding. It will help fill in any nutrients that may be missing from your diet.

For help planning a healthy vegetarian breastfeeding diet, see a registered dietitian or contact La Leche League, a nonprofit breastfeeding support group. (For more on a healthy breastfeeding diet, see "Best Breastfeeding Diet," page 166.)

Raising a vegetarian child

Any mother with a child who considers chicken nuggets to be an entire food group or whose primary vegetable intake comes from ketchup would scratch her head in wonder at the concept of raising a vegetarian child. But vegetarian, and even vegan, babies and children can get all the nutrients they need without meat or other animal foods.

A vegetarian baby follows the same first-year feeding schedule as a meat-eating baby. During the first six months of infancy, a baby needs only breast milk or formula. Soy formulas are available if you'd rather avoid cow's milk–based formulas. Beginning at around 6 months of age, babies begin eating grains, fruits, and vegetables. Most pediatricians advise adding meat, poultry, and fish to a baby's diet at 7 to 9 months of age. In lieu of those protein sources, however, you can feed vegetarian foods such as pureed tofu, cottage cheese, and pureed and strained beans, peas, chickpeas, and lentils.

At age 1, when babies usually transition from breast milk or formula to cow's milk, a vegetarian baby can continue to drink breast milk or switch over to soymilk or rice milk. Don't let uninformed people convince you that a child has to drink cow's milk in order to be healthy—as long as she eats a nutritious diet, she doesn't require cow's milk.

Toddlers are picky eaters in general, so if you're feeding your toddler vegetarian food only, talk with her doctor about supplements. Even meat-eating toddlers are at risk for vitamin deficiencies because of picky eating. It's tough to limit a toddler to vegan foods because the amount of plant foods they need for adequate calories and proper nutrition may be more than they can comfortably eat and digest. If you choose a vegan diet for your toddler, seriously consider seeing a registered dietitian for advice on food choices.

Children do not need meat, eggs, or cow's milk to grow up healthy. They do, however, need a varied diet full of nutritious foods. As with adults, special attention must be paid to a child's diet to make sure she's getting the calories, protein, calcium, vitamin B_{12}, iron, zinc, and other vitamins and minerals she needs for healthy growth. But that can be accomplished with nonanimal foods and, if the pediatrician recommends it, supplements.

Up until age 2, babies need plenty of fat in their diets because it contributes to brain development. Vegetarian diets tend to be lower in fat than diets that contain meat, so make sure your baby is getting the fat she needs. Some healthy sources of fat include mashed avocado, nut butters (for children over 1 year of age), and vegetable oils.

Older children sometimes decide to be vegetarians even though their families eat meat. Provided they approach vegetarianism in a healthy way, there's no nutritional reason not to support them. However, it can be more work for parents who have to put vegetarian meals on the table as well as meals with meat. Some families follow their older child's lead and become a family of vegetarians, or they increase their consumption of vegetarian meals.

If you decide to raise your child as a vegetarian, look for a pediatrician who supports your decision and has expertise in caring for vegetarian kids. Spending time with other vegetarian families can also help provide support, nutrition tips, food preparation ideas, and advice on how to raise a vegetarian child in a meat-eating world.

My Vegetarian Diet

Not sure you're getting the nutrients you need? Keep track of what you're eating each day with this chart.

Date _____

On most days, I eat the following:	S	M	T	W	Th	F	S
Number of servings of protein:							
Number of servings of whole grains:							
Number of servings of fruit:							
Number of servings of vegetables:							
Number of servings of dairy (if eaten):							
Number of servings of fat/oils:							
Did you get enough of the following nutrients today?							
Protein?							
Calcium?							
Vitamin D?							
Vitamin B_{12}?							
Iron?							
Water?							

Questions for my doctor or dietitian: _____

_____

_____

_____

_____

_____

_____

_____

_____

blood sugar problems
during pregnancy

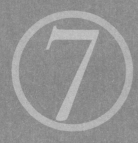

Gestational diabetes is one of the most common health complications of pregnancy. Your doctor will test you for it at the beginning of your 3rd trimester or earlier if you are at high risk of developing it. Although gestational diabetes may seem scary, it can be successfully treated and usually goes away after delivery. Your doctor may recommend diet changes and increased exercise to normalize your blood sugar, or you may need insulin shots. If you follow your doctor's advice—whether you have gestational diabetes or had diabetes prior to pregnancy—chances are good that you can have a normal pregnancy, an uncomplicated delivery, and a healthy baby.

Blood Sugar Problems

Gestational Diabetes

What it is

Gestational diabetes is a condition that occurs in a pregnant woman when her blood sugar is consistently higher than it should be. Gestational diabetes usually goes away when the woman gives birth. Your doctor will test you for gestational diabetes sometime between your 24th and 28th weeks of pregnancy. Although some women with gestational diabetes find that they are extremely hungry or thirsty, most have no symptoms of the condition.

To understand gestational diabetes, you'll have to recall a few things you learned in your high school biology classes. (Don't worry, there's no test at the end of the chapter.) When you eat food, your body either stores it as fat for future use or converts it to glucose. Glucose fuels your body, and many cells and tissues need it for energy. However, glucose requires insulin, a hormone secreted by the pancreas, to usher it into the cells. When your body doesn't make enough insulin or when insulin doesn't do its job properly, glucose accumulates in the blood. Left untreated, that extra blood glucose, which is also known as blood sugar, can cause damage over time.

People with diabetes—either gestational diabetes or diabetes that is unrelated to pregnancy—have too much glucose in their blood for one of two reasons: Either their pancreas fails to manufacture enough insulin or the insulin that their pancreas does secrete is not as effective as it should be in delivering glucose to the cells. (The latter is called insulin resistance

A note about diabetes

The nutritional recommendations and exercise advice in this chapter apply whether you have prediabetes, gestational diabetes, or type 2 diabetes. They will help you lower your blood sugar whether you were diagnosed with type 2 diabetes before pregnancy (which is referred to as preexisting diabetes) or with diabetes during pregnancy (gestational diabetes).

Type 1 diabetes, which is an autoimmune disease usually diagnosed in childhood, requires a somewhat different approach. Although diet and exercise are important, people with type 1 diabetes can't control blood sugar through diet and exercise alone. In type 1 diabetes, the body's own immune system attacks the pancreas, and the pancreas is unable to manufacture insulin. People with type 1 diabetes must have daily insulin injections in order to control their glucose levels.

because the body is resistant to the action of insulin, and therefore the pancreas has to pump out more and more of the hormone.) If insulin fails to bring glucose to your cells, then your cells can't get the energy they need from the food you eat.

Why pregnancy can cause it

During early pregnancy, your body produces a lot of insulin, and the insulin works well partly due to the high levels of estrogen. In the 2nd and 3rd trimesters, insulin continues to pour out, but the insulin doesn't work as effectively. That's because the placenta—a system of blood vessels and tissue that passes nutrients, blood, and water from you to your baby—makes certain hormones that prevent insulin from working as effectively as it is supposed to. This situation is called insulin resistance. To keep your metabolism working properly during the later stages of pregnancy, your body has to make three times or more its normal amount of insulin to overcome the action of those hormones from the placenta.

Most women's bodies manage to adapt and keep up with the increased demand for insulin during pregnancy, and their blood sugar levels stay in the normal range. But approximately 5 percent of pregnant women have bodies that can't keep up. By the 2nd or 3rd trimester, these women will develop gestational diabetes.

Fortunately, if you have gestational diabetes but keep your blood sugar in control, you likely will have an uncomplicated pregnancy and delivery.

Glucose challenge test

Sometime between your 24th and 28th weeks of pregnancy, your doctor will give you the glucose challenge test, or glucose load test (GLT), to determine whether you have gestational diabetes. However, if you are at high risk for developing gestational diabetes, your doctor may test your glucose at your first prenatal visit.

To take the glucose challenge test, you'll first have to ingest a significant amount of carbohydrate in the form of glucose, or simple sugar. In other words, you'll drink 50 grams of a very sweet solution. An hour later, a nurse will use a needle to take a small amount of blood from your arm in order to measure how much glucose, or sugar, you have in your blood. You don't have to fast before taking this test, although eating a large amount of food shortly before it could skew the results.

If the glucose challenge test shows an elevated blood sugar level, it doesn't necessarily mean you have gestational diabetes—only about one-third of women who test positive on the glucose challenge test actually have gestational diabetes. To be sure, your health care provider will schedule another visit and perform a fasting blood glucose test called the glucose tolerance test (GTT). This test often requires three days of eating an unrestricted diet (at least 150 grams of carbohydrates each day; ask your doctor for specific diet recommendations), followed by an overnight fast. You'll be asked to drink a 100-gram glucose solution and to stay at the doctor's office for 3 hours. Your blood

Gestational diabetes by the numbers

You are considered to have gestational diabetes if two of the four results of your 3-hour glucose tolerance test are equal to or higher than the levels recommended below. (**Note**: There is controversy in the field of diabetes in pregnancy about which set of numbers is considered "normal." Currently, the American College of Obstetricians and Gynecologists (ACOG) has not adopted one of the following over the other.)

Criteria based on the 1st International Gestational Diabetes workshop:

- A fasting blood sugar level of 105 mg/dL
- A blood sugar level at 1 hour of 190 mg/dL
- A blood sugar level at 2 hours of 165 mg/dL
- A blood sugar level at 3 hours of 145 mg/dL

Criteria based on the 4th International Gestational Diabetes workshop and supported by the American Diabetes Association:

- A fasting blood sugar level of 95 mg/dL
- A blood sugar level at 1 hour of 180 mg/dL
- A blood sugar level at 2 hours of 155 mg/dL
- A blood sugar level at 3 hours of 140 mg/dL

will be sampled right before you drink the glucose solution and then 1, 2, and 3 hours after you drink the solution. If two of the four samples show a high blood sugar reading, you'll be officially diagnosed with gestational diabetes. (For more information, see "Gestational diabetes by the numbers," above.)

Other tests

If you have gestational diabetes, your doctor may order additional tests throughout your pregnancy to check on your health and your baby's health. Your blood pressure and urine protein will be monitored regularly to detect hypertension, which is more common in women with gestational diabetes. You may have additional ultrasounds, particularly in the 3rd trimester, to be sure your baby is growing properly.

Your doctor may also order nonstress tests (NST) to monitor your baby's heart rate.

If you need to start insulin or glyburide (an oral drug to lower your blood sugar), you may have nonstress tests regularly late in the 3rd trimester.

Are you at risk?

Your chances of developing gestational diabetes go up if you have any of these risk factors:

- You have a parent or sibling who has diabetes.
- You are overweight.
- You had gestational diabetes during an earlier pregnancy.
- You have already given birth to a baby who weighed more than 9 pounds.
- You are a member of an ethnic group that has higher-than-average rates of

diabetes (Hispanic, African American, Native American, South or East Asian, Pacific Islander, or Indigenous Australian).

- You were told before pregnancy that you have prediabetes, which is also known as impaired glucose tolerance or impaired fasting glucose. Prediabetes is a condition in which blood glucose levels are elevated but are not high enough to be considered diabetes. (For more information, see "Prediabetes," page 109.)

Diabetes dangers

During pregnancy, excess blood sugar has the potential to harm you and your baby. For example:

- Women who have gestational diabetes also have an elevated risk of developing high blood pressure during pregnancy and preeclampsia (see "When swelling gets serious," page 123).
- Babies born to mothers with gestational diabetes are at increased risk of growing very big and having a birthweight of 9 pounds or more. This is called macrosomia, and it can make delivery more challenging for you and your baby.
- Because of their size, larger babies are more likely than smaller babies to require a cesarean delivery. They're also more likely to experience a birth complication known as shoulder dystocia, in which the baby's shoulders get stuck during delivery. Although in most cases the doctor can safely deliver a baby with shoulder dystocia, in rare cases it can cause complications in the mother

such as a severe vaginal or rectal tear. A baby with shoulder dystocia can suffer a broken clavicle or arm, a loss of oxygen, or neurological damage to the arm.

- Poorly controlled gestational diabetes also raises a baby's risk of death during the last four to eight weeks of pregnancy.
- These babies are also at risk for low blood sugar shortly after birth, heart problems, low calcium levels, low magnesium levels, jaundice, and breathing problems.
- Children of women with poorly controlled gestational diabetes are at increased risk of obesity, glucose intolerance, and developing diabetes in late adolescence and young adulthood.

Treatment and monitoring

Gestational diabetes sounds scary, and in fact, if it is not treated properly, it can be dangerous. However, there are several ways for pregnant women with gestational diabetes to reduce the chances that they or their babies will suffer any of the side effects of high blood sugar. The treatment goal is to keep their blood sugar within a healthy range. That can be done with diet modifications, exercise, medications, or a combination of all three. The medication may be injected insulin or glyburide, which is a pill.

If you are diagnosed with gestational diabetes, your doctor may refer you to an endocrinologist who specializes in the treatment of diabetes, a registered dietitian, and a diabetes educator (who is typically a registered nurse who has been certified in diabetes health education). Your doctor may suggest that you see an obstetrician who specializes in high-risk pregnancies.

During your pregnancy, your doctor will keep close tabs on your blood sugar levels and your weight gain. She will review your glucose recordings every week or two and make adjustments to your diet and exercise. You will also be taught how to monitor your blood sugar with home tests.

Daily monitoring. Women with gestational diabetes must test their blood at home several times a day to determine their blood sugar levels. You'll test your blood sugar level in the morning and before and/or after meals to see if it is within a desirable range. (Your doctor, dietitian, or diabetes nurse educator will tell you what your target range should be. See chart, page 107, for a general idea.) Each time, you'll prick your finger with a spring-loaded finger-stick device to obtain a small blood sample, which is placed on a strip and inserted in a meter that will measure the glucose level in your blood. At first you may find it daunting to prick your finger and squeeze out a drop of blood, but you'll probably get used to it within a couple of days. You'll track your numbers on a chart or in a computer program. You will also keep track of what you are eating and drinking in order to find correlations between your diet and blood sugar levels. Over time you'll gain a better understanding of what behaviors send up your blood sugar levels and what bring them down.

Drug therapy. If exercise and diet modifications don't get your blood sugar in control within two weeks or so, you may have to use medications. Approximately 40 percent of women with gestational diabetes require drug therapy. If you need insulin or glyburide, it does not mean that you "failed" in any way. Your body just needs extra help to handle the insulin resistance that develops as your pregnancy progresses.

Glyburide is a pill that increases insulin secretion. Recent studies show that glyburide lowers glucose adequately when started after 24 to 28 weeks' gestation. Some health care providers may start with glyburide if your glucose levels are only slightly high when you are eating a proper diet and exercising regularly.

If your fasting glucose is very high or all of your glucose levels after meals are high, many health care providers will start insulin injections. Insulin is safe for both you and your baby and has been used during pregnancy for many years. As your pregnancy progresses, you will likely need more insulin. This does not mean that you have type 1 diabetes or that your pregnancy is getting more dangerous.

It may be tricky to figure out what medications and how much medication works best for you, so it is important to check your glucose levels as often as your provider suggests—and to write down the results.

Giving yourself injections every day may sound intimidating, but don't worry. After proper training from a nurse educator, most people find that injections become simple and routine.

Injections are usually needed for only about three months.

Blood glucose targets for most women with gestational diabetes	
When you wake up in the morning:	Between 60 and 105 mg/dL
1 hour after a meal:	Less than 140 mg/dL
2 hours after a meal:	Less than 120 mg/dL

Your future diabetes risk

The good news is that gestational diabetes usually goes away after your baby is born. The bad news is that if you have gestational diabetes, you will be more likely to get type 2 diabetes later in life. (See "Type 2 Diabetes," this page.) You also will have a two in three chance of developing gestational diabetes during future pregnancies.

Your risk is especially high for developing type 2 diabetes if:

- You developed gestational diabetes before your 24th week of pregnancy.
- Your blood sugar level during pregnancy was consistently on the high end of the healthy range.
- Your blood sugar levels after your baby was born were higher than average.
- You are in the impaired glucose tolerance category after you deliver.
- You are obese.
- You have diabetes in your family.
- You belong to a high-risk ethnic group (Hispanic, African American, Native American, South or East Asian, Pacific Islander, or Indigenous Australian).
- You had gestational diabetes with other pregnancies.

Type 2 Diabetes

What is it?

A generation ago, type 2 diabetes was called "adult-onset diabetes" because it afflicted mostly older people. Today people of all ages develop it, including children and teens. Type 2 diabetes rates are skyrocketing among people of all ages because Americans are gaining weight, and being overweight is a major risk factor for diabetes. Two-thirds of American adults and 15 percent of American children and teens are now overweight or obese.

There is some good news about type 2 diabetes: Studies show that there are many things people can do to fight the disease. Recently a large study of people with prediabetes found that by making the right lifestyle choices—eating right, exercising, and losing a modest amount of weight—their chance of getting the disease diminished 58 percent. Likewise, research shows that those who already have type 2 diabetes can substantially cut their chances of developing other complications such as kidney or heart disease by controlling their blood glucose levels with medication.

Some 5.2 million people in the United States have type 2 diabetes but don't know it. People who go undiagnosed are more likely to develop the complications of type 2 diabetes because their blood sugar levels are out of control. Possible complications include cardiovascular disease, stroke, blindness, nerve damage, and kidney disease. Keeping blood sugar in control

is the best way to prevent the complications from progressing.

Once it is diagnosed, type 2 diabetes
is treated with medication, with
changes in lifestyle and diet, and often
with insulin injections.

Anyone who is at risk for diabetes
should be tested at least every three
years, including those who:

- Are 45 or over.
- Are overweight or obese.
- Have previously been identified as
  having impaired fasting glucose,
  impaired glucose tolerance,
  prediabetes, or borderline diabetes.
- Have a family history of diabetes.
- Are members of ethnic groups that
  have an elevated rate of diabetes
  (Hispanic, African American, Native
  American, South or East Asian,
  Pacific Islander, and Indigenous
  Australian).
- Have had gestational diabetes or
  have given birth to a baby weighing
  more than 9 pounds.
- Have any symptoms of diabetes
  (excessive thirst, frequent urination,
  unexplained weight loss, increased
  hunger, blurred vision, tingling or
  numbness in the hands or feet, slow-
  healing wounds, frequent infections,
  irritability, or unexplained fatigue).

Preexisting Diabetes

What is it?

Some women of childbearing age have
diabetes before pregnancy. This
is known as preexisting diabetes.
Preexisting diabetes is not the same as
gestational diabetes. Although both
conditions are the result of having too
much sugar in the blood, gestational
diabetes develops during pregnancy
and goes away after delivery.
Preexisting diabetes can develop at any
time, and after pregnancy it does not
go away.

Women with preexisting diabetes
can have healthy pregnancies provided
their blood sugar is under control
before the pregnancy begins.

Women who have poorly controlled
diabetes when they conceive are three
to four times more likely than women
without diabetes to have a baby with a
serious birth defect such as a heart
problem or neural tube defect (a brain
or spinal cord defect). They also have a
higher risk of miscarriage and stillbirth.
However, women with diabetes who
have their blood sugar well controlled
before conception are at no higher risk
than women without diabetes of having
a baby with a birth defect.

These risks make it extremely
important that women with preexisting
diabetes take folic acid supplements
before conceiving. (For more
information, see "Folic acid fights birth
defects," page 30.) Remember, these
birth defects occur before the 7th week
of pregnancy—often before a woman
even realizes she's pregnant. Women of
childbearing age who plan to get
pregnant or who are not using reliable
birth control should be especially
careful in controlling their blood sugar.

If you have preexisting diabetes
(either type 1 or type 2) and you plan
to have children, it's important to have
your blood sugar tested and under
control before you conceive. If

possible, talk with your doctor before getting pregnant.

The best conception time

When a woman with preexisting diabetes intends to conceive, her doctor may recommend a blood test to measure a substance called glycosylated hemoglobin (HbA1c). This test gives a helpful snapshot of how well blood sugar is controlled over several months, and it can be used to help a woman determine the best time to try to get pregnant.

Medication warning

If you have preexisting diabetes and take oral diabetes medications, you'll probably have to switch to insulin when you conceive. Scientists don't know for sure whether oral medications are safe in early pregnancy.

If you already use insulin, you may need a higher dose, especially during the 3rd trimester of pregnancy, because your body becomes more resistant to insulin during pregnancy.

Prediabetes

Cautions and concerns

People with prediabetes have blood sugar levels that are higher than normal but not high enough to merit a diagnosis of diabetes. (Prediabetes is also referred to as impaired glucose tolerance [IGT] or impaired fasting glucose [IFG]). If you are among the approximately 41 million Americans who have prediabetes, you're likely to develop type 2 diabetes in the future if you don't change your diet, weight, or exercise habits. People with prediabetes are 50 percent more likely than people with normal blood sugar to develop cardiovascular disease.

Normal fasting blood glucose for a nonpregnant adult is below 100 mg/dL. A person with prediabetes has a fasting blood glucose level between 100 and 125 mg/dL. If the blood glucose level rises to 126 mg/dL or higher, a person has diabetes.

What can you do if you have prediabetes? (Follow the suggestions in "Preventing type 2 diabetes," page 116.) Losing weight, eating a healthier diet, and exercising can actually bring your blood sugar levels back down into the normal range. Also, if you have prediabetes, do what you can to reduce other cardiovascular disease risk factors: Quit smoking, reduce saturated fat intake, and lower your blood pressure.

Pregnancy Diabetes Diet

Making smart choices

What you eat, when you eat, and how much you eat all have an impact on your blood sugar levels. Whether you have gestational diabetes, diabetes, or prediabetes, it's best for your health to try to keep your blood sugar levels relatively stable, but it can be tricky to do. That's why you should meet with a registered dietitian if you have diabetes. These health professionals provide education and guidance on all diet-related issues, including target weight gain, daily calorie goals, menu planning, meal scheduling, food choices, and recommended nutrient intake. A dietitian will help you understand why it is important to:

- Eat about the same amount of food each day.
- Eat a variety of nutritious foods each day.
- Eat about the same amount of carbohydrate-rich foods at about the same time each day.
- Eat a small meal or snack every 2 or 3 hours. Don't let yourself get too hungry and don't eat too much. See Chapter 15, "Light Mini Meals" (page 251), for great recipes.
- Eat your meals and snacks at about the same time each day.
- Avoid skipping meals or snacks.
- Exercise at about the same time each day.
- Limit your intake of sweets.
- Plan to eat a minimum of 175 grams of carbohydrates each day. For example, you may eat 30 grams at breakfast, 45 grams at lunch, 45 grams at dinner, and between 15 and 30 grams at each of two or three snacks.
- Limit your carbohydrate intake at breakfast. Your insulin resistance is highest at the beginning of the day, so eat no more than about 30 grams of carbohydrates at breakfast. That's the equivalent of about two slices of bread or two starch exchanges.
- Boost your fiber intake by eating more fruits, vegetables, whole grains, whole grain cereals, and legumes. (For delicious high-fiber recipes, see page 227.)
- Typically, dietitians recommend that

you eat 10 percent of your daily calories at breakfast, 30 percent each at lunch and dinner, and 10 to 15 percent from two or three snacks.

The truth about carbs

You may have heard that people with diabetes aren't supposed to eat starchy foods that are high in carbohydrates. That's outdated advice. Yes, it is true that limiting your intake of sweets and other carbohydrates is an important part of managing gestational diabetes because eating too many carbohydrates can cause your blood sugar to rise. However, drastically cutting carbohydrates or eliminating them from your diet completely is not a good idea. You and your baby need carbohydrates for energy. Also without enough carbohydrates your body will burn fat and produce ketones, which are potentially dangerous to your baby.

You and your dietitian will work together to find a balance between eating enough carbohydrates to get the energy and glucose you need and limiting the carbohydrates you eat to control your blood sugar level. In general, dietitians recommend that women with gestational diabetes consume a diet in which at least 40 percent of daily calories comes from carbohydrates, 20 to 30 percent comes from protein, and 30 to 40 percent comes from fats (with 10 percent or less coming from saturated fats).

Complex versus simple carbs. Include carbohydrates at each meal. Whenever possible, choose complex carbohydrates such as raw vegetables and fruits, legumes, and whole grain foods such as whole wheat bread or whole grain cereal. Your body breaks down these complex carbohydrates more slowly than the simple carbohydrates found in candy, sugar, white bread, and white pasta and other sweets and refined starches. As a result, glucose is released slowly and evenly into the bloodstream after you eat higher-fiber complex carbohydrates. Put simply, eat a sugary treat and glucose will be more rapidly dumped into your blood. Eat a slice of whole wheat bread and your blood sugar level will rise slowly and steadily, which is better for your health.

Fruits. Whenever possible, choose whole, raw, unprocessed fruits over processed fruit and fruit juices. For example, eating an apple causes a slow, steady increase in blood sugar, while eating applesauce, which is more processed than an apple, causes a spike in blood sugar. Drinking a glass of apple juice, which is highly processed (even if it's 100-percent fruit juice), can cause your blood sugar to skyrocket. Whole fruits are also more filling.

Meal planning

Most women with gestational diabetes are instructed to follow a meal plan to ensure that they get the nutrients and calories they need. There are two methods of designing a diabetes meal plan: the exchange system and carbohydrate counting.

The exchange system. In this system, people design their diet based on a series of exchanges. Each food is assigned to a certain category (starch, fruit, milk, vegetable, fat, protein), and you are permitted a certain number of

Example of a Healthy Meal Plan

Food	Carb	Pro	Fat
Breakfast:			
1 cup cooked cereal	30 g	3 g	—
½ cup fat-free milk	6 g	4 g	—
Boiled egg	—	7 g	5 g
1 tsp. margarine	—	—	5 g
Snack:			
1 small apple	15 g	—	—
1 oz. low-fat cheese	—	7 g	5 g
Lunch:			
2 slices whole wheat bread	30 g	6 g	—
3 oz. grilled chicken	—	21 g	9 g
2 cups salad	10 g	4 g	—
2 Tbs. dressing	—	—	10 g
1 cup skim milk	12 g	8 g	—
Snack:			
6 whole grain crackers	15 g	3 g	—
½ cup cottage cheese	—	14 g	6 g
Dinner:			
1 cup cooked wheat pasta	45 g	9 g	—
3 oz. lean ground beef or turkey breast	—	21 g	9 g
1 cup tomato sauce	10 g	4 g	—
1 cup side salad	5 g	2 g	—
2 Tbs. dressing	—	—	10 g
1 cup fat-free milk	12 g	8 g	—
Snack:			
12–15 grapes	15 g	—	—
Totals:	205 g	121 g	59 g
Calories: 1,835	820	484	531
% from:	45%	26%	29%

food exchanges for each meal. People using this system work with a registered dietitian to determine how many of each exchange they should eat each day and at each meal.

The "Healthy Eating Meal Plans," page 395, are based on this system.

Carbohydrate counting. In this eating plan, you are permitted a certain number of grams of carbohydrates per day, and you work with your dietitian to determine how many grams of carbohydrates you should eat at each meal and snack to keep your blood sugar in check. Many people find that carbohydrate counting is simpler than the exchange system, particularly now that food labels clearly list the number of grams of carbohydrates in foods.

The number of exchanges or grams of carbohydrates that you can eat each day or at each meal is determined by such things as your blood sugar levels, your weight, when and how much you exercise (since exercise lowers blood sugar), and whether you use insulin.

The menu on page 111 (see "Example of a healthy meal plan") is an example of a day's meal plan for a pregnant woman with gestational diabetes who needs between 1,800 and 1,900 calories a day. It shows how to get the right amount of protein, fat, and carbohydrates distributed throughout the day.

Calorie counts

Your dietitian will tell you how many calories you should eat each day. Eating a healthy amount of food is crucial in order for your baby to get the nutrients needed for development.

Eating too little food and restricting calories too much raises the ketone levels in your blood, and several studies have reported a relationship between elevated ketone levels and developmental delays in the children of mothers with gestational diabetes. (The recommendations may be different if you're obese; check with your health care provider.) Ketones are acidic chemicals that are released when you don't eat enough carbohydrate-containing food and your body has to go to fat stores for energy. Although it

Sugar-free doesn't mean calorie-free

Everything from candy and cookies to soft drinks comes in sugar-free varieties. This is great for people with any kind of diabetes who are trying to limit their sugar intake. If you use these foods, use them in moderation. And remember that sugar-free doesn't always mean calorie-free. For example, some hard candies that are sugar-free contain 50 calories for a three-piece serving. Although calorie-free sweeteners such as aspartame, saccharin, sucralose, and acesulfame-K won't increase your blood sugar levels, low-calorie sweeteners known as sugar alcohols (xylitol, mannitol, and sorbitol) do increase your blood sugar level slightly. (For more information, see "Common Artificial Sweeteners," page 81.) If you want to include sugar-free foods in your diet, go ahead and do so, but be sure to check the food label for calorie information and fat content.

The glycemic index

With all the buzz about low-carbohydrate diets in the past few years, you may have heard about something called the glycemic index. Although low-carb diets are falling out of favor—and well they should, since they are not healthy—the glycemic index is actually a handy tool for figuring out which carbohydrates are the best ones to include in your diet.

First, a definition: The glycemic index is a ranking of carbohydrate foods that is based on how they release glucose into your blood. For example, a highly processed, sugar-coated cereal, which causes a large, rapid dump of glucose into the blood, is said to be high on the glycemic index. By contrast, a bowl of whole grain cereal, which releases a slow, steady stream of a smaller amount of glucose into the blood, is low on the glycemic index.

The GI scale goes from 0 to 100. (The GI of pure glucose is 100.) Under 55 is considered low, 55 to 70 is medium, and over 70 is high. A food's GI is determined by many factors, including its carbohydrate content; how much fiber, protein, and fat it contains; what form it is in (apple versus applesauce versus apple juice); and how it was prepared (raw versus cooked).

You don't have to keep track of GI numbers in order to make smart choices. Just keep this list in mind when choosing your foods:

- Low-GI foods include high-fiber cereals, many fruits and vegetables (but not potatoes), and many legumes, including black beans, lentils, garbanzo beans (chickpeas), and kidney beans.
- Medium-GI foods include grains such as barley, bulgur, oatmeal, brown rice, whole grain breads, and whole grain pasta.
- High-GI foods include potatoes (baked or french fried), white flour, white rice, candy, sugary beverages such as soda, sweetened fruit juice, and refined cereals.

But no matter what the GI numbers, always remember that keeping track of the total amount of carbohydrate in your diet is the most important tool in blood sugar management.

sounds like fat-burning would be a good idea, during pregnancy it isn't because ketones may be harmful to your baby.

Your doctor may test your blood for ketones or may want you to monitor the ketones in your urine each day with a home test. (If your doctor wants you to do home-testing, she'll write a prescription for the test, which you can buy at a drugstore.) If your ketone levels are too high, your dietitian help you make changes in your diet.

Consistency is critical

Eating a consistent diet is critical when you have gestational diabetes because very high blood sugar spikes (hypergly-cemia) or very low blood sugar drops (hypoglycemia) are not good for your baby. If you get sick with the flu or experience pregnancy-induced nausea and vomiting, try to have juice, soup, or crackers if you can't stick with your everyday diet. If you do finger-prick blood sugar testing, continue to do so and call your doctor if you vomit more than once or have diarrhea for more than 6 hours.

Why Exercise Matters

Get moving!

Moderate physical exercise has been shown to lower blood sugar. When you exercise, your muscles need energy, which comes from the glucose in your blood. Regular exercise allows your body to use blood sugar without extra insulin. Unless a pregnancy complication such as placenta previa keeps you from exercising, you should start or continue an exercise program if you are diagnosed with gestational diabetes.

Any kind of exercise helps: yoga, swimming, walking, jogging, working out on an exercise machine, or anything else that gets you moving. (For more information see Chapter 9, "Keeping Fit During Pregnancy," page 133.) Aim for 30 to 60 minutes of exercise a day.

One note of caution: Excessive exercise can use up too much blood sugar, leaving you with hypoglycemia, or low blood sugar. (Exercise of 30 to 60 minutes a day won't cause low blood sugar.) Hypoglycemia can cause

dizziness, sweating, heart palpitations, and hunger. If you experience any of these symptoms, stop exercising and test your blood sugar. If it is 70 or below, eat one of the following foods immediately: two or three glucose tablets, 4 ounces of fruit juice, 4 ounces of sugary soda, 8 ounces of milk, five or six pieces of hard candy, or 1 to 2 teaspoons of sugar or honey. (If you exercise outdoors or away from home, carry glucose tablets or hard candy with you.) Test your blood sugar again after 15 minutes to determine whether it has returned to normal. As soon as possible, have a balanced snack with some carbohydrate, fat, and protein. A great choice is four to six whole grain crackers with 1 ounce of hard cheese. Eat a small snack if your blood sugar is below 100. And no matter what your blood sugar, be sure to drink plenty of water before, during, and after exercise.

Fact or fiction? Since my blood sugar levels are normal, I don't have to worry about how much sugar I eat.

Fiction. It's fine to eat some sugar, honey, molasses, brown sugar, and other sugary sweets, but loading up on them is a bad idea even if your blood sugar is normal. Sweets contain a lot of empty calories and not much in the way of nutrition, and they contribute to weight gain and dental cavities. Plus, up-and-down blood sugar levels can trigger nausea and make you hungry. If you're craving something sweet, have a piece of fruit. You'll at least get some fiber and nutrients with your sugar fix.

Alert: Watch for swelling

Some swelling is normal during pregnancy, but if you find that you are developing rapid swelling, particularly in your hands and face, call your doctor right away. You may be developing preeclampsia, a sudden increase in blood pressure after the 20th week of pregnancy. Women with gestational diabetes are at elevated risk of developing preeclampsia. Left untreated, preeclampsia can lead to serious complications for mother and baby. (See "Swelling," page 122, for more information.)

Delivery and Beyond

During delivery

If you have diabetes of any kind, your blood sugar levels will be monitored closely during delivery. If you need insulin, you'll be given an injection or will receive it intravenously. After your baby is born, you will deliver the placenta, which caused insulin resistance. When the placenta is gone, gestational diabetes usually goes away.

Some women with gestational diabetes find that their blood sugar returns to normal shortly after delivery; others find that it takes several weeks for levels to normalize. A small number of women continue to have high blood sugar and are diagnosed with nongestational diabetes.

If your blood sugar is normal at your six-week visit, your diabetes is considered resolved. Your doctor will recommend a 2-hour glucose test and blood tests every one to three years, depending on your risk factors.

Your new baby's health

Your baby's pediatrician will pay close attention to your baby's growth and development. Chances are, your baby will be fine, especially if you kept your blood sugar in control during pregnancy. You might want to just forget about your gestational diabetes after your baby's birth, but don't forget to mention it to any doctors that your child sees during infancy and throughout childhood.

Breastfeeding

Women with gestational diabetes absolutely can breastfeed. Be prepared for a delay, however, because women who have gestational diabetes sometimes find that their milk takes five or six days to come in rather than the more typical three or four days.

Until your blood sugar levels stabilize after birth, you will have to continue to take special care of yourself and pay close attention to keeping your blood sugar in the healthy range. You'll have to be careful to eat and drink enough to maintain your milk supply but not eat so much that you send your blood sugar levels through the roof.

If you plan to breastfeed, discuss it ahead of time with your dietitian and diabetes nurse educator. Line up knowledgeable support people before delivery. Ask your baby's pediatrician to refer you to a lactation consultant with gestational diabetes training or contact La Leche League, a nursing support organization. Whether or not you have gestational diabetes, if you're a first-time mother, you may be well served by taking a breastfeeding class. Most hospitals and obstetrician offices offer classes or can tell you where to find them in your area. (For more information, see Chapter 11, "Breastfeeding," page 161.)

Preventing type 2 diabetes

If you had gestational diabetes, your risk of developing type 2 diabetes is elevated. Fifty percent of women with gestational diabetes develop diabetes by age 50. After your baby is born, you can reduce your risk of developing type 2 diabetes by taking these steps:

Watch your weight. It's best if you can get down to your ideal weight (see "Body Mass Index" chart, page 45). If you can't, even losing a small amount of weight can make a difference. For example, if you weigh 200 pounds, losing 10 to 14 pounds reduces your chances of getting type 2 diabetes.

Exercise. Aim for at least 30 minutes of activity most days of the week.

Eat right. Follow a diet that includes whole grains, legumes, fruits, and vegetables and the recommended balance of carbohydrates, protein, and fat. And have hope: Research suggests that making healthy lifestyle changes such as these may reduce the incidence of future diabetes by as much as 58 percent.

special
diets

Many things may lead you to a special diet during pregnancy. Dietary changes can improve pregnancy complications such as heartburn, constipation, and swelling. Other health concerns such as celiac disease, high cholesterol, high blood pressure, or lactose intolerance may dictate special diets to help you and your baby remain healthy. Special diets may also come into play if your religious traditions include fasting or if you underwent weight-loss surgery. This chapter describes how to make the best food choices that will satisfy your special dietary needs in each of these situations.

Special Diets

Heartburn

A common problem

Heartburn, unfortunately, is common during pregnancy. To understand why, you need to understand why heartburn occurs. When you swallow food, it travels down your esophagus and into your stomach. In your stomach, very strong acids break down the food, digesting it so the body can use it. These acids are kept in the stomach by the lower esophageal sphincter (LES), a ring of muscle at the bottom of the esophagus. Sometimes, though, food and stomach acid leak back or are pushed into the esophagus, causing a burning pain in the throat or chest known as heartburn. Other names for heartburn are indigestion, acid indigestion, reflux, and gastroesophageal reflux disease (GERD). Although it causes burning pain in the chest, heartburn actually has nothing to do with your heart.

Pregnancy hormones can relax the LES, making it less effective at preventing the contents of the stomach from entering the esophagus. Also, as your baby grows larger inside you, your uterus can push up into the stomach, squashing it and forcing food and stomach acids out of it. (Pregnancy heartburn is more common in the 2nd and 3rd trimesters.) Finally, because your entire digestive system slows down during pregnancy, food stays in your stomach a lot longer than when you're not pregnant, which may cause heartburn.

Prevention techniques

Heartburn occurs more often when your stomach is full, so the best advice for preventing heartburn is to avoid overfilling your stomach with food or drink. Heartburn prevention is yet another good reason to eat five or six small meals a day while you're pregnant—when you do this, your stomach never gets very full.

Here are some other things you can do to prevent and cope with heartburn:

- Take small bites and chew your food well.
- Eat slowly.
- Don't drink during meals. Sip what you need to moisten your food, but no more. Large amounts of liquid can expand your stomach and cause some of its contents to push back into the esophagus. Drink your liquids an hour or so after eating meals and snacks.
- Avoid foods that trigger your heartburn. Listen to your body when it comes to determining trigger foods. The foods that set off an attack of heartburn are different for

different people. Common trigger foods include citrus fruits, tomatoes, vinegar, mint, food and beverages that contain caffeine (caffeine stimulates the production of excess stomach acid), chocolate (a chemical in chocolate called theobromine can irritate the stomach), and foods that are very spicy or fatty.

- Wait an hour or more after eating before napping or going to bed. Lying down with food in the stomach can allow stomach contents to seep into the esophagus. If you can't wait an hour to nap, sleep sitting up in a reclining chair.
- Sleep with the head of your bed elevated. Stuff a few towels or a board between the mattress and box spring or prop yourself up with pillows. This helps keep stomach acids in the stomach.
- Avoid drinking through straws because it can cause you to swallow air, which aggravates heartburn.
- Chew with your mouth closed to avoid swallowing air.
- Wear loose clothing that doesn't cinch your waist or tighten around your stomach.
- Experiment with carbonated beverages such as seltzer. Although some people find that the bubbles in carbonated drinks trigger heartburn, others find that drinking bubbly water or soda causes them to burp, which releases air from the stomach and relieves feelings of pressure.
- Don't gain more than the recommended amount of weight. Excess fat around the abdomen can put pressure on the stomach.
- Include protein in meals and snacks. Protein puts pressure on the LES and helps keep it closed.

Safe medications

Before pregnancy you may have reached for an over-the-counter antacid during bouts of heartburn. Are they safe during pregnancy? Yes, provided you use them sparingly and wisely. Over-the-counter antacids such as Mylanta, Maalox, Rolaids, and Tums can relieve the pain of heartburn. If you use them excessively, however, they can reduce the absorption of nutrients, particularly iron.

Read the label before you take an antacid. Most over-the-counter brands use different combinations of three elements—magnesium, calcium, and aluminum—along with hydroxide or bicarbonate ions that neutralize acid in the stomach. Magnesium can cause diarrhea and aluminum can cause constipation, so avoid those ingredients if you're having trouble with diarrhea or constipation. Although calcium can cause constipation in some people, it's a better choice than aluminum or magnesium mixtures because it adds to your daily calcium intake. Follow the directions on the label and don't take more than the recommended number of tablets.

Other heartburn medications, both prescription and over-the-counter, include H2 blockers (Tagamet, Pepcid, Axid, Zantac), proton pump inhibitors (Prilosec, Prevacid, Protonix, and Nexium), and prokinetics (Urecholine and Reglan). Although some of these medications are considered safe during

Fact or fiction? Eating peppermint candy or chewing peppermint gum relieves heartburn.
Fiction. Peppermint triggers heartburn in many people. However, chewing nonmint gum may be a good idea—a new study shows that chewing it after a big meal can reduce acid levels in the esophagus and may help prevent gastroesophageal reflux disease. If you notice heartburn worsening with gum chewing, you may be swallowing too much air.

pregnancy, it's best not to self-medicate. If your heartburn fails to respond to diet changes or over-the-counter antacids, talk with your doctor before taking anything stronger.

Constipation

The basics

About half of all women become constipated sometime during pregnancy. Constipation causes less-frequent bowel movements—as few as three a week. (However, when determining whether you're constipated, don't use that as a rule. The range of normal varies widely, from three times a week to several times a day. There is no "right" number of bowel movements—when you have constipation, you simply have fewer than your normal number of bowel movements.)

You're more likely to be constipated during pregnancy for several reasons. The hormones that relax your muscles so that your baby can ease out of your uterus also relax the digestive system. The muscle contractions that move food through your digestive system also slow down during pregnancy. This slowing down gives your body extra time to extract the maximum amounts

of nutrients from the food you eat, but it can also contribute to constipation.

The iron in prenatal vitamins can contribute to constipation as well. Dehydration, even if a mild case, can also slow down your stools. And during the latter part of pregnancy, your baby may press on your intestines, making passage more difficult.

It's important to take constipation seriously during pregnancy because chronic constipation can lead to painful, itchy hemorrhoids, as well as anal fissures, which are small tears in the skin around the anus. If your constipation lasts more than a week, alert your health care provider.

Prevention tips

Here are some ways to prevent and treat constipation:

Stay hydrated. Drink water, fruit juice, milk, decaffeinated tea, and decaffeinated coffee. Sip on water in between meals and snacks. If plain water tastes terrible to you, add lemon, lime, or orange slices to flavor it or try soda water.

Eat a high-fiber diet. Be sure you're getting at least 25 grams of fiber a day. To meet your fiber needs, eat extra fruits and vegetables in addition to whole grains because fruits and vegetables contain water. Your body needs both soluble and insoluble fiber for proper intestinal movement. (For more fiber information, see "Carbohydrates," page 19.)

Increase fiber gradually. Don't go from cornflakes to Kashi overnight—adding too much fiber to the diet too quickly can cause, rather than relieve, constipation. Add about 3 grams a day and be sure to increase your water intake too because fiber absorbs lots of water as it works its way through your intestines.

Choose "wet" fruits and veggies that contain a high percentage of water and avoid bananas, which are binding and can contribute to constipation. (See "Juicy fruits and veggies," right.)

Eat dried plums. That's probably what your grandmother would recommend, and it's good advice because dried plums (also called prunes) are a natural laxative. Eat a few prunes or drink a glass of prune juice.

Add fiber with fiber supplements. Try Benefiber, Metamucil, or Citrucel. Follow the directions on the container to use these products as a fiber supplement rather than a laxative.

Take your time. Having a bowel movement can take a few minutes and rushing it increases the risk of hemorrhoids.

Go when you feel the urge. People who routinely ignore the urge to have a bowel movement may stop feeling the urge, which can lead to constipation.

Exercise. As you get moving, so do your intestines—exercise spurs muscle contractions, which move food through your body. Try walking, swimming, riding a stationary bicycle, or prenatal yoga. Deep breathing and certain yoga positions act as a kind of internal massage that can help kick-start your intestines. If you take prenatal yoga classes, ask your instructor about constipation-prevention poses.

Stay away from oils and herbal remedies. Home remedies are not as safe as you may think. Mineral oil can decrease nutrient absorption, and castor oil can cause contractions. As for herbal remedies such as senna, most are untested and their safety during pregnancy has not yet been determined, so avoid them.

Talk with your doctor about taking iron supplements with stool softeners. Some iron supplements contain stool softeners. Iron can cause constipation,

Juicy fruits and veggies

These fruits and veggies are at least 90 percent water (by weight) and are sometimes described as wet. Eating them can help boost your daily fluid intake.

Broccoli
Cantaloupe
Cauliflower
Eggplant
Iceberg lettuce
Sweet pepper
Radishes
Spinach
Zucchini
Grapefruit
Tomatoes
Strawberries
Celery
Watermelon
Cucumbers
Red and green cabbage

A guide to constipation medication

"Laxative" is the general term for any constipation-relieving aid. Laxatives fall into several categories, which include the following:

Fiber/bulk-forming. This category contains psyllium husk, which is a soluble fiber, not a chemical stimulant. It helps increase the stool's bulk and helps the colon to hold and absorb more fluid. Metamucil is a fiber/bulk-forming laxative that you can use for constipation or as a fiber supplement. (The directions on the package give dosage directions for each.)

Stool softeners. These medications (such as Colace) draw more liquid into the colon to help soften hard stools, thus making them easier to pass and reducing strain.

Saline laxatives. These medications contain nonabsorbable ions from magnesium (magnesium citrate, for example), which remain in the colon and cause fluid to be drawn in, thus softening the stool. Milk of Magnesia is a popular saline laxative. These laxatives also have mild stimulating effects on the colon.

Stimulants. This type of medication causes the muscles of the small intestine and colon to move their contents more rapidly. Chronic use of any stimulant has the greatest potential for overuse or dependency. Long-term use may worsen the condition. Ex-Lax and Senokot are two stimulants.

but stool softeners make the stool easier for the body to pass. However, you should take a stool softener only if your doctor recommends it.

Swelling

Pregnancy problems

It's normal to have some swelling during pregnancy. As your baby grows and your pregnancy progresses, your blood volume increases by 50 percent. The amount of water in each of your body's cells increases too, so it's no surprise that you may experience some swelling, particularly in your extremities (feet, legs, hands, and arms), where blood can pool.

Swelling is more common in the summer, particularly in humid weather. Swelling is usually nothing more than an inconvenience. The exception is when it's a symptom of preeclampsia; see "When swelling gets serious," opposite page.

Treatment

The best way to cope with swelling is to stay active, avoid standing for long periods of time, and put your feet up when you can (this encourages blood to drain out of your feet and legs). If you can't get up and walk, do foot rotations to pump up the circulation in your feet.

Believe it or not, drinking adequate water can help with swelling too. To figure out how much water you should be drinking, divide your weight by two. That number is how many ounces of water to drink each day.

Salt: Stay or go?

You may think that you should cut salt out of your diet if you are having trouble with swelling. Although excessive salt intake isn't a good idea during pregnancy, neither is a drastically low-salt diet. During pregnancy, sodium helps you maintain a healthy blood pressure. It also plays a part in muscle and nerve development. If you develop swelling, aim to eat an average amount of salt. Eat some salty foods, but don't go overboard with the salt shaker.

Eat potassium-rich foods because a shortage of potassium can contribute to swelling. Foods that are high in potassium include apricots, bananas, milk, broccoli, cantaloupe, prunes, spinach, sweet potatoes, beans, lentils, almonds, and peanuts. Avoid caffeine because it can make swelling worse.

High Cholesterol

Issues during pregnancy

You've probably heard all sorts of bad things about cholesterol, but the truth is that cholesterol is necessary during pregnancy. Your baby needs cholesterol for healthy development. It helps build cell membranes, develop the brain, and manufacture hormones in your baby's body.

What is cholesterol? It's a fatlike substance in your blood. Two kinds of blood cholesterol exist: LDL, which is known as "bad" cholesterol because it can damage your arteries, and HDL, which is known as "good" cholesterol because it boosts heart health by carrying excess blood cholesterol out of the body. A healthy goal is to maintain high HDL levels and low LDL levels.

When swelling gets serious

Some swelling in pregnancy is normal, and elevating your feet or cutting down on very salty foods can reduce swelling. However, substantial swelling could be a sign of preeclampsia, a potentially dangerous condition that has nothing to do with salt intake. Preeclampsia affects about 5 percent of pregnant women, usually during the first pregnancy, and it's more common in women who are over 35, overweight, or carrying multiples.

If you have preeclampsia, you will develop high blood pressure and there will be protein in your urine. (That's why your doctor measures your blood pressure.) Other signs may include significant swelling of the hands and feet, sudden weight gain of a pound or more a day, blurred vision, severe headaches, dizziness, and intense upper abdominal pain.

Preeclampsia is dangerous because it can slow your baby's growth and increase the chances of the placenta separating from your uterine wall. In rare cases preeclampsia develops into eclampsia. This condition causes convulsions, which may lead to stroke, coma, or even the death of the mother in rare cases.

Call your doctor immediately if you develop symptoms of preeclampsia. Although the only way to cure preeclampsia is by delivering the baby, sometimes health care providers will monitor you at bed rest for weeks before preeclampsia worsens.

During pregnancy, your body makes most of the cholesterol your baby needs, so you don't need to eat extra. Since your baby needs extra cholesterol for healthy growth, your body will boost production and the cholesterol levels in your blood will go way up during pregnancy. If you have a cholesterol blood test while you're pregnant, the levels may be as much as 60 percent higher than before pregnancy. (Because of this, just about any pregnant woman who has a blood cholesterol test will have "high" cholesterol. If you started pregnancy with high cholesterol levels, they'll soar even higher while you're pregnant. Then, after pregnancy, they'll return to prepregnancy levels.)

Because cholesterol levels go up substantially during pregnancy, the best way to get an accurate postpartum blood cholesterol reading is to wait at least six weeks after delivery to have a blood cholesterol test. But don't worry, this condition is temporary for most pregnant women.

Cholesterol 101: Should I avoid eggs?

Eggs are an excellent pregnancy food. They are a rich source of protein, B vitamins, and iron. For people who don't eat fish, eggs can be a great source of omega-3 fatty acids (if they are eggs laid by hens that are fed flaxseed).

But eggs also contain saturated fat and cholesterol. If you have normal cholesterol levels and a low risk of heart disease, eating three or four eggs a week is fine. (Do limit the butter, bacon, and other high-fat foods that often accompany eggs, however.)

If you have elevated cholesterol levels and are at an elevated risk of heart disease, the American Heart Association (AHA) recommends that you further limit your egg intake. A large whole egg contains about 213 milligrams of cholesterol, which is about 71 percent of the daily recommended limit (300 milligrams) for healthy people and too much for those with certain risk factors who have a daily recommended limit of 200 milligrams. Extra-large and jumbo eggs contain even more cholesterol.

If you enjoy eggs and would like to include them in your diet—whether or not you have high cholesterol—keep these AHA tips in mind:

- If you eat a whole egg, avoid or limit other sources of dietary cholesterol and saturated fat that day.
- Choose small or medium eggs, rather than large, extra large, or jumbo. Small eggs have about 157 milligrams of cholesterol, and medium have about 187 milligrams.
- Egg whites have no cholesterol. Use two egg whites, or one egg white plus 2 teaspoons of unsaturated oil, in place of one whole egg in cooking. When making scrambled eggs or omelets, use one whole egg and several egg whites. You can buy refrigerated cartons of egg whites in many grocery stores.
- Use cholesterol-free egg substitutes in omelets, in scrambled egg dishes, and in baking.

Fact or fiction? Only foods high in cholesterol can raise blood cholesterol.
Fiction. If you have high cholesterol, you should pay attention to how much fat a food has in addition to how much cholesterol it contains. Eating foods that have high amounts of cholesterol, including fatty meat, eggs, and whole-fat dairy products, can raise your blood cholesterol. But it is the saturated fats in these foods that have the most dramatic effect on your blood cholesterol level, not the cholesterol itself. If you have high cholesterol, read food labels so you can avoid saturated fat, trans fat, and cholesterol.

Dangers and medications

When there is too much LDL cholesterol in your blood, it builds up on the walls of your arteries. Over time, this buildup can cause what's known as hardening of the arteries, a condition in which blood flow to the heart is slowed down or blocked because arteries have become narrowed. If the blood supply to a part of the heart is completely cut off, a heart attack occurs. Having high LDL cholesterol levels in your blood is a major risk factor for heart disease, which is the number-one killer in the United States.

If you are on cholesterol-lowering drugs and you want to conceive, don't discontinue them without your doctor's supervision, but do call your doctor immediately to discuss how to get off the drugs. These medications may cause birth defects even before you know you are pregnant.

Keeping it in check

Although you shouldn't take cholesterol-lowering drugs during pregnancy, you can take several steps to keep blood cholesterol levels in check during pregnancy:

Watch your diet. Eat a diet that is low in saturated fat, trans fat, and cholesterol. Animal foods (meat, butter, whole milk, and egg yolks) contain saturated fat and cholesterol. Limit yourself to 300 milligrams a day of cholesterol (200 milligrams if you already have a known blockage in your arteries) and keep your saturated fat intake at 7 percent of calories (about 15 grams a day). There is no recommended safe intake of trans fats, so avoid them as much as possible. Trans fats are found in processed foods such as packaged cookies and crackers, fast-food french fries, and other high-fat snack foods.

Watch your weight. People who are overweight tend to have high cholesterol. Losing weight can raise your HDL (good cholesterol) levels and lower your LDL (bad cholesterol) and triglycerides (another kind of fatlike substance in the blood that increases the risk of heart disease). Pregnancy is no time to diet, and losing weight during pregnancy is not safe for your baby (see "Dieting during pregnancy," page 56). But you can be heart-healthy by trying not to gain excess weight while you're expecting.

Get moving. Exercise can help lower your LDL and raise your HDL cholesterol levels.

Plant sterols and margarines

You may have noticed advertisements for margarines, such as Benecol and Take Control, that contain plant sterols—or, if you had high cholesterol before getting pregnant, you may already include these margarines in your diet. Plant sterols are compounds that are found naturally in many plant foods and vegetable oils and in much higher amounts in plant sterol margarines. Evidence suggests that eating these margarines can lower LDL cholesterol levels by 10 to 15 percent.

But is it safe to use these margarines while you're pregnant? The answer is maybe. No research has concluded that plant sterol margarines are unsafe during pregnancy, but there is no evidence that they are safe either. Some researchers have raised concerns that because plant sterols block the body's ability to absorb cholesterol from other foods that are eaten, they may also inhibit the body's ability to absorb fat-soluble vitamins such as vitamins A, E, and D, which could rob your baby of necessary nutrients and also leave you short of vitamins you'll need during breastfeeding. Other researchers, however, point out that vegetarian women eat substantial amounts of naturally occurring plant sterols without putting their pregnancies in danger.

Until a definitive answer is found, a cautious approach is to limit your use of plant sterol margarines during pregnancy unless your doctor recommends otherwise.

Eat more fiber. Foods that contain soluble fiber (oats, oranges, pears, Brussels sprouts, carrots, dried peas, and dried beans) can lower LDL levels in the blood.

Your Bed Rest Diet

When you're stuck in bed

If you're experiencing a pregnancy complication such as bleeding in late pregnancy or preeclampsia, your health care provider may tell you that you need to reduce your activity or stay in bed for long periods of time. Reducing your activity level may require you to make some changes in your diet, including the following:

Calorie intake. If you go from being active to spending most of your day lying on a bed or sofa, your calorie needs will decrease.

Fiber. When you slow down, so do your intestines. Be sure to eat plenty of high-fiber foods and drink lots of water to avoid getting constipated. (For more constipation-prevention ideas, see "Prevention tips," page 120.)

Sit up after eating. Being on bedrest increases your chances of developing heartburn, so be sure not to lie down after you eat.

Get whatever exercise you can. Talk with your doctor about exactly what activity is allowed. Even if you are confined to bed, it may be OK for you to do ankle circles, biceps curls, leg lifts, or other exercises that you can do while lying down. These exercises can burn calories and help you maintain muscle tone.

Watch your boredom eating. Being bored is a major cause of mindless eating. Pay attention to whether you eat out of boredom. If you do, look for other ways to alleviate the tedium of bedrest.

Choose convenience foods carefully. If you can't cook, you may have to rely on convenience foods. Try to choose premade salads, vegetable-based soups, and other healthy choices rather than high-fat, high-calorie, high-salt take-out food. If you rely on commercially made frozen dinners, choose varieties that are low in salt and fat. Better yet, ask friends and relatives to fill your freezer and refrigerator with nutritious home-cooked dinners.

Avoid caffeine. Some women find they have trouble sleeping while on bedrest because of a lack of activity. Caffeine only makes it worse.

Make sure you're getting enough calcium. Bedrest can cause bone loss because exercise helps keep bones strong. Minimize the damage with a calcium-rich diet.

Get support. The Sidelines National Support Network (www.sidelines.org) provides excellent information, advice, and support for pregnant women on bedrest.

Lactose Intolerance

Pregnancy issues
Getting ample calcium during pregnancy is important for your baby and for your bone health. Dairy foods are the richest source of calcium, and three servings a day are recommended.

If all that milk gives you stomach and intestinal discomfort, it may be that you are lactose intolerant.

Lactose intolerance is the inability to digest significant amounts of lactose, a kind of sugar found in milk. Intolerance occurs due to a shortage of the enzyme lactase, which breaks down the sugar in milk so it can be absorbed into the bloodstream. When there is not enough lactase to digest the amount of lactose consumed, gas, bloating, nausea, cramps, and diarrhea can occur within 30 minutes to about 2 hours after consuming a lactose-containing food.

Some 30 million to 50 million Americans are lactose intolerant. Certain ethnic and racial populations are more widely affected than others. As many as 75 percent of all African Americans and American Indians and 90 percent of Asian Americans are lactose intolerant. The condition is least common among persons of northern European descent.

The severity of symptoms of lactose intolerance varies from person to person. Some people with lactose intolerance can eat cheese and yogurt but have trouble with milk. That's because a serving of milk contains more lactose (11 grams per cup) than ice cream (6 grams in a half-cup serving), yogurt (5 grams in a one-cup serving), cottage cheese (2 to 3 grams in a half-cup serving), or Swiss cheese (1 gram in a 1-ounce serving).

Although milk and foods made from milk are the only natural sources, lactose is often added to prepared foods. People with very low tolerance for lactose should know about the many food products that may contain even small amounts of lactose, such as bread and other baked goods; processed breakfast cereals; instant potatoes; instant soups; breakfast drinks; margarine; nonkosher lunch meats; salad dressings; some candies and other snacks; mixes for pancakes, biscuits, and cookies; and powdered meal-replacement supplements. Be careful, too, because some products labeled "nondairy" may include ingredients that are derived from milk and therefore contain lactose. This includes items such as powdered coffee creamer and whipped toppings.

When you're looking at food labels to determine whether a food contains lactose, don't just look for milk or lactose in the ingredients. Check to see if the food contains whey, curds, milk by-products, dry milk solids, or nonfat dry milk powder. If any of these are listed on a food label, the product contains lactose.

In addition, lactose is used as the base for more than 20 percent of prescription drugs and about 6 percent of over-the-counter medicines, including some medications for stomach acid and gas. However, these products typically affect only people with severe lactose intolerance.

You can still get all the calcium you need if you are lactose intolerant. A variety of lactose-free milk products are available in most grocery stores. If you don't consume any milk or milk products, you can get calcium from a variety of other sources, including calcium-fortified orange juice and calcium-fortified soymilk. (For more information on nonmilk calcium sources, see "Calculating Calcium," page 33, and "Plant Sources of Calcium," page 91.)

Religious Diets

Fasting and kosher meals

Some religions require its followers to fast or eat a special diet. If you are having an otherwise healthy pregnancy, and if you are gaining an adequate amount of weight, it's fine to fast on holidays such as Yom Kippur or during Lent or Ramadan. (Check to see if pregnant women are exempt from fasting rules.) If you fast, try to decrease your activity that day and be sure to drink plenty of water.

If you will be fasting for more than a day or two, such as during Ramadan, it is best to consult a registered dietitian for specific and personalized recommendations. The dietitian can help you ensure that you're meeting the nutritional needs of pregnancy during this potentially restrictive period.

You should not fast if you are not gaining enough weight or if you have gestational diabetes or other nutrition-related health issues.

Jewish women who follow a kosher diet needn't worry. A kosher diet can be balanced and perfectly healthy during pregnancy.

Celiac Disease

A digestive disease

Celiac disease, or celiac sprue, is a digestive disease that damages the small intestine and interferes with absorption of nutrients from foods. People with celiac disease can't tolerate gluten, a protein found in wheat, rye, and barley. Gluten is also an ingredient added to some vitamins and medicines.

When people with celiac disease eat gluten, their immune system responds in a way that damages or destroys the villi, which are fingerlike protrusions that line the small intestine. You need healthy villi in order to absorb nutrients properly. Without them, you can become malnourished even if you eat ample amounts of food.

People with celiac disease must completely avoid gluten in order to heal existing damage to the intestine and prevent further damage. In fact, a gluten-free diet is the only treatment for celiac disease.

Following a completely gluten-free diet during pregnancy is crucial. If you eliminate gluten completely, you can have as healthy a pregnancy as women without celiac disease. If you don't, your body may not be absorbing nutrients properly, which may mean your baby is not getting the nutrients he needs. Also, babies of mothers with undiagnosed or uncontrolled celiac disease are three times more likely to suffer from intrauterine growth restriction—which means they don't grow at the normal rate inside the uterus. There is also an increased risk of low or very low birthweight, preterm birth, and cesarean delivery.

And be warned: If you have celiac disease and you're not eating a gluten-free diet, you and your baby may be malnourished even if you don't have any of the symptoms of celiac disease. Common symptoms include gas, abdominal bloating, muscle cramps, tooth discoloration, chronic diarrhea, and chronic constipation.

Eating gluten-free

Fortunately more and more gluten-free products are appearing on grocery store shelves. Gluten-free bread, pasta, and cereals can be made with potato, rice, soy, amaranth, quinoa, buckwheat, or bean flour. As awareness of celiac disease increases, more gluten-free choices are becoming available.

Following a gluten-free diet is a challenge, particularly when you eat in restaurants or at a friend's house. If you need help planning your diet, meet with a registered dietitian and join a celiac disease support group such as the Celiac Disease Foundation (www.celiac.org) or the Celiac Sprue Association of the USA (www.csaceliacs.org).

Prenatal vitamins

In addition to eliminating gluten from your diet, be sure you take prenatal vitamins so you'll get any vitamins and minerals that are lacking in your diet. While it may seem like women with celiac disease are at a higher risk of having a child with a neural tube defect (both because their bodies are less able to absorb folic acid and other vitamins and because they don't eat grains that are fortified with folic acid), medical research doesn't seem to support this association. The recommendation for women with celiac disease is to get adequate amounts of folic acid from supplements (800 micrograms to 1,000 micrograms a day).

It's best for all women, particularly those with celiac disease, to start taking prenatal vitamins containing folic acid three to six months before conceiving because the neural tube closes so early in pregnancy. (Call the vitamin manufacturer to ensure the supplement you take is indeed gluten-free.) Continue to take a daily multivitamin after you give birth to keep up with the increased nutrition demands of breastfeeding and to prepare your body once again if you plan to get pregnant anytime soon.

After Weight-Loss Surgery

Issues to consider

Weight-loss surgery has become more common during the past few years. It is possible to get pregnant and have a healthy baby after weight-loss surgery, but you'll have to take some special steps to ensure good health.

Weight-loss surgery promotes weight loss by restricting food intake, limiting absorption of calories and nutrients, or

Eating during labor

You may think that eating will be the last thing you'll want to do during labor, but the fact is, unless you have a very short labor, you'll need to eat and drink.

In past decades, doctors disallowed eating and drinking during labor. They believed it was better for a woman to have an empty stomach because it would reduce the chance that she would vomit and inhale (aspirate) stomach contents into her lungs while under general anesthesia, possibly causing a life-threatening pneumonia.

Today general anesthesia is rare, and improved anesthesia techniques make it far less likely that aspiration will occur. What's more, many women find that labor is more difficult and they have less energy if they are hungry.

If you're not hungry, don't force yourself to eat. But do try to sip fluids or suck on ice chips so you don't become dehydrated.

Most doctors and midwives recommend that laboring women drink clear liquids such as water, tea, broth, sports drinks, or clear low-acid fruit juices (apple, white grape, cranberry), as well as light, easily digested snacks such as saltine crackers, graham crackers, toast, nonfat yogurt, fresh fruit, or freezer pops. Avoid anything acidic, such as orange juice, in case you vomit (when vomited, acidic foods can cause an unpleasant burning feeling in the throat). It's also best to avoid large meals like pasta with meatballs, which may create quite a mess if you vomit in active labor.

Don't get anxious about vomiting during delivery. Most women don't. Plus, unless you had a large meal right before going into labor, it's likely that not much will come out.

Eating after a vaginal delivery

It's fine to have something to eat shortly after your baby is born. In fact, some women find that the exertion of labor and delivery leaves them with a ferocious appetite. No matter how hungry you are, however, it's best to start small with a light snack such as tea and toast or half a sandwich. If that sits well, eat more, but don't load up with filling, high-fat food because it may make you feel nauseated. Be sure to keep drinking water or other fluids to prevent postpartum constipation and to help establish your milk supply for breastfeeding.

both, depending on the type of operation. People who have weight-loss surgery are advised to take vitamin supplements for the rest of their lives, and this is especially important during pregnancy. The nutrients they are most likely to lack include iron, calcium, vitamin B_{12}, and folic acid. Be sure to tell your obstetrician that you had weight-loss surgery and to discuss what supplements you should take.

Ideal conception time frames

The year or two after weight-loss surgery is usually a time of major weight loss. Having a healthy pregnancy is much more difficult if you're also losing weight, so you should conceive no sooner than 12 to 18 months after weight-loss surgery. If you get pregnant earlier than that, your baby may have an elevated risk of intrauterine growth restriction (not growing adequately in the uterus), or being born small. You may experience anemia or bleeding in your stomach or intestines. If your weight-loss surgery included the implantation of a gastric band, it may need to be adjusted, so be sure to check with your surgeon.

On the positive side, if you've had weight-loss surgery and have lost a significant number of pounds, you have lowered your risk of developing gestational diabetes and high blood pressure, and you are less likely to need a cesarean delivery or to have a very large baby. In general, women who have had weight-loss surgery and are at a healthy weight have fewer pregnancy-related complications than obese women.

Surgery concerns

Pregnant women who have had recent weight-loss surgery must watch out for something called "dumping," which can occur if you eat certain foods. For example, some women find that if they have something sweet they soon feel crampy, nauseated, dizzy, sweaty, and flushed. Women who have dumping may not be able to tolerate the drink that's part of the 1-hour glucose challenge test, which is normally given between the 24th and 28th weeks of pregnancy. If that is the case, these women may have a periodic fasting and 2-hours-after-meal glucose test to determine if they have gestational diabetes. Discuss with your doctor which screening options are best for

Fact or fiction? Too much salt in the diet during pregnancy causes hypertension. **Fiction.** Although excess salt can exacerbate high blood pressure if it was a preexisting condition in the mother, it cannot cause it.

you. (For more information, see "Blood Sugar Problems During Pregnancy," page 101.)

Remember, if you remain overweight or obese even after your weight-loss surgery, your health care provider may order a 1-hour glucose loading test during your 1st trimester. This way, if you have pregestational diabetes, you can start treatment with insulin early in your pregnancy.

Hydrating issues

Women who have had weight-loss surgery may also find that they vomit often. Frequent vomiting makes it hard to stay hydrated and to absorb nutrients from food, so be sure to let your doctor know if you can't keep food down.

Eating enough calories

Serving sizes must always remain small after weight-loss surgery, making it a challenge to get enough calories when you're pregnant. Even if you're still overweight or obese, your baby needs extra calories to grow properly. Not all of the dietary recommendations for pregnant women apply to those who have had weight-loss surgery. For example, instead of small snacks spread throughout the day, some surgeons encourage their patients to eat four higher-protein mini meals a day to get the proper nutrition while reducing the risk of excess empty calories and weight regain. Check with your doctor and a registered dietitian to see what intake pattern may be best for you.

Eating after a cesarean delivery

It's generally fine to sip on clear liquids a few hours after your baby is born, as long as you had spinal or epidural anesthesia (not general anesthesia). If clear liquids stay down without nausea, your health care provider will likely allow you to eat light snacks soon after.

You may notice during the day or two after cesarean delivery that your belly has blown up as if you were pregnant again. Fear not, it is just gas, which accumulates when your intestines are not moving at their normal speed. It is a temporary reaction of the intestines to manipulation during surgery and to medications given around the time of surgery. Walk around and resume your normal eating pattern slowly until you are passing gas.

keeping fit
during pregnancy

When your mother was pregnant, her doctor probably told her to take it easy. He certainly didn't tell her to go jogging. Today doctors know that exercise is beneficial during pregnancy. Unless you have certain medical conditions, exercise poses no risk to your baby. How much and how hard you exercise depends on your fitness level before conceiving. If you've never exercised before, now is not the time to train for a marathon. But with your doctor's approval you can walk, swim, do prenatal yoga, take low-impact aerobics classes, lift weights, and work out with exercise machines. You'll benefit your health and that of your baby, and you may even make your labor easier.

Keeping Fit During Pregnancy

Benefits of Exercise

It's great to be active

Exercise is one of the best things you can do for yourself while you're pregnant. In addition to helping you feel better, it also gives you a sense of control over a body that is changing—and getting larger—every week. Exercise releases endorphins, the feel-good brain chemicals that give runners a high. Exercise also offers the following benefits:

- Reduces your chances of developing pregnancy-related annoyances such as backaches and constipation.
- Aids in weight control and reduces body fat.
- Improves circulation, which helps prevent constipation, varicose veins, leg cramps, and hemorrhoids.
- Helps prevent gestational diabetes. Or if you have gestational diabetes, exercise keeps it in control.
- Helps keep blood sugar levels in check. This is particularly important for women with gestational diabetes, but women with normal blood sugar benefit too because rising and falling blood sugar levels can leave you feeling fatigued.
- Energizes you. Some women find that it gives them more energy than a nap.
- Helps you sleep better. Pregnant women sometimes have trouble sleeping, particularly during the latter part of pregnancy. Exercise helps you relax, which can make it easier for you to sleep.
- Builds muscle, which makes it easier for your body to support the additional weight of pregnancy.
- Reduces swelling and bloating.
- Improves your posture, which reduces your chances of developing aches and pains during pregnancy.
- Prepares you for labor and delivery. Fit mothers have shorter labors, fewer medical interventions, and less fatigue during delivery. Exercise also builds endurance, which comes in handy during labor.
- Eases the discomforts of pregnancy and increases your overall health. Exercise also reduces the risk of chronic disease such as heart disease, high blood pressure, type 2 diabetes, and arthritis. It helps build and maintain strong bones and may reduce bone loss after age 30. It keeps muscles and joints strong. It boosts mood; reduces anxiety, tension, and depression; and helps you feel more resilient in the face of stressful situations.

Who shouldn't exercise

Not everyone should exercise during pregnancy. It's important to check with your doctor to see if it's safe for you. Certain health conditions make exercise risky during pregnancy. Unless your doctor gives you the OK, the American College of Obstetricians and Gynecologists recommends avoiding exercise if you have any of the following conditions:

- Significant heart disease
- Restrictive lung disease
- Incompetent cervix (a condition in which the cervix is weak and cannot adequately hold the baby in the uterus)
- Preterm labor (labor before week 37)
- Bleeding from the vagina during the 2nd or 3rd trimesters
- Preeclampsia
- Placenta previa (a condition in which the placenta lies low and covers all or part of the cervix)
- Ruptured membranes

Smart Exercise Choices

Three kinds of fitness

Fitness is broken into three major categories. The best exercise programs incorporate activities that improve all of them.

1. Cardiovascular fitness. Walking, running, cycling, and swimming are examples of cardiovascular workouts that get your heart pumping and your blood flowing. These workouts, which strengthen your heart and your lungs, are also known as aerobic exercise. During pregnancy, cardiovascular fitness helps keep you energized and gives you the endurance you need to get through labor and delivery.

2. Muscular strength. If you have muscular strength, your muscles have the ability to exert force. You use your muscular strength when you lift a bag of groceries or carry a suitcase. You can strengthen your muscles by lifting weights or simply by using your own body as resistance. For example, you can work your hip muscles by lying on your side and lifting your leg. Muscle-strengthening exercises also strengthen bones. Having muscular strength during pregnancy makes it easier for you to carry extra weight without straining your back.

3. Flexibility training. Stretching and doing yoga make you more flexible. They lengthen your muscles and allow your body to move through its full range of motion. Being flexible makes it easier to move your larger-than-usual body comfortably during pregnancy.

Walking

Walking is an excellent pregnancy exercise. You can do it anytime, anywhere, at any intensity, and for any amount of time. You can walk inside (on a treadmill or track, or in a mall) or outside (in your neighborhood, along the beach, at a park, or on an outdoor track). You can walk alone or with friends. You can carry along a personal stereo and listen to music, the news, or a book on tape. You can walk on flat paths or up steep roads. It requires no expensive gym membership and, aside from a good pair of walking shoes, no special equipment.

Best Pregnancy Activities		
Activity	**Benefits**	**Cautions**
Walking	Builds cardiovascular fitness, strengthens lower-body muscles, improves feeling of well-being, burns calories.	Start with a pace and distance that is comfortable and easy to do; increase intensity gradually. Follow safety recommendations when walking outdoors (see "Exercise dos and dont's," page 137).
Pilates	Builds core strength (abdominal muscles, back muscles), puts minimal pressure on your back, and is helpful postpartum when you're trying to lose weight and build muscle tone.	Fine during the 1st and 2nd trimesters. During the 3rd trimester, be careful not to lie flat on your back. Use a wedge-shape pillow instead. Pilates can be vigorous, so don't start it during pregnancy unless your instructor is aware that you're pregnant.
Running	Builds cardiovascular fitness and burns calories.	As your pregnancy progresses, running may become less comfortable. For example, you may leak urine because of pressure on your bladder. Monitor how you feel and switch to short runs, slower runs, or walking if you feel uncomfortable. An elliptical exercise machine is a good substitute for running.
Free weights	Build strength throughout your body.	Use common sense. Don't overextend yourself by lifting heavy weights. Proper lifting form is more important than ever, so use a spotter or schedule a session with a personal trainer who can evaluate your form.
Swimming	Builds cardiovascular strength and endurance without straining your joints or back.	Don't swim if your water has already broken.
Yoga	Increases flexibility and muscle tone.	Be careful not to overstretch because during pregnancy ligaments are loose and overstretching can injure them. Stick to yoga classes designed for pregnant women if you've never done yoga before.
Exercise machines	Provide cardiovascular workout indoors.	Recumbent bike, treadmill, and elliptical trainer are fine. Avoid rowing machines unless you're in excellent shape and have used them before.
Exercise classes	Depending on the type of class, can provide cardiovascular workout, strength training, and/or flexibility training. Water aerobics are particularly good during pregnancy because water supports your belly and reduces injury risk.	Aerobics classes are fine if they match your ability level (opt for low- or medium-impact aerobics classes). During the 3rd trimester you may be clumsy and less balanced, so be extra careful doing anything that could cause a fall if you lose your balance, particularly if you do step aerobics.

Activity	Benefits	Cautions
Dance classes (ballet, modern dance)	Provide an energizing workout that works the cardiovascular system, increases flexibility, and tones muscles.	Keep in mind that your center of gravity changes as your pregnancy progresses, and you may lose your balance or trip more easily. You may also feel less comfortable doing certain moves when you get larger.
Sit-ups	Tone the abdominal muscles, which takes pressure off the back.	As pregnancy progresses your abdominal muscles stretch out, so you may have trouble isolating your abdominals and sit-ups may become less effective.
Stretching	Lengthens muscles and improves flexibility and range of motion.	Don't overstretch because during pregnancy ligaments are loose and overstretching could injure them.
Stability ball	Offers a variety of ways to stretch and build strength.	Be cautious using a stability ball, especially if you've never used one before. Avoid doing any moves that could cause you to fall off the ball and land on your belly. Remember that pregnancy affects your balance.
Exercise videos or DVDs	Offer a variety of workouts that you can do at home, often without needing equipment.	Choose videos made for pregnant women and tailored to your level of fitness.

Swimming

Swimming is great for pregnant women. When you're in the water it's easy to forget about those 25 or 30 extra pounds you're carrying. Swimming builds endurance and exercises your heart, but it is gentle on your joints. If you swim, remember two important things: Drink plenty of water and don't let yourself get overheated. When you're in water you're less likely to notice the signs of overheating or dehydration, so be extra aware of your fluid intake and body temperature.

More ways to move

Another way to work exercise into your life is to make your daily routine more active. Walk to the store instead of driving. Go for a stroll with a friend you haven't seen in a long time rather than going out to dinner. Park your car farther away from your destination. Skip the elevator and take the stairs. These are quick, easy ways to get your blood pumping.

Safety and Your Baby

Exercise dos and don'ts

Take these safety tips to heart:

DO watch your positions. Avoid lying on your back during your 3rd trimester. The weight of your growing baby can press on a large blood vessel, which can reduce blood circulation to your uterus.

DON'T get too adventurous. Running, aggressive racquet sports, and intense strength training are recommended only for women who have experience doing them before pregnancy.

DO watch your step. The extra weight you're gaining shifts your center of gravity forward and can affect your balance. Be careful when doing anything that requires balance.

DON'T walk or run on bumpy terrain. Walking, running, or hiking on unstable ground can lead to falls and injuries because your ligaments are more relaxed during pregnancy. Opt for smooth sidewalks, trails, and pathways and keep your eyes peeled for sticks, rocks, and other things that might trip you.

DON'T walk on roads if you can avoid it. Whenever possible, walk on sidewalks, paths, and trails rather than roads. If you must walk on a road, walk on the left side, facing traffic. If you walk at night, wear a reflective vest over your jacket so oncoming cars can see you.

DON'T walk outside when it's dark because you're more likely to trip on unnoticed roots, rocks, or uneven sidewalks. If you do walk at night, though, carry a flashlight. It will help drivers see you, and it will help you avoid tripping over things.

DON'T walk in isolated areas. Tell someone where you are going and be aware of your surroundings.

DON'T use a personal stereo when walking in traffic.

DO watch for hypoglycemia (low blood sugar) if you have gestational diabetes. (For strategies to prevent hypoglycemia, see "Get moving!" page 114.)

DON'T get overheated. A body temperature over 102.6 degrees F is not good for your baby, particularly during the 1st trimester, when extreme heat may contribute to birth defects. However, there have been no reports that increased body temperatures due to exercise cause birth defects. For your comfort, work out in a well-ventilated room and consider running a fan or air-conditioner. When it's hot outside, either exercise in an air-conditioned area or exercise early in the morning or late in the evening when it's cooler outside.

DO drink plenty of water or other fluids before, during, and after exercise. (See "What should you drink while exercising?" page 147.)

DON'T overstress your back. Avoid positions and exercises that require extreme bending of your back because they put extra stress on your abdominal

Exercises to avoid during pregnancy

The following exercises are not safe for pregnant women:
- Contact sports such as football or soccer
- Horseback riding
- Waterskiing. A fall could be incredibly dangerous.
- Scuba diving (it can cause gas bubbles to form in your baby's blood)
- Any activity that could put you at risk for an abdominal injury (including ice hockey, kickboxing, and soccer). Even a minor injury to your abdomen could harm your baby.

When to stop exercising

The American College of Obstetricians and Gynecologists recommends that you stop exercising and call your doctor immediately if you experience any of the following symptoms:

- Bleeding from your vagina
- Sudden or severe pain in the abdomen or vagina
- Shortness of breath
- Contractions that continue for 30 minutes after you exercise
- Dizziness
- Unexplained or severe headache
- Chest pain
- Muscle weakness
- Calf pain or swelling
- Preterm labor
- Decreased movement of your baby
- Leakage of fluid from your vagina
- Blurred vision

muscles (which are already being stretched by your growing baby) and compress the joints in your spine.

DO pay attention to air quality. During ozone alerts or days when the air quality is bad, avoid outdoor activity, especially if you have respiratory disease.

DON'T exercise intensively if you're having trouble gaining adequate weight. Save those valuable calories for your baby instead.

DO call for help if you need it. If you trip and fall and feel you may have hurt yourself, don't try to walk home. Call someone to pick you up, or if you think you may be badly hurt, call an ambulance. Don't take a chance.

DO carry identification when you exercise outdoors and, if possible, a cell phone programmed with emergency phone numbers.

DON'T exercise too close to bedtime

if you have trouble sleeping. Not everyone has this problem, but for some people, exercising within 3 or 4 hours of bedtime keeps them from falling asleep.

DON'T hold your breath while exercising. Sometimes people focus so much on their activity that they forget to breathe deeply. Fill your lungs with deep breaths. If you lift weights, exhale while you lift and breathe in when you stop. This is important all the time but especially during pregnancy, when improper breathing could make you feel light-headed.

DON'T launch a weight-lifting regimen during pregnancy. You can lift weights if you were doing it for some time before conceiving and know how to do it safely. If you do lift weights, avoid lifting heavy weights over your head and stay away from motions that may strain your lower back muscles.

DO relax after a workout with a dip in the pool, but stay out of the hot tub, whirlpool, or sauna because they can overheat your body.

DO exercises that strengthen your abdominal muscles, but only with pregnancy-safe abdominal exercises. (Ask your health care provider for suggestions.) Strong abs help support your baby without putting excessive strain on your back. They also help you push your baby out during labor.

The right intensity

How much, how long, and how intensely should you exercise? The answer varies from person to person, but you should be cautious not to overexert yourself. That's because when you exercise, your muscles need more oxygen. In order to deliver the oxygen the muscles need, your body diverts oxygen away from other areas.

Provided you've got your doctor's permission to exercise, use these general guidelines to plan your pregnancy workout routine:

- If you were sedentary before conceiving, start slowly with a gentle exercise such as walking. As you become fitter you can increase both the duration and intensity of your workouts.
- If you exercised moderately before conceiving, keep up the good work.

Provided you're doing activities that are considered safe during pregnancy, you can stay the course. You may feel like reducing your intensity as your pregnancy progresses and you get larger, but until then, you can do whatever you did before you conceived.

- If you exercised strenuously before conceiving, you may have to rein yourself in a bit, especially if you take part in activities that are not safe during pregnancy. Talk with your doctor about designing a fitness plan that is vigorous but safe for you and your baby.

Measure your intensity

Exertion is the amount of effort you put into your workout. To be sure that you're not overexerting yourself, you can measure your exertion, or intensity level, in two ways: by using the "talk test" or by tracking your heart rate.

The talk test. With the talk test, you should be exercising enough to feel like you're exerting yourself, but not so hard that you can't talk. You should be able to hold a conversation while you exercise without gasping for breath. If you can't talk, you're exercising too hard. If it's easy to chat a mile a minute, you can push your intensity up a notch.

Heart-rate monitoring. Some people prefer to use heart rate monitors and

How to measure your heart rate

- Press two fingers (not your thumb) on your wrist or neck to find your pulse.
- Count the number of pulse beats at your wrist or neck for 15 seconds.
- Multiply that number by four to get beats per minute.

Health alert: hiking during pregnancy

It's fine to hike when you're pregnant, but you should avoid going higher than 6,000 feet above sea level. Oxygen is limited in high altitudes, and in these locations your baby may not get enough. Get down that mountain quickly if you experience nausea, headache, and other symptoms of altitude sickness.

other fitness gadgets to measure their exertion. If tracking your heart rate motivates you, by all means, go for it. With heart-rate tracking, the goal is to get your heart rate into a target zone and to keep it there for at least 20 minutes. Exercising at this intensity helps strengthen your heart—it's what delivers the cardiovascular benefits of exercise. Your target zone is 70 percent of your maximum heart rate. To find your target heart rate, follow these simple steps:

1. Subtract your age from 220 to find your maximum heart rate.

2. Multiply that number by 0.7 to find your target heart rate.

So, for example, if you're 30 years old, your target heart rate is 133 (220 - 30 = 190; 190 × 0.7 = 133 beats per minute).

Traditionally, pregnant women have been advised to keep their heart rate under 140 beats per minute. However, doctors today don't give pregnant women any heart rate restrictions. What's most important is that you listen to your body. If you are struggling at 130 beats per minute, decrease your intensity until you feel more comfortable.

Limitations by trimester

Where you are in your pregnancy also helps determine how intensely you should exercise.

During the 1st trimester, the major impediments to exercise are fatigue and nausea. Nobody feels like exercising when they're exhausted and nauseated. If you feel terrible, skip a workout, but if you're only moderately sick or tired, see if a short walk helps. Some pregnant women find that gentle exercise energizes them and chases away feelings of nausea. However, don't exercise if nausea, vomiting, and food aversions are impeding your ability to gain weight.

You may find that the smell of the locker room at the gym is too much to bear. In that case, take your power walking outside. Some women want to exercise even while nauseated, which is fine. Just keep in mind that some exercise (such as the elliptical machine) is no good for a queasy stomach. Instead, explore a different type of exercise. A lap or two in the pool may take your mind off your nausea and vomiting.

If you did abdominal exercises before you conceived, you can continue to do them through your 1st trimester and into the 2nd. Later in your pregnancy, however, abdominal exercises may be less beneficial. If your abdominal muscles are stretched out by a 3-pound baby, it is difficult to locate which muscles should be contracting while exercising.

During the 2nd trimester, exercise should get easier. Your nausea will probably abate, and your energy will return. Although you'll be getting larger, you'll still be able to do many of the activities you did before pregnancy. Make the most of the energy burst and consider adding stress-relieving yoga or tai chi to your exercise routine.

During the 3rd trimester, exercise becomes more difficult. Your belly seems to get in the way of everything, and you tire easily. You also need to go to the bathroom more often, so if you're exercising outdoors, be sure to plan your route accordingly. Activities that you could do effortlessly may become more difficult during the 3rd trimester. Follow your body's wisdom and reduce exercise intensity. Don't stop moving altogether because now is when exercise helps you the most. Activities like yoga decrease your stress level, gentle back stretches after a brisk walk relieve low-back pain, and swimming relaxes all your muscles and your hip joints.

Avoid unsafe exercises, and modify any moves that require you to lie on your back.

Some women are bothered by leaking urine while exercising. Wear a pantyliner while exercising and do Kegel exercises (see page 150).

Structuring a Program

Aerobic workouts

Here's how to structure a 30- to 40-minute aerobic exercise session:

Warm up. Start with 5 to 10 minutes of gentle motion: walking, slow jogging in place, or whatever will prepare your body for the workout to come. This allows your body a few minutes to warm up gradually. During your warm-up, your heart rate, pulse, breathing rate, and body temperature increase. If you skip this step and start exercising intensely right away, you force your body to make all of these changes very quickly.

Pick up speed. This is the meat of your workout, the time when you push yourself. Don't push too much—if you can't talk while you're exercising, you're pushing too hard. Keep it up for 20 to 30 minutes.

Do intervals. If you find yourself getting tired, vary your pace by using a technique called interval training. Alternate bursts of exertion with recovery time. For example, during a 30-minute workout, try alternating 1 minute of fast walking with 2 minutes of slow walking. Over time, as you become more fit, you'll be able to lengthen the speedy parts of your session and decrease the recovery time.

Add intensity. When you're ready, you can turn up the intensity of your workout by going farther, moving faster, or staying at it longer. If you walk or jog, look for a hill to climb or increase the incline on your treadmill. Remember to intensify your workout

Fact or fiction? It's better to jog than to walk.

Fiction. Walking briskly can burn as many calories as a leisurely jog. Plus, walking is easier on your knees.

gradually and only when your body is ready.

Cool down. End your workout with 5 to 10 minutes of slow walking and gentle stretching. This allows your muscles to cool down gradually. Stopping abruptly can cause dizziness.

Four-week walking plan

It takes about a month to establish a fitness habit. If you're a new walker, try the following four-week get-started plan. At the end of the four weeks, continue walking every day for at least 30 minutes.

Week 1: Start small. Walk 10 minutes a day for seven days. That helps you get into the habit of doing it on a daily basis. Walk comfortably and enjoy yourself. Your job this week is to start building a walking habit, not to walk a marathon distance. Focus on your posture: Walk tall and hold in your abdominal muscles.

Week 2: Walk 15 minutes a day every day. This week, focus on taking a stride that is a comfortable length. Push off with your back foot and roll from heel to toe as your foot lands on the ground.

Week 3: Walk 20 or 25 minutes a day. This week, put some push into your pace. Start with five minutes of comfortable walking. Then, midwalk, strive for shorter, quicker steps. Slow down if you're out of breath. End your walk with a 5-minute cooldown of slow,

comfortable walking and some stretching, such as the shin stretch (while standing on one foot, trace circles in the air with the toe of your other foot, then switch feet) and the hamstring stretch (bend your left knee, extend your right leg in front of you, stretch, then switch).

Week 4: Increase the time to your goal of 30 minutes a day. Get your arms involved. Bend them at a 90-degree angle at the elbows and pump them gently as you walk. Every few minutes, speed up your pace for 20 quick steps, then slow back down.

Watch your posture. As you walk, pay attention to your technique and posture. Walk tall with your head up and eyes forward. Keep your back straight, your shoulders low and relaxed, and abdominal muscles contracted gently. Bend your arms at a 90-degree angle at the elbow, tracing an arc with your hands from your hip to your chest. Hold your hands in loose fists. Choose a stride length that is comfortable. Walk naturally—striding in an unnatural way pushes your body out of alignment and can lead to soreness or injuries. Land on your heel and roll forward to push off from the ball of your foot. As you walk, breathe rhythmically and mindfully. When walking up hills, lean forward slightly.

Use a pedometer. The President's Council on Physical Fitness and Sports

Fact or fiction? It's not safe to run during pregnancy.

Fiction. If you're in the habit of running for exercise, you have no health problems or pregnancy complications, and your doctor says it's OK, there's no reason to stop running during pregnancy. You can do a few things to make it safer. For example, replace your running shoes more often than you usually would to ensure adequate support and run on soft surfaces rather than hard roads. If you weren't a runner before your pregnancy, now's not the time to start. Choose walking and save the running for after your baby is born.

recommends setting a walking goal of 10,000 steps a day, or about 5 miles. If you're in good shape starting your pregnancy, this is a good goal to aim for during pregnancy. The easiest way to reach 10,000 steps a day is to use a pedometer that counts every step and every "bout" of exercise throughout the day. Inexpensive pedometers are available that count every step, which includes walking down the hall at work, climbing stairs instead of taking the elevator, walking to the bus stop, and so on. With a pedometer, you may discover that you're walking more than you realize.

Researchers say people with pedometers are more likely to stick to their fitness programs than those who don't use pedometers because they have a concrete goal that is easy to measure. Many clinics and doctors' offices give their patients a pedometer because they find it is a very effective way to get people moving.

Walking 10,000 steps a day is not realistic for everyone. To figure out what goal is good for you, wear a pedometer for a few days to determine how many steps you ordinarily take. Make that number your benchmark.

Then, each week or two, add 500 steps a day to your benchmark. If you find that it's tiring to meet your new goal, back it up 500 steps a day until you become fitter.

To accumulate steps during the day, look for ways to walk a few extra paces here and there. Here are some smart, simple suggestions:

- At work, use the restroom on a different floor.
- Every hour, take a 2- to 5-minute break. Stand up and walk around or go up a flight of stairs.
- Invite a group of coworkers to start a lunchtime walking group.
- Take messages to coworkers instead of emailing them.
- Carry letters or parcels to the post office or overnight delivery box rather than having them picked up.
- Exercise while you watch TV. Whenever a commercial comes on, get up and walk around the house until the program comes back on.
- Park the car in the spot farthest from the grocery store entrance.

Buying a pedometer. You can buy a pedometer at a sporting goods store, discount store, or online for $15 to $40. If you spend more, you can get one

Fact or fiction? You should avoid exercise if you have a head cold.

Fiction. You may not feel like exercising, but if you have a simple case of the common cold, it's fine to exercise. However, skip your workout if you have a fever over 100 degrees F, chest congestion, or anything more serious than a cold.

with extra features, such as a heart rate monitor, a clock, or a stopwatch, but those things are unnecessary if all you need is a step counter.

Building a strong back

Throughout your pregnancy, it's important to build and maintain back strength. Doing so will help prevent the low-back pain that is common among pregnant women and also will give you the muscle you'll need to lift a baby seat out of the back of the car without rupturing a disk. Ask your health care provider to recommend back strengthening exercises that are safe during pregnancy.

What's the "right" time?

What's the best time of day to exercise? There's no right or wrong time. It's all about personal preference and what fits into your schedule. A morning workout wakes you up and energizes you for the day ahead. A late-afternoon workout helps you get your muscles in motion after a day at work. Some people enjoy exercising in the evening.

The best time for you to exercise is the time that you can commit to. The fewer interruptions, the more likely you are to stick to your program.

For New Exercisers

Getting started

If you've never exercised before, getting started may seem difficult. You may feel intimidated or embarrassed. It's normal to feel that way, but if at all possible, try to overcome your discomfort. If you can't do it for yourself, do it for your baby.

Before you take a single step or swim a single lap, you have to get your mind in the right place for exercise. That's why the first part of any exercise program is to make a commitment. Promise yourself that you'll make exercise a priority in your life. For some, a visual reminder can offer

Walk away from diabetes

Exercise—both before and during pregnancy—is a fantastic way to reduce your risk of gestational diabetes, according to a study published in April 2004 in the *American Journal of Epidemiology*. The study found that compared with inactive women, women who spent more than 4.2 hours per week engaged in physical activity before and during pregnancy had a 70 percent lower risk of gestational diabetes.

Talk to Yourself

Having trouble convincing yourself to exercise? The next time you make excuses, use these facts to talk yourself into exercising.

When you think …	tell yourself …
I'm too exhausted to exercise.	Exercise gives me energy.
Exercise makes me tired.	That can be the case when someone first starts exercising. But as I become fitter and my heart and muscles become stronger, I'll feel less tired after workouts.
I can't afford to join a gym.	Walking outdoors costs nothing. All I need is a good pair of walking shoes.
I'm too out of shape to exercise.	Even the most sedentary person can exercise. Even if I start out with just 5 minutes of walking a day, I'm taking steps toward a healthy pregnancy.
I don't have time to exercise.	If I don't have a 30-minute block of time for exercise, I can break it up into three 10-minute chunks.
It will hurt.	If I start slowly and increase intensity gradually, I shouldn't feel any soreness.
I don't have the right clothes for exercise.	I can walk in anything that feels comfortable.
It's too hot or unsafe for me to exercise outside.	I can exercise indoors. (You can take an exercise class, join the YWCA, check with your local high school to see if the indoor track is open to the public, or walk in a mall. Many malls have walking programs and admit walkers before the mall opens. Some even have incentive programs and prizes.)
Exercise is boring.	If I try different activities and classes, maybe I'll find one I enjoy. (Vary your activities—swim one day, walk the next, do yoga the next.)

incentive. If it helps, write yourself a letter or sign a contract and post it in a place you'll see every day. Once you've committed yourself to exercising, follow these steps to get your fitness regimen off the ground:

Begin slowly. If you have been sedentary, begin with 5 to 10 minutes of walking each day. Each week, add 5 minutes to your daily walk time. Within five or six weeks you'll be walking half an hour a day, and within 12 weeks you'll be logging an hour every day. Aim for 30 to 60 minutes each day.

Don't do too much too soon. Gradually increase your time spent exercising. Resist the temptation to go all-out and push yourself to your limit the first day. If your workout leaves you feeling sore and exhausted, you're less likely to stick with it.

Don't overdo it. When pregnant, never exercise to the point of exhaustion or breathlessness. Stop before you do too much.

What should you drink while exercising?

It's important for everyone to stay hydrated during exercise, but it's even more important during pregnancy, when dehydration could lead to light-headedness, fatigue, and eventually constipation. Your body is about two-thirds water, and it needs constant replenishment to function well. Exercise increases your body's need for fluids because when you sweat you lose water.

Don't rely on thirst to tell you when to drink. By the time you're thirsty, you might already be dehydrated. Have a drink about 20 minutes before you exercise, every 20 minutes during your workout, and when you end your exercise session. If it's warm or windy outside, drink a little more.

Be on the lookout for the signs of dehydration: feeling dizzy or light-headed, having a sticky dryness in your mouth, and passing dark-colored urine. If you experience any of these dehydration symptoms, stop exercising and get something to drink immediately. And swimmers, don't forget to drink during your water workouts. You may not feel thirsty, but you still need to stay hydrated.

Although there are many sports drinks to choose from, water is usually your best bet if you exercise moderately. It hydrates without sugar and excess calories. Sports drinks are recommended for intense workouts of 90 minutes or more. These drinks provide carbohydrates for quick energy and electrolytes (body chemicals that are found in sweat).

Work exercise into your schedule. Once a week, grab your calendar and figure out what time you'll exercise each day during the following week. Write it down in your date book and take it as seriously as you do a doctor's appointment.

Be patient. It may take some time to notice results.

Set aside a regular time for exercise. If you work out at the same time every day, you never have to think about when you're going to exercise.

Make it a daily event. For best results, plan to do at least some exercise every day of the week.

Exercise with a friend. Your workouts will seem to go faster when you have have a friend exercising with you. Exercise with the same person every day or line up different people for each day of the week.

Get support. Even if they can't be out there exercising with you, friends and family can offer moral support.

Set realistic goals. Then reward yourself with something special when you achieve them.

Write it down. Keeping a log is a great motivator.

Have fun. You're more likely to stick with it if you enjoy it, so pick an activity you like.

Listen to your body. Slow down if you feel out of breath, light-headed, or tired.

The Right Gear

Dressing for exercise success

Put yourself on the road to exercise success by dressing properly for whatever activity you choose. Wear clothing that fits well, is comfortable, and gives you the freedom to move. Follow these tips:

- Wear shoes that are comfortable and the right fit for your feet. Your shoes should also adequately support your ankles and your arches and be designed for the particular activity.
- Replace your shoes every 6 months or 500 miles, whichever comes first.
- Wear socks made from acrylic or an acrylic blend because they won't retain moisture as cotton and wool often do. Excess moisture can lead to blisters and other foot problems.
- Remember that your feet may get larger during pregnancy, and it's not a good idea to stuff your feet into too-small shoes. If your shoes feel tight, buy new ones.
- Wear a supportive sports bra. As your pregnancy progresses your breasts will get larger and, most likely, more sensitive. A good sports bra will keep them comfortably in place.
- Wear exercise clothing that makes you feel confident.
- If you swim, you may need to buy a new bathing suit. Look for maternity suits or just go up a size or two in regular suits. Choose a suit with straps that don't fall down or press into your skin.
- To avoid catching athlete's foot or other contagious conditions, wear water shoes to and from the pool, in the locker room, and in the shower.
- Dress in layers. If you get too warm, you can remove a layer and cool off.
- If you're walking outdoors, check the thermometer and dress as if it's 10 degrees cooler than it actually is. Begin your walk going with the wind (rather than against it, which makes you feel colder). As you warm up and cool down, you can remove or add layers as needed.
- Wear light colors in summer (they reflect the sun's rays) and dark clothes in winter.
- Don't forget a hat. In cold weather, you'll lose a lot of body heat through your uncovered head. A hat can also shield you from the sun's rays.
- Never wear rubberized or plastic clothing that interferes with evaporation of perspiration. It can cause you to overheat.

Choosing good walking shoes

- Shop in a shoe store with knowledgeable salespeople. If they suggest you walk in a shoe designed for another sport, pick a new store.
- Invest in good walking shoes, not running shoes. Walking shoes are specially designed for walking. If you walk in running shoes, their overly cushioned heels, which are perfect for the high-impact action of running, could cause your toes to slap down as you walk. That can lead to shin soreness.
- Choose a walking shoe with good support, a moderate amount of cushioning (more if you're overweight), a roomy toe box, and a

low, beveled heel that accommodates
the heel-to-toe roll of walking.

- Have your feet measured every time
you buy new walking shoes.
- Try on shoes after you've exercised,
when your feet are their largest.
Wear the socks that you walk in.
- Make sure the shoe fits in the heel.
Many women choose shoes that are
too small so the shoes won't slip off
their heels as they walk, but that's
not a good idea. If you try on a shoe
that fits well in the toe box but not
the heel, pass it up for a style that
fits in both places.

Kegel exercises

Kegels are an exercise that you can do anytime. These exercises, which are named after the doctor who discovered them, help strengthen the pelvic floor muscles (the muscles that support the bladder, urethra, uterus, and rectum and control urination). The pelvic floor muscles are attached to the pelvic bone and act like a hammock, holding the organs in place. Strong pelvic floor muscles make delivering a baby slightly easier and help prevent urinary incontinence. As your uterus grows larger and the weight of the baby presses down on the pelvic floor muscles, they may weaken.

Pelvic floor exercises can help strengthen those muscles. Here's how to do Kegels:

1. Tighten the pelvic floor muscles. Do what you would do if you wanted to stop the flow of urine while urinating.

2. Hold the muscles tight, then release.

Choose a Kegel counting strategy. You can hold the muscles tight for a count of four, then release for a count of four, and repeat that sequence for several minutes. Or you can hold the muscles tight for up to 10 seconds, release, and repeat 10 times several times a day.

When you do Kegels, keep these tips in mind: As you tighten the pelvic floor muscles, try not to tighten other muscles (abdominals, for example). The exercise is more effective if you can isolate your pelvic floor muscles and work them. Also, even though a Kegel is the same action as stopping urine flow, it's best not to do Kegels while you're urinating because doing so can cause incomplete emptying of the bladder and, in turn, infections of the bladder and urinary tract.

A good way to remember your Kegels is to do them at the same time each day or while you're doing a certain activity. For example, you can do them every morning before you get out of bed or whenever you're stopped at a red light.

eating well
after baby arrives

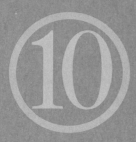

Eating a nutritious diet is as important after delivery as it was during pregnancy. Nutritious foods will help your body heal and, if you're breastfeeding, help nourish your baby. Although rapid weight loss isn't safe during the first few weeks after you deliver, you can take healthy steps through diet and activity to start shedding those pregnancy pounds. This chapter tells you what to eat during the first few postpartum weeks, how much, and which nutrients are particularly important. How can you start to regain your prepregnancy body? Read on for the answers to all of your questions.

Eating Well After Baby Arrives

New mothers have a tough act to follow. Magazine covers and television talk shows feature celebrities who are back in their bikinis and low-cut jeans within weeks of having a baby. Don't let these reports convince you that you've failed if you're not down to your prepregnancy weight before your six-week checkup—or even within six months. It took you nine months to gain that weight, and it's not unusual for it to take just as long to lose it. Losing weight too quickly may not be good for you or for your baby, if she's breastfeeding. If you exercise and stick to a smart eating plan (not a "diet"), you'll get rid of the extra pounds.

0–6 Weeks After Delivery

Expected weight loss

During the first few weeks after your baby is born, you'll lose about 15 to 20 pounds. That weight consists of your baby, the placenta, amniotic fluid, and the fluid that was needed to increase your blood volume. Most of what remains is fat, which does not disappear as easily. If you gained 25 to 30 pounds, you're left with 5 to 15 pounds of extra fat. If you gained excess weight—40, 50, 60 pounds or more—most of that extra weight is squirreled away in your fat cells.

Your new fat cells

Fat stores help your body make breast milk for your baby. Not only do your fat cells get bigger during pregnancy, but new research suggests you actually may grow *more* fat cells. The evolutionary explanation for these cells is that they help protect you and your baby from famine by allowing your body to efficiently hoard saved energy. Today in the United States, however, famine's not much of a concern—but obesity is. Unfortunately, adding all those fat cells and eating a typical American diet can make it hard to lose weight. No matter how much you diet or exercise, those extra fat cells are yours forever. You can reduce their size though.

Rather than cursing your body for holding on to its fat stores, try to look at your weight gain in a more accepting way. Sure, it's a pain that you'll have to work off 10 or 15 pounds (or more) of fat, but while you're burning up miles on the treadmill or forgoing chips and cookies, think about how amazing it is that your body was able to create and carry your baby. When you're tempted to criticize yourself because you can't slim down quickly, try to be compassionate instead. Your body deserves your respect and kindness, rather than anger and disapproval.

Weight Loss

Setting realistic goals

If you're not nursing, you can start to
work off that weight by cutting calories
and increasing activity beginning at
about six weeks postpartum. (If you're
breastfeeding and eager to lose weight,
you shouldn't cut calories. In fact,
you'll have to add calories in order to
have an adequate milk supply. See
"Best Breastfeeding Diet," page 166.)

Don't lose weight too quickly
though. The best way to slim down is
through slow, steady weight loss of
about a pound a week if you're
breastfeeding and 1 to 2 pounds a week
if you're not. If you're losing more than
that, you should add more calories back
in to your diet.

"Wait a minute," you may be
thinking. "One to 2 pounds a week? If
I lose that slowly, it will take me
forever to shed these extra pounds."
True, it may take a while, but slow
weight loss is healthy weight loss, and
it is also more likely to be permanent
weight loss.

Try to have realistic expectations
about how much you'll lose, how
quickly you'll lose, and how long it
might take to get back into your tight
jeans (or even your *loose* jeans). If you
anticipate that it could take several
months to reach your goal, you won't
be disappointed when you get on the
scale and the numbers have barely
budged. Don't be discouraged—if you
eat right and exercise, you will lose
those extra pounds.

The right calorie counts

The first step down the road to weight
loss success is to figure out how many
calories you should consume each day.
Start by using the calorie calculator
(see "Your Calorie Needs," page 160)
to determine how many calories you
would need in order to maintain your
prepregnancy weight. Then adjust it
according to these recommendations:

**During the first six weeks after
giving birth,** it is recommended that
you eat the same amount of calories
that you did during pregnancy so your
body is able to recover from childbirth.
(It also takes about six weeks for the
uterus to shrink down to its normal
size.) So continue to eat what you did
when you were pregnant, which is
about 300 calories more than your
prepregnancy intake.

After the first six weeks—and after
you've seen your doctor for your six-
week checkup—you'll need to add or
subtract calories, depending on
whether you're breastfeeding:

- If you are not breastfeeding, return
  to your prepregnancy calorie count.
  On average, nonpregnant women
  need about 1,800–2,200 calories
  daily, but your number could be
  higher or lower based on your height
  and weight and your activity level.
- If you're breastfeeding, add an
  additional 200 calories a day to the
  amount you ate during pregnancy, for
  a total of 500 calories more than
  before pregnancy. (For more
  information, see "Calorie counts,"
  page 166.)

Fad diets and pills

Sure, you'd lose weight fast if you cut down to 1,200 calories a day. But that could be harmful. After pregnancy, you need to build up your nutrient stores, and if you don't eat enough food, you can't get the nutrients your body needs. It's fine to cut out junk food, but don't cut out the healthful foods—fruits and vegetables, legumes, lean meat or meat substitutes, and nonfat dairy products—you need to heal your body. (For specific serving recommendations, see Chapter 1, "A Healthy Everyday Diet," page 9.)

Avoid fad diets and very low-carbohydrate diets such as Atkins and South Beach. Although fad diets help some people lose weight, they do so by eliminating groups of food that your body needs, especially after giving birth. Low-carbohydrate diets tend to be too low in phytochemicals, antioxidants, fiber, and minerals and too high in protein. Some nursing mothers find that low-carbohydrate diets decrease their milk supply. Plus, most low-carbohydrate diets are nearly impossible to follow in the long term.

Avoid all diet pills and supplements, especially when you're breastfeeding, because no controlled studies have been done to test for safety. Most contain caffeine as the primary ingredient to help curb appetite, and because they are not controlled by the U.S. Food and Drug Administration, their labels may not accurately reflect what is in the pill.

Diet programs

Diet plans that integrate education and support into their programs can be a good way to lose weight. These plans—Weight Watchers is a good example—use real food and teach real eating skills. You can also get education and support from a registered dietitian, who can meet with you and help you determine what you should eat and how many calories you should consume. If you are not breastfeeding, it is fine to go back to a balanced diet plan when you are ready.

What about diet plans that require you to eat special foods? Some plans sell you the food you need, and others rely on liquid meals or meal-replacement bars. These plans are fine (albeit expensive) provided they don't incorporate drugs or herbs and if they encourage the use of real food in addition to their shakes and bars. If you go on one of these diets, it's a good idea to review with a registered dietitian how to utilize the products in a healthy, balanced way.

When you're thinking of following a certain diet plan, you want to choose one that will help you lose weight safely and permanently. You can judge diet plans by asking yourself these five questions:

- Does it promote a weight loss of greater than 1 or 2 pounds a week? Losing more than 2 pounds a week may not be safe. Plus, you may lose more muscle and water than fat. Slower weight loss is more likely to result in permanent weight loss.
- Does it sound too good to be true? (It probably is!)

- What are the credentials (if any) of the people running the program?
- Does the plan include all food groups? (If not, think again. Could you live forever without a slice of bread?)
- Could you live and eat this way for the rest of your life?

Permanent and successful weight loss involves a lifestyle change and not just a short-term diet. If the answer to the last question is "no," you run the risk of facing another cycle of the dieting roller coaster.

The healthiest way to lose weight is by curbing calories and gradually adding exercise into your life. Eat less and exercise more. It's not a sexy message, but it works.

An "energized" diet

During the next few months, you need lots of energy to care for your newborn. Exercise and sleep give you energy, but there will be days when you don't get much of either. So it's important to eat an energizing diet. Here's how:

- Eat ample calories. If you don't eat enough food, you will not have the energy and stamina you'll need to take care of your baby. Know your target daily calorie intake and aim to stay as close to it as possible.
- Get the nutrients you need. Your postpartum body has special nutrient needs, particularly if you're breast-feeding (see "Postpartum Nutrients," right). Vitamin and mineral shortages can contribute to a feeling of tiredness and lethargy.
- Eat foods that fuel. A diet rich in lean protein, complex carbohydrates, and fresh fruits and vegetables will keep you energized.
- Limit candy, cookies, and other sweets. True, they give you an immediate sugar rush, but shortly after, blood sugar levels plummet and you may feel more fatigued than before. If you crave sweets, eat fresh fruit.
- Drink plenty of water. Even mild dehydration can take the wind out of your sails.
- Eat small, frequent meals and snacks. Big, heavy meals weigh you down and make you sleepy. Plan on having five or six mini meals that consist of 300 to 400 calories each.
- Don't count on a caffeine buzz. It doesn't last long, and when it leaves, you feel even worse.

When you're not losing weight

If you're eating properly and getting enough rest and you still feel like you have no energy, talk to your doctor. Postpartum conditions, including inflammation of the thyroid, postpartum depression, postpartum anxiety, and anemia, can cause feelings of lethargy. These conditions can also interfere with weight loss, so if you're not losing weight despite your efforts to eat well and exercise, your doctor may be able to help you figure out why.

Postpartum Nutrients

Your body's changing needs

Although most of your vitamin and mineral needs stay about the same after pregnancy, a few do change.

Here's a recap of the nutrients you'll need more—or less—of after your baby is born.

More iron, then less iron. Your iron stores may be low, especially if you lost blood during delivery, so you may need extra iron shortly after your baby is born. However, after six weeks or so your iron requirement goes down, especially if you're breastfeeding (see "Iron," page 167). In short, your postpartum daily iron needs are:

- 27 milligrams during pregnancy and for six weeks after delivery
- 9 milligrams (beginning six weeks postpartum) if you are breastfeeding, then 18 milligrams when you wean your baby from breastfeeding and begin to menstruate again
- 18 milligrams (beginning six weeks postpartum) if you aren't breastfeeding your baby.

Less folic acid. The folic acid recommendation after pregnancy goes down from 600 micrograms to 500 micrograms if you're breastfeeding. If you're not breastfeeding, your needs go down to 400 micrograms. Count on getting 400 micrograms from your prenatal vitamin (you should keep taking it until your six-week checkup) and the remaining 100 micrograms, if you're breastfeeding, from food. (See "When should I stop taking prenatal vitamins?" page 158).

More zinc if you're breastfeeding. Zinc needs go from 8 milligrams before pregnancy to 11 milligrams during pregnancy to 12 milligrams if you are breastfeeding. They return to 8 milligrams after your six-week checkup (if you're not breastfeeding) or after weaning (if you are breastfeeding). Your body absorbs only 20 percent of the zinc in foods, so it's important to get enough.

More vitamin B_{12}. Your daily vitamin B_{12} needs go from 2.4 micrograms before pregnancy to 2.6 micrograms during pregnancy to 2.8 micrograms while breastfeeding. They go back down to 2.4 micrograms after your six-week checkup (if you're not breastfeeding) or after weaning (if you are breastfeeding). If you eat meat, you should have no problem getting the vitamin B_{12} you need. If you are a vegan, consider taking a B_{12}

Keep eating fiber

During delivery, the muscles that keep your digestive system moving often get stretched and strained, and it may take them a few days to get back into the groove. Drugs and anesthetics take a toll on your intestines too. Add to that dehydration, inactivity, and a lack of fiber—all of which happen during delivery—and you're likely to end up with postpartum constipation.

After delivery, focus on eating fiber-rich food (high-fiber cereal, fresh fruit, fresh vegetables, whole grain bread, beans) and drinking plenty of water. If you're still backed up, use a stool softener or a mild laxative, but for only a few days. As soon as you can manage it, get up and move around. Even if you only walk around the house or yard, moving your body will help move your bowels too.

supplement on a regular basis.

Plenty of water. You need lots of fluid postpartum for two reasons: First, constipation is common after delivery, and drinking plenty of water and other fluids (along with eating a diet rich in fiber) can help keep you regular. Second, you lose a lot of fluid during delivery, and drinking water can help restore your body's fluids to their normal levels and ward off dehydration. Drink water, decaffeinated tea or coffee, and 100-percent fruit juice. You can also add water to your diet by eating fruits and vegetables that have a high water content (see "Juicy fruits and veggies," page 121). Finally, if you're breastfeeding you need even more water (see "Boost your milk supply," page 171).

Postpartum Exercise

Smart strategies

Take time before your baby is born to plan your postpartum workout strategy so you can hit the ground running, so to speak, after you have your baby. You can start doing gentle activity, such as walking, shortly after giving birth— perhaps even in the hospital, if you feel up to it and your doctor approves. As you feel better, you can gradually increase your exertion, although it's best to hold off on vigorous exercise until you get your doctor's OK at your six-week checkup. If you notice excessive bloody discharge after you exercise during the first few weeks postpartum or feel tremendous pelvic pressure, you're doing too much.

Once you're ready to move around more, here are some ways to get the most out of exercise. (For more tips, see Chapter 9, "Keeping Fit During Pregnancy," page 133.)

Exercise every day. Even if it's just a walk to the mailbox and back, plan to do something every day. Studies show that daily exercise brings success. Overweight mothers who exercise daily a year after the birth of their first child are, on average, 12 pounds lighter than overweight mothers who rarely work out, according to a 2002 study from Cornell University.

Enroll in a postpartum exercise class. Many hospitals, YWCAs, health clubs, and community centers offer mommy-and-me classes taught by trainers who have experience with postpartum exercise. Don't wait until your baby is born to sign up for a class because they often fill up fast. Exercise classes are a great way to get to know other women with new babies too.

Line up some babysitting. When friends and relatives ask if there's anything they can do to help you out during the first few months after your baby arrives, ask them to babysit while you exercise. Or offer to swap babysitting duties with another new mom. Even a half hour will give you time to go for a walk or a jog. Check out your gym or YWCA too. Some offer on-site babysitting, although they may not take very young infants.

Check out exercise videos. See what postpartum tapes and DVDs are available at your library and video store.

Set up a home gym. If you can afford it, having a treadmill or stationary cycle

When should I stop taking prenatal vitamins?

Doctors generally suggest that if you aren't nursing you continue to take your prenatal vitamin for six weeks postpartum, then switch to an ordinary multivitamin (or go off supplements completely). If you are breastfeeding, you may stay on your prenatal vitamin until your baby is six months old (that's when your baby will start eating solid foods in addition to breast milk), then switch to a regular multivitamin. Or you may switch to a multivitamin as soon as you run out of your prenatal vitamins, as you likely will not need the extra iron a prenatal vitamin contains.

If you plan to get pregnant again within a year or so, stay on your prenatal vitamins to ensure that you are getting enough folic acid and iron. Your stores of folic acid might be low, and if you don't rebuild them you increase your risk of having a baby with a neural tube defect. Similarly, your risk of anemia may increase without the supplemental iron a prenatal vitamin provides.

in your house, along with some free weights and exercise balls, can make it easy to get in a workout without leaving the house.

Buy or borrow a good walking stroller and frontpack. With the right equipment, you can take your baby along on walks.

Make plans with an exercise buddy. Do you know another new mother who wants to work out? Create a buddy system. On nice days, the two of you can walk together with your babies in strollers. On inclement days, you can take turns watching the babies while the other one goes to the gym, takes an exercise class, or pulls on a cozy raincoat or snow parka and braves the elements. (As long as you're properly dressed, walking in rain or snow can actually be quite invigorating.)

Special Concerns

If you had gestational diabetes

If you were diagnosed with gestational diabetes, it will likely go away after you deliver your baby and the placenta. Although some women experience ups and downs in their blood sugar level the first few weeks postpartum, most find that their blood sugar returns to normal. (If it doesn't, you may have developed actual diabetes, not the pregnancy-only kind.)

Healthy eating and postpartum weight loss are very important if you've had gestational diabetes because about 50 percent of women with gestational diabetes go on to develop type 2 diabetes by age 50.

To decrease your risk of developing type 2 diabetes, try to reach and maintain a healthy body weight. If you are overweight or obese, even modest weight loss—just 5 percent to 10 percent of your weight—can reduce

Will I get my body back?

You can return to your prepregnancy weight and fitness level, but that doesn't necessarily mean you'll be the exact same shape and size that you were before conceiving. Your body changes during pregnancy, and sometimes the changes are permanent. Your hips may be a bit wider than they were before, your waist may be a little thicker, your feet may be bigger—even your breasts may have changed size and shape, requiring you to go up or down a cup size when you buy bras.

The great news is that if you exercise, you can regain or even improve upon all of your prepregnancy strength, flexibility, stamina, and tone. You may even get some parts of your body back, depending on what activities you do, your genetics, and what kind of body you had to start with.

your chance of developing type 2 diabetes sometime in your life by 20 to 50 percent.

The best way to lose weight healthfully is to follow an eating plan that is similar to the one recommended for gestational diabetes (see Chapter 7, "Blood Sugar Problems During Pregnancy," page 101). Distributing calories, carbohydrates, fat, and protein throughout the day helps keep blood sugar levels stable, and, as a result, you'll eat less. (See "Your Calorie Needs," page 160, or ask a registered dietitian how many calories you should consume each day.) If using artificial sweeteners helps you, go ahead and use them moderately.

If you had gestational diabetes during this pregnancy, there's a 30 to 65 percent chance you'll develop it again in your next pregnancy. Again, you can reduce your risk of a second bout of gestational diabetes by eating right between pregnancies, losing weight (since high stores of body fat affect insulin sensitivity), and exercising. Even if you don't lose weight, mild to vigorous exercise after delivery can cut your risk of developing type 2 diabetes by 30 to 50 percent. If you have your obstetrician's OK, go ahead and get 30 minutes a day of moderate exercise most days of the week.

Your Calorie Needs

The Healthy Eating Meal Plans (see page 395) are a great tool that can help you easily keep track of what you eat. Each day of the meal plan is broken down into three meals and a minimum of two snacks. You can spread the food out through the day however you like; the checklists are simply a guide. They give you an idea of the portion sizes and types of foods to have at each meal. Before you decide which meal plan is right for you, you'll need to determine the calorie range that meets your needs. There are a couple of ways you can do this:

1. Use the "Your calorie calculator" section on page 50. The formula will give you an idea of how many calories you needed to maintain your prepregnancy weight. During pregnancy, you would add 300 calories a day (or 500 calories a day if you are pregnant with twins). If you already delivered your baby, see the general guidelines, below, for weight loss.

2. Use the general guide, below, to find which calorie range is best for you.

If you are ...	... start with this meal plan
Six weeks postpartum and not breastfeeding	1,600 calories
Six weeks postpartum and breastfeeding	1,800 calories
Pregnant and beginning your pregnancy at a healthy weight, with a BMI of 18.5–25	2,000–2,200 calories
Pregnant and beginning your pregnancy overweight, with a BMI greater than 25	1,800 calories
Pregnant and beginning your pregnancy underweight, with a BMI of less than 18.5	2,400 calories
Pregnant with twins	2,400 calories

Remember that these meal plans are simply a tool. They are meant not to be a strict diet but to provide a sense of what a calorie-controlled and nutritionally balanced day can look like. Your own sense and weight-gain pattern will be your best guide to your daily intake.

Breastfeeding

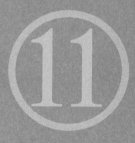

Breastfeeding is the best way to feed your baby. Breast milk provides a balance of nutrients that matches an infant's requirements for growth and development better than any formula can. Your breast milk actually varies in composition based on what your baby needs at different times in her infancy. Shortly after your baby is born, for example, your breasts secrete fluid called colostrum, which provides her with substances that protect from infection. Whether you breastfeed or formula feed is a personal choice. Rest assured that if you opt to feed with formula, your baby will still get the nutrition she needs.

Breastfeeding

Infant formula was first created in the 1800s for babies who were not breastfed by their mother or by a wet nurse. Back then it was a godsend because many babies who could not breastfeed eventually died. Those who were fed cow's milk developed health problems and vitamin deficiencies because unprocessed cow's milk has more protein than a new baby's kidneys can handle and it lacks other nutrients babies need.

Over the years, manufacturers have improved the recipe for baby formula in a constant attempt to emulate breast milk. During the 1960s and 1970s, many doctors became convinced that formula was superior to breast milk, and they advised their patients not to breastfeed. Since then, research has uncovered many ways in which breast milk is superior to formula, and doctors heartily endorse breastfeeding as the best way to nourish your baby.

It's a Great Choice

Benefits to baby

If you're not convinced that breast is best for your baby, take a look at this long list of the important benefits of breastfeeding:

Provides easily digested nutrition. Breast milk is easier for a baby to digest than formula and milk from other animals because it contains just the right amount of protein, fat, carbohydrates, vitamins, and minerals in an easily digestible form.

Reduces your baby's chance of developing an infection. Human milk contains antibodies and other ingredients that fight infection. Studies show that compared with formula-fed babies, breastfed babies are less likely to develop diarrhea, respiratory tract infections, ear infections, pneumonia, urinary infections, necrotizing enterocolitis (a gastrointestinal infection), and several kinds of bacterial infection.

May make your baby smarter. Studies show that breastfed babies have higher IQs than formula-fed babies—on average, eight IQ points higher.

Reduces your baby's risk of chronic disease in childhood and adulthood, including celiac disease, inflammatory bowel disease, some kinds of cancer, allergies, and asthma. Adults who were breastfed have lower cholesterol levels (both total cholesterol and LDL or bad cholesterol) on average than adults who were fed formula.

May help your baby stay lean. A 2006 Harvard study found that the longer babies breastfeed, the lower the likelihood they'll be overweight later in life. The study found that each four-month increase in breastfeeding was linked to a 6 percent dip in the risk of becoming overweight by adolescence. Another study published in 2006 found that even one month of breastfeeding reduces the risk of being overweight by 4 percent, and breastfeeding through 9 months of age reduces the risk of being overweight in the future by 30 percent. (It is not known whether the positive effect continues to rise beyond the ninth month of breastfeeding since the study did not consider breastfeeding beyond this point.) Scientists don't know why breastfeeding helps prevent excess weight gain. However, they suspect that breast milk somehow affects the areas of the brain that control appetite and body weight.

Helps your baby's jaws and teeth develop normally. This in turn helps facilitate speech development.

Reduces diabetes risk. Breastfeeding cuts your new baby's chances of developing diabetes.

Is always safe and fresh. Moreover, when you breastfeed, there's no need to mix formula and wash bottles.

Benefits to you
Your baby isn't the only one who will benefit from breastfeeding—it does your body good too. Breastfeeding has the following benefits:

Helps your body recuperate from delivery. Breastfeeding increases levels of oxytocin, a hormone that stimulates uterine contractions. This reduces blood loss and helps the uterus return to its normal size.

Keeps periods from resuming. Breastfeeding postpones the beginning of ovulation and the return of your menstrual period, although you can't count on breastfeeding as a form of contraception.

Makes you feel good. Breastfeeding gives many women a feeling of increased self-confidence and closeness with their babies.

Cuts cancer risk. Breastfeeding may reduce your risk of breast cancer and ovarian cancer.

Has a beneficial effect on blood sugar and insulin resistance. Breastfeeding lowers blood glucose levels and reduces your risk of developing diabetes later in life, especially if you had gestational diabetes.

Improves bone density and reduces your risk of developing osteoporosis. In fact, studies show that bone density in breastfeeding women may surpass prepregnancy rates. Scientists aren't sure why this is so, but they suspect that during pregnancy the body becomes more efficient at extracting calcium from food.

Saves money. Even if you rent or buy a breast pump, you can save hundreds of dollars if you nurse for a year rather than buy formula. You may also save money on health care: Medical care expenditures (doctor visits, hospitalizations, and prescription medications) are about 20 percent lower for fully breastfed infants than for infants who were never breastfed.

How long should I breastfeed?
The American Academy of Pediatrics, the American Dietetic Association, and many other health organizations

recommend breastfeeding for one year. That means exclusive breastfeeding for 6 months and breastfeeding along with appropriate solid foods from ages 6 to 12 months and beyond.

The benefits of breastfeeding are dose-related. In other words, the longer you breastfeed, the more likely you and your baby are to receive breastfeeding's health benefits.

Nursing for 6 months or a year—or more—is not something that every woman can do. It's important to remember that any amount of breast-feeding is better than none. Deciding whether to breastfeed doesn't have to be a black-and-white decision: You don't have to forgo breastfeeding completely because you don't think you can do it for months and months. Commit to it for a short time, then decide whether you want to continue.

If at all possible, try to breastfeed for the first few weeks. During that time, your baby will receive some of the most important health-protecting nutrients. The first fluid your breasts will produce is colostrum, which contains extremely valuable ingredients that help your baby's body fight infection.

Although health organizations recommend breastfeeding exclusively for the first six months, supplementing with an occasional bottle of formula is fine. Yes, exclusive breastfeeding is best, but if a formula bottle here and there makes it possible for you to continue nursing, it's worth it.

Feeding Challenges

Support means success

Breastfeeding isn't always the easiest choice of feeding methods. If you breastfeed your baby, you're on feeding duty 24-7 (unless you use a breast pump to express your milk and bottle-feed it to your baby another time). Breastfeeding problems can arise: Your baby may have trouble latching on, or you may develop a painful breast infection or a plugged milk duct. You can usually solve these problems with the advice and support of a lactation consultant or nurse who specializes in breastfeeding issues. Once you and your baby have established a solid nursing routine, breastfeeding usually proceeds comfortably.

The best way to ensure breastfeed-ing success is to gather support even before your baby is born.

Take a breastfeeding class. Contact your local hospital about schedules.

Line up a lactation consultant. To find one in your area, check with your pediatrician or contact the International Lactation Consultant Association at www.ilca.org or 919-861-5577 for a referral.

Choose a pediatrician who fully supports breastfeeding.

Talk with your family about your choice. Your mother may have given birth at a time when formula was believed to be the better option, and she may advocate formula feeding over breastfeeding. Talk with family members so they understand why you want to breastfeed: because there is extensive evidence that breastfeeding is best for your baby's health. Your partner may not understand the value of breastfeeding, and he may feel jealous and left out of the intimate time breastfeeding will give you and your baby. Assure him that he can be a part of the feeding experience. He can be with you and your baby while you breastfeed, and after four weeks, you can express your breast milk and he can feed it to your baby in a bottle.

Contact an organization that helps breastfeeding women. The following are excellent sources of information and advice:

- La Leche League is an international nonprofit, nonsectarian organization dedicated to providing education, information, support, and encouragement to women who want to breastfeed. All women interested in breastfeeding are welcome to attend local chapter meetings or to call a group leader for breastfeeding help. Contact: www.lalecheleague.org or 800-LALECHE (847-519-7730). Or consult La Leche League's *Breastfeeding Answer Book* (available from bookstores or from La Leche League's website).
- The African-American Breastfeeding Alliance is committed to raising the number of African-American women who breastfeed by offering support and educational materials to women and their families. Contact: www.aabaonline.com or 877-532-8535.
- Medela International is a company that sells high-quality breast pumps. Medela's website is a good source of information about pumping and storing breast milk and can refer you to where to buy a pump in your area. Contact: www.medela.com or 800-435-8316.
- Avent is another company that sells quality pumps and has a helpful website. Contact: www.aventamerica.com or 800-542-8368.

Common problems

Problems do sometimes arise during nursing. You may experience sore nipples, plugged milk ducts, or mastitis (a breast infection), or your baby may have trouble latching on, sucking, or gaining weight. Nearly all nursing problems can be solved with the help of an experienced lactation consultant or nurse who specializes in breastfeeding support. (Many pediatricians' offices have a nurse on staff who specializes in lactation issues.)

When it's not an option

A small number of women should not breastfeed because it could harm their babies. Do not breastfeed if you:

- Are infected with HIV.
- Have tuberculosis that has not been treated.
- Are receiving certain cancer treatments.
- Smoke, abuse alcohol, or use street drugs.
- Are taking certain medications that can pass into your breast milk and harm your baby. (Certain antidepressants, cardiovascular medications, immunosuppressants, and some other types of medication are safe to take while breastfeeding. Check with your doctor.)

- Have a baby with galactosemia, a rare genetic disorder of carbohydrate metabolism.
- Have a baby with PKU (phenylketonuria), a rare genetic disorder of protein metabolism. You still may be able to breastfeed while following a special diet and supplementing with a special formula for the baby. Discuss your options with your doctor and pediatrician.

Additionally, women who have had breast surgery (breast reduction, breast augmentation with implants, and biopsies) may or may not be able to breastfeed, depending on whether the surgery severed milk ducts.

Babies with cleft lips or palates may or may not be able to breastfeed, depending on whether they can latch on.

Best Breastfeeding Diet

Why your diet is key

When you're breastfeeding, your baby gets all of her nutrition from you, which means it's crucial that you eat a healthy diet. Much of the same advice that applies during pregnancy continues to make sense during breastfeeding. Eat plenty of fruits, vegetables, whole grains, and beans, along with fat-free dairy and lean meat.

Calorie counts

Your calorie needs increase when you breastfeed. During pregnancy, you need 300 calories a day more than before pregnancy. That number goes up to 500 extra calories daily when you're breastfeeding exclusively. Here's the reasoning behind that recommendation:

The average breastfeeding woman makes about 25 ounces of milk each day. To do so she needs about 640 extra calories—500 from her diet and 100 to 150 from stored fat.

If you are breastfeeding exclusively and not supplementing your baby's diet with formula, add 500 calories a day while you are nursing until your baby starts eating solid foods (and less breast milk).

If you are supplementing with formula, reduce your calorie intake accordingly. For example, if you are feeding half breast milk and half formula, reduce your extra calorie need by half (250 calories instead of 500).

Breastfeeding by the numbers

- Seventy percent of mothers in the United States breastfeed during the first few weeks postpartum.
- Thirty-six percent of mothers in the United States are still breastfeeding six months after their child's birth.
- Fewer than 20 percent of mothers in the United States are still breastfeeding 12 months after their child's birth.
- Globally, 79 percent of infants are breastfed for 12 months.

The right calories

The extra 500 calories should come from healthy foods. (Don't you wish the recommendation were to have 500 calories' worth of cookies, cake, chips, and ice cream each day?) The healthiest ways to spend those extra 500 calories are with an extra piece of fruit or serving of vegetables (for vitamins, minerals, and fiber), an extra glass of fat-free milk (for calcium and fluid), an extra slice or two of whole wheat bread or beans (for vitamins, fiber, and energy-rich carbohydrates), and an extra serving of lean meat or meat substitute (for protein).

You may be tempted to cut down on calories to speed up weight loss. That's not a good idea because if you don't take in enough calories, you may have trouble making enough milk for your baby. Plus, it's tough to get all of the nutrients you and your baby need from a low-calorie diet. It's fine to lose about a pound a week while breastfeeding, but more than that may affect your milk supply.

Your Nutrient Needs

Many of your nutrient needs are the same as they were in pregnancy, but a few change. Here are some nutrients to be aware of:

Iron

Concern: Right after giving birth, your iron stores may be low, particularly if you lost blood during delivery. However, your iron needs diminish after about six weeks, especially if you

breastfeed, because you probably won't get your period, and monthly bleeding is the primary cause of iron loss in women of childbearing age. The iron content of breast milk is fairly low and very easy for your baby to absorb (this is known as "high bioavailability"), so not much is needed

Bottom line: Continue to take your prenatal vitamin for six weeks postpartum. It will deliver the 27 milligrams a day of iron you need. Beginning at six weeks postpartum, your iron need goes down to 9 milligrams.

Often breastfeeding women are told to continue taking a prenatal vitamin until six months postpartum, but switching to a multivitamin instead may be perfectly fine for you. If you're unsure what's best for your situation, ask your health care provider and dietitian. (For more information, see "When should I stop taking prenatal vitamins?" page 158.)

When you wean your baby from breastfeeding, your iron requirement goes back to the prepregnancy level of 18 milligrams.

Folic acid

Concern: It's important to get enough folic acid while breastfeeding because you have to maintain your own reserves while providing adequate supplies for your baby.

Bottom line: Ensure adequate folic acid intake by taking a supplement or eating foods rich in folic acid, such as fortified breakfast cereals, spinach, navy beans, and orange juice. If there is any chance of your getting pregnant again, take a supplement that provides 400 micrograms of folic acid daily.

Zinc

Concern: Zinc needs are slightly higher for a new mother who is breastfeeding than for one who is formula feeding.

Bottom line: Boost intake of zinc with high-zinc foods such as beef, wheat germ, crab, wheat bran, and sunflower seeds.

Vitamin B$_6$

Concern: Your vitamin B$_6$ requirement is slightly higher during breastfeeding than during pregnancy.

Bottom line: Up your intake of vitamin B$_6$ by including chicken, pork, peanut butter, black beans, and fortified cereals in your diet.

Vitamin B$_{12}$

Concern: This is usually more an issue for mothers who don't eat animal products, although your needs will increase slightly while breastfeeding.

Bottom line: If you are a vegan, a vegetarian who shuns all animal food, you may need to take a B$_{12}$ supplement while you breastfeed. (If you took a B$_{12}$ supplement during pregnancy, keep taking it while you're nursing.) Failing to get enough vitamin B$_{12}$ while you're breastfeeding could cause permanent nerve damage in your baby, so this is an important issue if you are a strict vegetarian.

Vitamin D

Concern: If you don't get enough vitamin D from sunlight or food, your baby may be short on vitamin D too.

Bottom line: Keep your vitamin D stores well stocked by drinking vitamin D-fortified milk and getting about 10 minutes of sunlight each day. The American Academy of Pediatrics recommends giving exclusively breastfed babies vitamin D supplements (see "Supplements," below), starting before the baby is 2 months old.

Carbohydrates

Concern: The recommended carbohydrate intake increases from 175 grams in pregnancy to 210 grams while breastfeeding.

Bottom line: Eat foods that are high in healthy complex carbohydrates, such as fruit and whole grain breads and cereals. Also, keep in mind that many dairy products have carbohydrates as well. For instance, milk has about 12 grams of carbohydrates in an 8-ounce serving.

Supplements

Does your baby need them?

If you eat a healthy diet, your breast milk will likely contain all of the nutrients your baby needs. In some cases, supplements are still necessary:

Vitamin D: The American Academy of Pediatrics (AAP) recommends all infants get at least 200 International Units (IU) of vitamin D per day beginning in the first two months of life. For babies who are exclusively breastfed, this needs to come from supplementation.

Breastfeeding may lower your risk of diabetes

Breastfeeding your baby can substantially cut your risk of developing type 2 diabetes later in life, according to a 2005 study conducted by researchers at the Harvard School of Public Health. The study found that each year a woman breastfeeds cuts her risk of type 2 diabetes by 15 percent. Why? Researchers don't know for sure, but they suspect it is because breastfeeding improves insulin sensitivity and glucose tolerance. In other words, it helps your body use insulin more effectively and keep blood sugar in balance.

In addition, the AAP recommends that an intake of 200 IU of vitamin D per day be continued throughout childhood and adolescence. Vitamin D supplements are available over the counter in drugstores.

Why is it important? If a baby doesn't get enough vitamin D, she is at risk of developing a bone-softening disease called rickets. Your body manufactures vitamin D in the presence of sunlight, but if you live in an area that doesn't get much sun, you have to rely on food for vitamin D. Not many foods contain this vitamin. Primary sources include egg yolks, saltwater fish, and vitamin D-fortified milk. So it's easy to be deficient, and if you are deficient, so is your breast-feeding baby.

You are especially likely to be short of vitamin D if you aren't getting adequate vitamin D in your diet, don't get much sunlight, have dark skin, or cover up with clothing or sunscreen when you're outdoors.

Vitamin B_{12}: If you are a breastfeeding vegan and don't take vitamin B_{12} supplements, your baby may not be getting enough B_{12} from your breast milk even if you show no signs of deficiency. Be sure you're getting

enough vitamin B_{12} from your diet (see "Vitamins," page 21 for B_{12} sources) or take supplements.

Iron: Breast milk alone may not provide enough iron for premature newborns, infants whose mothers have low iron stores, and infants older than 6 months. Talk with your pediatrician about whether your baby should have supplemental iron. When you begin feeding your baby solid foods at 6 months or so, be sure to choose a cereal that is fortified with iron.

Your Baby's Reactions

Diet and colic

You might have read that some of the foods you eat—including Brussels sprouts, cow's milk, and garlic—have the potential to cause fussiness and colic in your breastfeeding baby. Often colic has no known cause, although some babies get relief when their mothers avoid foods that commonly cause allergies.

What is colic? The word *colic* is not an actual medical term. It's really a catchall word used to describe an infant's unexplained fussiness, crying, and screaming. Approximately

28 percent of infants have colic, which tends to begin between the third and sixth weeks of life and is characterized by more than 3 hours a day of crying. Colic symptoms usually peak at about 6 weeks of age and improve gradually over the following weeks.

Colic and your diet. The foods you eat might bother your baby. If your baby develops a skin rash, gas pains, or diarrhea, or if she cries more often than she used to, talk with your baby's pediatrician or a registered dietitian about what changes you should make in your diet.

Keep in mind, though, that the majority of mothers eat a wide range of foods, including "gassy" vegetables and pungent spices, and their babies are just fine. (See "Do food sensitivities cause colic?," below.)

Food records. If you suspect that something you are eating may be causing your baby distress, use a food record to keep track of all of the foods you eat each day, and in what amount. Use the "Baby's Sensitivities During Breastfeeding" fill-in food records (see page 180) or make your own. The key to success is to be as specific and precise as possible so you can correlate your infant's symptoms and your food intake. Write down what you eat at every meal and snack. If you notice that your baby is extra fussy, note it in your food record. Over time, you may notice that fussing is associated with a certain food. Or you may figure out that you can eat a small amount of an offending food without bothering your baby, but not a large serving. Once you identify a suspect food, leave it out of your diet for two weeks to see if your baby's symptoms improve.

You may be tempted just to cut out entire categories of food—all of the gassy cruciferous vegetables such as broccoli and Brussels sprouts, for

Do food sensitivities cause colic?

Until recently scientists disagreed over whether hypersensitivity or allergy to food in the mother's diet caused colic in infants. A study published in the November 2005 issue of the journal *Pediatrics* went a long way toward answering that question.

The study looked at the diets of 90 colicky babies who breastfed exclusively. (The babies ranged in age from about 3 to 9 weeks.) One group of mothers excluded the most common allergy-causing foods—cow's milk, eggs, peanuts, tree nuts, wheat, soy, and fish—from their diet. The women in the other group continued to eat these foods.

After seven days, researchers measured the babies' fussiness and crying for 48 hours. They found that the babies whose mothers avoided the highly allergenic foods fussed and cried 21 percent less than those whose mothers ate the foods.

If your baby has colic, eliminating highly allergenic foods from your diet may ease your baby's discomfort (and make life easier for you too). You may be able to introduce them back into your diet after several weeks or months because most babies with colic outgrow it (with or without changes in their mothers' diet) by the time they're 3 months old.

Can I eat fish while I'm nursing?

Fish is an excellent source of protein and omega-3 fatty acids. However, because fish may contain contaminants such as mercury, you should continue your pregnancy precautions while breastfeeding. (See "Fish Facts," page 77.)

- Avoid shark, swordfish, mackerel, and tilefish, which are more likely than other fish to contain mercury.
- Eat up to 12 ounces a week of other kinds of fish, with a maximum of 6 ounces of canned tuna per week.
- Check with your local health department about eating locally caught fish. If no fish advisories are available, limit intake of locally caught fish to 6 ounces per week and consume no other fish in that same week.

example—without investigating whether they actually bother your baby. This is a mistake because cruciferous vegetables are nutritional powerhouses that are chock-full of vitamins, minerals, and compounds believed to help prevent cancer. Giving them up unnecessarily robs you and your baby of an important source of nutrients.

If you find yourself cutting out more than a few foods, talk with your baby's pediatrician. Some babies are very sensitive and their moms must follow exceptionally restricted diets that avoid many vegetables, soy, eggs, milk, and other important foods. This is rare, but it does occur. If it happens to you, ask for a referral to a registered dietitian who can help you build a healthy diet without the offending foods. Doing so is a complicated task that is best done by a professional.

Cutting out favorite foods is frustrating, but keep in mind that it is only temporary. As your baby gets older and his gastrointestinal system matures, the foods may stop bothering

him and you may be able to reintroduce them into your diet.

Boost your milk supply

Your body can make all of the milk needed by your baby (or babies). However, certain things—for example, becoming dehydrated—can compromise your milk supply. Keep your milk flowing by following these guidelines:

Drink plenty of water. Fill up a quart bottle of water and carry it around with you. If you drink a tall glass of water every time you nurse, you'll be well hydrated since new babies breastfeed 8 to 12 times a day. Aim to drink 13 cups of fluid (water, juice, milk) each day. If you drink alcohol, do so only in moderation (see "Common Questions," page 177).

Consume enough calories. Although you might be tempted to make substantial cuts in your calorie intake in order to lose weight, highly restrictive diets can backfire by slowing down your milk supply. Cut out sweets and fatty snacks, but eat a healthy diet that includes ample calories.

Nurse frequently. The more your baby nurses, the more milk your body makes. To make breastfeeding easier at night, have your baby sleep in a cradle near your bed.

Pump frequently. If you express breast milk at work, do so every three hours in order to keep up your supply.

Avoid drugs that decrease milk supply. These include oral contraceptives that contain estrogen and moderate or large amounts of alcohol.

Be cautious with herbs. Friends may recommend herbs to use to increase your milk supply. Fenugreek, blessed thistle, and alfalfa are some of the herbs traditionally recommended for boosting breast milk volume. However, a lack of scientific research into the safety and efficacy of these herbs during lactation makes it a good idea to ask your health care provider first.

Going Back to Work

You can still breastfeed

You may think you have to stop nursing when you go back to work. In fact, returning to work is the number one reason women stop breastfeeding. But millions of women find they can express their milk at work so that it can be fed to their babies at a later time. If you think your workplace doesn't support nursing mothers, talk with someone in human resources—the company may have more support in place than you realize.

Expressing your milk

All you need to express milk at work is a private room for pumping, a comfortable chair, an outlet (if you're not using a manual or battery-operated pump), a small table for your breast pump, and a place to wash your hands. You can refrigerate the milk you pump or place it in a cooler with ice packs. Some breast pump bags contain an insulated section that has room for an ice pack and several bottles of milk.

It's best to express your milk every three hours or so. If you express less frequently, you risk having your milk supply drop off. Your breasts work on a supply-and-demand basis: The more milk you breastfeed or express, the more milk your breasts make. On the flip side, if you nurse or express less often, it sends a message to your breasts that your baby needs less milk and that your breasts don't need to produce as much.

Breast pumps. You have several kinds of breast pump to choose from. A manual pump requires you to squeeze a bulb-type device to operate it. An electric or battery-operated pump costs more but is much faster.

Before choosing a pump, think about how much you'll use it. If you plan to nurse for a year and are going back to work full-time, investing in a good pump with a handy carrying case is the best idea. If you're staying home with your baby and will need to pump only occasionally, a manual pump will be fine. (You can also express milk with your fingers, but this method is time-consuming. Using a pump is faster and much easier.)

Breast milk storage time limits

Like regular milk, breast milk can spoil. Use these guidelines from La Leche League to determine how long you can safely store breast milk:

- At room temperature (66–72 degrees) for 10 hours
- In the refrigerator (32–39 degrees) up to eight days
- In a freezer compartment contained within a refrigerator up to two weeks
- In a self-contained freezer, either on top of or on the side of the refrigerator, for three to four months
- In a deep freezer for six months to one year

Some lactation consultants have pumps available for rental. If you rent a pump, be sure to get a brand-new set of plastic pump shells, tubing, and bottles. Or ask a friend if you can borrow or buy her breast pump. Although using a rented or second-hand pump is fine (your milk doesn't touch the pump itself), the items that come in contact with your milk should be new for sanitary reasons.

You can buy a breast pump at a baby-supply store, a pharmacy, or a department store for under $50. Or you can buy one through your hospital, a breastfeeding organization, or a lactation consultant for about $200. The kinds available in stores tend to be less expensive than (and not as good as) the professional-quality pumps. Inexpensive pumps may cause more discomfort than a better pump.

Practice makes perfect. Begin practicing pumping a few weeks before you go back to work. Pump your breasts after feeding your baby and save the milk for a bottle-feeding. You can introduce a bottle of pumped breast milk when your baby is about 3 to 4 weeks old. If you wait much longer than that, your baby may refuse bottles. Continue to feed your baby with a bottle once every day or two so she continues to accept it.

At work, pump your breasts at the same times you would feed your baby if you were at home. To facilitate letdown of your milk, think about your baby or look at a picture of her. Plan to set aside the same amount of time for pumping that you would spend nursing. If you'd like to speed things up, buy or rent a pump that expresses both breasts at once. The first few times you use a double pump it can be tricky, but you'll get the hang of it soon enough. Pump milk into a sterile container and write the date on it so you can keep track of how old it is.

When you are finished pumping, wash your equipment with soap and water and let it air dry. You can store your milk in glass or hard plastic containers or in plastic storage bags that are designed for freezing breast milk and fit directly onto your breast pump. (See "Breast milk storage time limits," above.)

Thaw frozen milk by running warm water over it or put the milk in a pan of warm water on the stove. Never put breast milk in the microwave. Once it's defrosted you can store it in the refrigerator, but you shouldn't freeze it again. Don't be alarmed if the milk separates while in the refrigerator or freezer—that's entirely normal.

Supplementing with formula

In a perfect world you would give your baby breast milk only and not a drop of formula would pass his lips. But let's face it, you don't live in a perfect world, and supplementing with formula is common when moms return to work. Formula is the next-best food for babies, and unless your baby has unusual allergies or health problems, giving an occasional formula bottle is fine. If you supplement with formula, keep these guidelines in mind:

- Wait until he's older than 4 weeks. You and your baby should have a successful, well-established nursing routine in place before giving any kind of bottle.
- To preserve your milk supply, keep formula feedings to a minimum. Or pump your breasts and store your extra milk in bottles when your baby is drinking formula.

- If your baby has no health concerns, use a formula derived from cow's milk. If it causes wheezing, fussiness, or coughing, it may mean he has trouble digesting milk protein, so try a soy formula instead.
- Always choose an iron-fortified formula.
- Follow the recommendations on the formula container regarding mixing and storage. If you use a concentrated or powdered formula that must be mixed with water, be sure to add the proper amount of water.
- Your baby may not like the taste of formula and may refuse to feed, especially if you're feeding him. He may be more receptive if someone other than you feeds him formula bottles instead. A baby senses his mom and will naturally want to nurse, but he won't have this reaction with another person and will be more likely to take the bottle.

The exercise/breast milk myth

For many years, researchers believed that lactic acid—a harmless substance that muscles make during exercise—gave breast milk an unpleasant taste that caused babies to reject their mother's breasts after a workout. That theory has been largely disproved, and most mothers have no trouble breastfeeding even immediately after an intense workout. Although it's unlikely, if you find that your baby refuses to eat after you work out, try leaving more time after exercise for lactic acid levels to go down. Cooling down for 5 or 10 minutes after a workout is a good idea even if your baby doesn't mind the taste of your post-exercise milk because it allows your muscles to cool off and your heart rate to return to normal.

> **Fact or fiction?** It's possible to breastfeed twins and triplets.
>
> **Fact.** The thought of nursing two or more babies may seem astonishing, but the truth is, many mothers of multiples manage nursing just fine. If you have twins and are otherwise healthy, you should be able to make enough milk for both. Plenty of women breastfeed their twins exclusively—their breasts respond to the demand and increase their supply. Breastfeeding triplets is a bit trickier, however—some women find that with triplets, some supplemental bottles are necessary. If you breastfeed multiples, be sure to add an extra 300 to 500 calories a day to your diet for each baby.

Exercise

Smart precautions

It's perfectly safe for nursing mothers to exercise. Exercising tones your muscles, strengthens your heart, and helps you lose pregnancy weight. It also can be a wonderful break from a busy, stressful day.

Begin with gentle activity and slowly increase your exertion over time. Hold off on vigorous exercise until your six-week doctor checkup. Listen to your body in terms of exercise intensity. If it feels like you're doing too much—or if you notice more bloody discharge after you exercise—you're probably doing too much too soon. You can start with gentle activity, such as walking, shortly after giving birth. As you feel better, you can gradually increase your amount of exertion.

As a nursing mother, you can do just about any exercise you did before pregnancy. There are some guidelines and tips to keep in mind, however:

Drink extra water. The more you exercise, the more water you need. And that's in addition to the 9 to 10 cups of water you should drink each day while breastfeeding. Add a cup of water for every 20 minutes of activity, and more if it's very warm or if you sweat a lot. (Keep in mind that during the first few weeks postpartum, it's not unusual to sweat a lot even if you don't usually perspire much. It's one of your body's ways of eliminating the excess fluid you needed when you were pregnant.)

Wear the right bra. Choose a sports bra that supports you adequately and comfortably without pressing or binding your breasts. Pressure on your breasts can cause plugged milk ducts and breast infections. Some women find it more comfortable to wear two sports bras for extra support.

Avoid high-impact activities. Jumping around may be painful, so opt for low-impact exercises that minimize the movement of your breasts.

Nurse before working out. Exercising with empty breasts is much more comfortable than exercising with full breasts. Even when they're empty, your breasts will likely be bigger than they were before pregnancy, and that may take some getting used to.

Avoid activities that expose your breasts to potential injury. Skip contact

Fact or fiction? If you get pregnant again, you'll have to stop breastfeeding.
Fiction. If you're having an otherwise healthy pregnancy, you can continue to breastfeed. Many mothers nurse one baby or toddler while expecting. Breastfeeding may bring on uterine contractions, but these are harmless, provided you are not at high risk for preterm delivery. If you breastfeed while pregnant, make sure that you and your breastfeeding child are gaining adequate amounts of weight. Once your new baby is born, you can choose to wean your older child or nurse them both. This is called tandem nursing, and if you eat a healthy diet and drink plenty of water your body should be able to make enough milk for both children.

sports or wear protective gear. Breast injuries are painful and can impact your milk supply.

Avoid moves that require you to lie on your chest. The pressure could cause ducts to become plugged.

Refuel after burning calories. If you exercise intensely, you may need to up your calorie intake. Keep an eye on the scale: If you're losing more than a pound a week, eat more.

Don't overtire yourself. Exhaustion can take a toll on your milk supply.

Common Questions

Q. Can I drink caffeinated coffee and tea while breastfeeding?

A. Yes, in moderation. The caffeine in up to 3 cups of coffee a day is fine for most babies. Drinking more than 3 cups a day can overstimulate your baby. If you notice your baby is sensitive to the caffeine in your diet—if she appears unusually wide-eyed or won't sleep—cut back for two weeks and see if things improve. Keep in mind that the amount of caffeine in breast milk peaks about an hour after consuming a caffeine-containing food.

Q. Can I drink alcohol while breastfeeding?

A. Yes, if it's just a little. Having an occasional drink is believed to be safe. However, having more than that can affect your ability to nurse effectively—it can interfere with your breasts' ability to let down milk (the process that brings milk from the glands to the nipple, where your baby can access it). To minimize the amount of alcohol in your body, time your glass of wine or beer so that 2 hours can pass between drinking and nursing. And pay attention to how your baby reacts. Some babies feed less after mom has a drink because the alcohol leaves an unpalatable taste in the milk.

Q. Will drinking a beer before nursing increase my milk supply?

A. No. Although one drink won't diminish your milk supply, it won't boost it either. A larger amount of alcohol will decrease your milk supply, so limit yourself to no more than two drinks in one sitting.

Q. Can my baby develop an allergy to my milk?

A. No, although she may be bothered by substances in the food that you eat that pass into your milk. If your baby is inexplicably fussy or gassy; if she develops diarrhea, a rash, or patches of dry skin; if she pulls her knees to her chest while crying or passes green stools with mucus, she may be reacting to something in your diet. Spicy foods, foods that cause gas (such as cabbage or beans), and dairy products are common culprits. If you eliminate antagonizing foods from your diet, your baby's discomfort should disappear and the problem will go away. (See "Diet and colic," page 169.)

In rare cases, babies may develop galactosemia, an inability to break down the lactose (milk sugar) in your breast milk. Babies who develop this rare condition must be fed plant-based formula (such as soy) or galactose-free formula.

Q. Do you have to drink milk to make milk?

A. No. Although dairy foods are a rich source of calcium, you don't have to drink milk while breastfeeding. You do need to drink plenty of fluids to maintain your milk supply, and you also need to make sure you get 1,000 milligrams of calcium each day. But your calcium doesn't have to come from dairy. You can get it from other sources such as calcium-fortified orange juice, calcium-fortified soy products, and supplements.

Fact or fiction? You should not breastfeed if you have a cold because your baby could catch it.

Fiction. Common illnesses such as cold, flu, or diarrhea can't pass to a baby via breast milk. In fact, it's quite the opposite: When you are sick, your body creates protective antibodies that pass to your baby in your breast milk. Those antibodies help keep her from getting what you have.

Books about breastfeeding

These books are excellent resources for nursing mothers:
- *The Breastfeeding Answer Book* by La Leche League
- *The Womanly Art of Breastfeeding* by La Leche League
- *Breastfeeding Made Simple: Seven Natural Laws for Nursing Mothers* by Nancy Mohrbacher and Kathleen Kendall-Tackett
- *The Breastfeeding Book: Everything You Need to Know About Nursing Your Child from Birth Through Weaning* by Martha Sears and William Sears
- *The American Academy of Pediatrics New Mother's Guide to Breastfeeding* by Joan Younger Meek
- *The Black Woman's Guide to Breastfeeding* by Katherine Barber
- *The Nursing Mother's Companion* by Kathleen Huggins
- *Breastfeeding for Dummies* by Sharon Perkins and Carol Vannais

Q. Does breastfeeding accelerate weight loss?

A. Maybe, maybe not. Women have long been told that breastfeeding is one of the best ways to lose the weight gained during pregnancy. Unfortunately, there isn't much in the way of proof behind this promise. In fact, two recent studies found that there is no connection between breastfeeding and postpartum weight loss—mothers who fed with formula lost weight at the same rate as those who breastfed.

Q. Is it safe for me to take herbal supplements and remedies when I'm breastfeeding?

A. So little research has been done on herbs and breastfeeding that it's best to avoid herbs while you're nursing. Drinking herbal tea in moderation is fine, as is using herbs in cooking. However, be sure to check the label of herbal teas to see if there is a warning against drinking them while breastfeeding. Some herbs, such as sage, peppermint, chickweed, lemon balm, oregano, thyme, sorrel, yarrow, parsley, and black walnut, can decrease milk supply if taken in large amounts. (Don't worry about the oregano you add to your spaghetti sauce or the peppermint candies you like to eat.)

Some herbs are potentially harmful to you and your baby, so avoid them completely. They include bladder wrack, buckthorn, chaparral, coltsfoot, dong quai, elecampane, ephedra (also known as ma huang or ephedra sinica), ginseng, Indian snakeroot, kava kava, petastites root, rhubarb, star anise, tiratricol, uva ursi, and wormwood.

Food and breastfeeding interactions

Most women will be able to eat and drink what they like (see "Your Baby's Reactions," page 169) while breast-feeding their babies. But rarely a specific food or protein that you eat may trigger anything from fussiness to a full-blown allergic reaction in your baby. If you suspect this may be the case, arrive fully armed at your next doctor's appointment. Before cutting out a variety of healthy and likely

innocent foods from your breastfeeding diet, fill in charts like the ones on the following pages for a week to see if you discover any true correlations between what you are consuming and your infant's symptoms. (The chart below is a sample.) This way, you will keep your intake varied as long as possible, and you will have concrete information to share with your pediatrician.

Baby's Sensitivities During Breastfeeding—Sample Chart				
Time/Meal	Amount	Food/Beverage	Breastfeeding Time/Duration	Baby's Symptoms
9 a.m.	2 slices 2 slices 1 cup	Whole wheat bread Low-fat cheddar Fat-free milk	10 a.m., 15 minutes each side	Wheezing/congestion 1 hour afterward
11 a.m.	2 tablespoons	Almonds	noon, 15 minutes each side	No symptoms
2 p.m.	1 large 2 teaspoons 3 ounces ½ cup 1 cup	Green salad Oil and vinegar Grilled salmon Brown rice Seltzer water	2 p.m., 15 minutes each side	Wheezing/congestion 1 hour afterward

Baby's Sensitivities During Breastfeeding				
Time/Meal	Amount	Food/Beverage	Breastfeeding Time/Duration	Baby's Symptoms

Baby's Sensitivities During Breastfeeding				
Time/Meal	Amount	Food/Beverage	Breastfeeding Time/Duration	Baby's Symptoms

Baby's Sensitivities During Breastfeeding				
Time/Meal	Amount	Food/Beverage	Breastfeeding Time/Duration	Baby's Symptoms

Baby's Sensitivities During Breastfeeding				
Time/Meal	Amount	Food/Beverage	Breastfeeding Time/Duration	Baby's Symptoms

resources

For more information about the many important topics covered in this book, tap into these reputable sources.

Resources

American Academy of Family Physicians
Information on mother/baby health
P.O. Box 11210
Shawnee Mission, KS 66207
800-274-2237
www.aafp.org

American Academy of Pediatrics
Children's health topics, clinical resources, and research
141 Northwest Point Boulevard
Elk Grove Village, IL 60007
847-434-4000
www.aap.org

American College of Allergy, Asthma, and Immunology
Information about allergies/asthma
85 West Algonquin Road, Suite 550
Arlington Heights, IL 60005
847-427-1200
www.acaai.org

American College of Obstetricians and Gynecologists (ACOG)
Information on obstetrics and gynecology issues, research, publications, lists of providers
409 12th Street, SW
P.O. Box 96920
Washington, DC 20090
202-638-5577
www.acog.org

American Diabetes Association
Information on gestational, type 1, and type 2 diabetes
1701 North Beauregard Street
Alexandria, VA 22311
800-342-2383
www.diabetes.org

American Dietetic Association
Information on food and nutrition and referrals to registered dietitians in your area
120 South Riverside Plaza, Suite 2000
Chicago, IL 60606-6995
800-877-1600
www.eatright.org

Environmental Protection Agency
Information about which fish are safe to eat and other environmental/food safety issues
Fish Advisory Program
U.S. Environmental Protection Agency
Office of Science and Technology (4303T)
1200 Pennsylvania Avenue, NW
Washington, DC 20460
www.epa.gov/ost/fish

Environmental Working Group
Information on pesticides and other
environmental toxins
1436 U Street, NW
Suite 101
Washington, DC 20009
202-667-6982
www.ewg.org

Genetic Alliance
Resources and information about genetic
diseases and testing
4301 Connecticut Avenue, NW
Suite 404
Washington, DC 20008-2369
202-966-5557
www.geneticalliance.org

International Childbirth Education
Association and Book Center
Information on childbirth and
childbirth educators
P.O. Box 20048
Minneapolis, MN 55420
952-854-8660
www.icea.org

March of Dimes
Information on pregnancy, genetics, birth
defects, preterm birth, and more
1275 Mamaroneck Avenue
White Plains, NY 10605
914-428-7100
www.marchofdimes.com

Medem Online Medical Library
Physician websites and referral lists,
online medical library
649 Mission Street, 2nd Floor
San Francisco, CA 94105
877-926-3336
www.medem.com

National Diabetes Information
Clearinghouse
Information on diabetes and how to
manage it from the National Institute
of Diabetes and Digestive and Kidney
Diseases (NIDDK)
1 Information Way
Bethesda, MD   20892-3560
800-860-8747
www.diabetes.niddk.nih.gov

National Highway Traffic Safety
Administration
Information on child safety seats
NHTSA Headquarters
400 Seventh Street, SW
Washington, DC 20590
888-327-4236
www.nhtsa.gov

National Institute of Child Health and
Human Development (NICHD)
Information related to the health
of children and families, including
information on gestational diabetes
P.O. Box 3006
Rockville, MD 20847
800-370-2943
www.nichd.nih.gov

National Institute for Occupational
Safety and Health
Workplace safety and health information
Hubert H. Humphrey Building
200 Independence Avenue, SW
Room 715H
Washington, DC 20201
800-356-4674
www.cdc.gov/niosh

Special Supplemental Nutrition Program for Women, Infants, and Children (WIC)
Government agency: provides food for low-income women and children
3101 Park Center Drive
Alexandria, VA 22302
703-305-2746
www.fns.usda.gov/wic/

State Children's Health Insurance Program (SCHIP)
Information for pregnant women without health insurance
7500 Security Boulevard
Baltimore, MD 21244
877-267-2323
www.cms.hhs.gov/schip/

Feeding Options

African-American Breastfeeding Alliance
Resources and support for African-American mothers who breastfeed
P.O. Box 117
Joppa, MD 21085
877-532-8535
www.aabaonline.com

International Lactation Consultant Association
Breastfeeding information, lactation consultants, books about nursing
1500 Sunday Drive, Suite 102
Raleigh, NC 27607
919-861-5577
www.ilca.org

La Leche League
Breastfeeding information, nursing support groups, lactation experts
1400 N. Meacham Road
Schaumburg, IL 60173-4808
847-519-7730
www.lalecheleague.org

Medela
Breastfeeding pumps and other nursing products
1101 Corporate Drive
McHenry, IL 60050
800-435-8316
www.medela.com

National Women's Health Information Center
Information on all women's health topics from the U.S. Department of Health and Human Services
8270 Willow Oaks Corporate Drive
Suite 301
Fairfax, VA 22031
800-994-9662
www.4woman.gov/breastfeeding

U.S. Food and Drug Administration Center for Food Safety and Applied Nutrition
Regulates the manufacture of infant formula
5100 Paint Branch Parkway
HFS-555
College Park, MD 20740
888-SAFEFOOD
www.cfsan.fda.gov/~dms/inf-toc.html

healthy and
quick recipes

You can eat healthy both during and after your pregnancy with the simple yet flavorful and nutritious recipes in this section of the book. Some are high in specific nutrients to help you get just what you need each day. Other recipes provide quick, convenient foods for when you're on the go or when you don't feel like making a big meal. You'll also find some recipes to make ahead and freeze before your baby arrives, so dinner will be ready when you need it.

Recipes

high-calcium recipes

12

A diet high in calcium is important for everyone, yet few women get the recommended amount. During pregnancy, your developing baby needs calcium to grow strong bones and teeth, so make sure you get enough from the foods in your diet. Here you'll find some delicious high-calcium recipes your whole family will enjoy.

Mighty Mac and Cheese `670 mg calcium`

Prep: 30 minutes Bake: 25 minutes Stand: 5 minutes Oven: 350°F Makes: 4 servings

1⅓ cups dried corkscrew pasta or elbow macaroni (about 5 ounces)

¼ cup nonfat dry milk powder

¼ cup finely chopped onion

2 tablespoons all-purpose flour

¼ teaspoon salt

1½ cups reduced-fat or fat-free milk

10 slices reduced-fat American cheese (7 ounces), torn

6 flavored crisp breadsticks, such as cheese or garlic, coarsely crushed (1 ounce total)

1. Cook pasta according to package directions. Drain; set aside.

2. Meanwhile, in a medium saucepan stir together the milk powder, onion, flour, and salt. Gradually stir in the milk until mixture is smooth. Cook and stir over medium heat until thickened and bubbly. Reduce heat to low. Add the cheese, stirring until melted. Stir in the pasta. Spoon mixture into a 1½-quart casserole.

3. Bake, uncovered, in a 350° oven about 25 minutes or until hot and bubbly, stirring once and topping with crushed breadsticks after 15 minutes of baking. Let stand 5 minutes before serving.

Nutrition Facts per serving: 344 cal., 10 g total fat (5 g sat. fat), 33 mg chol., 889 mg sodium, 44 g carbo., 1 g fiber, 20 g pro.
Exchanges: ½ Milk, 2½ Starch, 1½ Lean Meat, ½ Fat

Ravioli with Sweet Peppers 320 mg calcium

Start to Finish: 20 minutes Makes: 4 servings

1 9-ounce package refrigerated light cheese-filled ravioli

$^2/_3$ cup chopped red sweet pepper

$^2/_3$ cup chopped green sweet pepper

1 medium carrot, cut into thin bite-size strips

$^1/_3$ cup chopped onion (1 small)

2 cloves garlic, minced

1 tablespoon olive oil

1 cup chopped tomato (2 medium)

$^1/_4$ cup reduced-sodium chicken broth or vegetable broth

3 tablespoons snipped fresh basil or 2 teaspoons dried basil, crushed

1. Cook pasta according to package directions; drain. Return pasta to saucepan; cover and keep warm.

2. Meanwhile, in a large nonstick skillet cook sweet peppers, carrot, onion, and garlic in hot oil over medium-high heat about 5 minutes or until vegetables are tender. Stir in tomato, broth, and basil. Cook and stir about 2 minutes more or until heated through.

3. Add vegetable mixture to the cooked pasta; toss gently to combine.

Nutrition Facts per serving: 280 cal., 9 g total fat (4 g sat. fat), 26 mg chol., 381 mg sodium, 39 g carbo., 2 g fiber, 14 g pro.
Exchanges: 2 Vegetable, 2 Starch, ½ Lean Meat

Corn and Tomato Pudding `300 mg calcium`
Prep: 20 minutes Bake: 30 minutes Oven: 375°F Makes: 6 servings

3 tablespoons snipped dried
  tomatoes (not oil pack)

4 eggs

1½ cups reduced-fat or fat-free
  milk

1 tablespoon snipped fresh basil
  or 1 teaspoon dried basil,
  crushed

4 cups torn whole wheat English
  muffins or dry French bread*

1½ cups fresh or frozen whole
  kernel corn

1 cup shredded reduced-fat
  cheddar cheese or Monterey
  Jack cheese (4 ounces)

  Thin tomato wedges (optional)

1. In a small bowl soak the dried tomatoes in enough hot water to cover for 10 minutes; drain.

2. Meanwhile, in a medium bowl beat together eggs, milk, and basil; set aside. In a 2-quart square baking dish toss together drained tomatoes, torn English muffins, corn, and cheese. Carefully pour egg mixture evenly over the muffin mixture.

3. Bake in a 375° oven about 30 minutes or until a knife inserted near center comes out clean. Cool slightly. If desired, serve with tomato wedges.

*Note: You'll need about 5 cups fresh bread cubes to make 4 cups dry cubes. Cut bread into ½-inch slices; cut into cubes. Spread in a single layer in a shallow baking pan. Bake in a 300°F oven for 10 to 15 minutes or until dry, stirring twice; cool. (Bread will continue to dry and crisp as it cools.) Or let bread cubes stand, loosely covered, at room temperature for 8 to 12 hours.

Nutrition Facts per serving: 268 cal., 9 g total fat (4 g sat. fat), 160 mg chol., 393 mg sodium, 31 g carbo., 3 g fiber, 17 g pro. **Exchanges:** 2 Starch, 1½ Medium-Fat Meat

Bean and Rice Stuffed Peppers 340 mg calcium

Prep: 15 minutes   Cook: 6 to 6½ hours (low) or 3 to 3½ hours (high)   Makes: 4 servings

4 small to medium green, red, and/or yellow sweet peppers

1 cup cooked converted rice

1 15-ounce can chili beans with chili gravy

1 cup shredded Monterey Jack cheese (4 ounces)

1 15-ounce can chunky tomato sauce with onion, celery, and green pepper

1. Remove tops, membranes, and seeds from sweet peppers. In a large bowl stir together rice, beans, and ½ cup of the cheese. Spoon the rice mixture into the peppers. Pour tomato sauce into the bottom of a 5- to 6-quart slow cooker. Place peppers in cooker.

2. Cover and cook on low-heat setting for 6 to 6½ hours or on high-heat setting for 3 to 3½ hours. Transfer peppers to a serving plate. Spoon tomato sauce over peppers and sprinkle with the remaining cheese.

Nutrition Facts per serving: 323 cal., 11 g total fat (5 g sat. fat), 25 mg chol., 918 mg sodium, 41 g carbo., 9 g fiber, 16 g pro.
Exchanges: 2 Vegetable, 2 Starch, 1 High-Fat Meat, ½ Fat

Cheesy Lasagna 390 mg calcium

Prep: 30 minutes Bake: 25 minutes Stand: 10 minutes Oven: 375°F Makes: 8 servings

12 ounces lean ground beef

½ cup chopped onion (1 medium)

½ cup finely chopped carrot
    (1 medium)

2 cloves garlic, minced

1 15-ounce can Italian-style
    tomato sauce

1 6-ounce can tomato paste

½ cup water

¼ teaspoon black pepper

9 dried lasagna noodles

1 egg, beaten

1 15-ounce carton light ricotta
    cheese or low-fat cottage
    cheese, drained

    Nonstick cooking spray

1 cup shredded part-skim
    mozzarella cheese (4 ounces)

¼ cup grated Parmesan or
    Romano cheese

1. For sauce, in a large saucepan cook beef, onion, carrot, and garlic over medium-high heat until meat is brown and vegetables are tender. Drain off fat. Stir in the tomato sauce, tomato paste, water, and pepper. Bring to boiling; reduce heat. Simmer, covered, for 10 minutes, stirring occasionally.

2. Meanwhile, cook the lasagna noodles according to package directions. Drain; rinse with cold water. Drain well; set aside. For cheese filling, in a small bowl stir together the egg and ricotta cheese.

3. Lightly coat a 2-quart rectangular baking dish with cooking spray. Layer 3 noodles in the prepared baking dish. Spread with a third of the cheese filling. Top with a third of the sauce and a third of the mozzarella cheese. Repeat layers twice. Sprinkle with Parmesan cheese.

4. Bake, covered, in a 375° oven for 20 minutes. Uncover and bake for 5 minutes more or until heated through. Let stand for 10 minutes before serving.

Nutrition Facts per serving:: 299 cal., 10 g total fat (5 g sat. fat), 73 mg chol., 514 mg sodium, 28 g carbo., 3 g fiber, 25 g pro.
Exchanges: ½ Vegetable, 1½ Starch, 3 Lean Meat

Double Corn Tortilla Casserole `360 mg calcium`

Prep: 20 minutes Bake: 40 minutes Stand: 5 minutes Oven: 325°F Makes: 4 servings

Nonstick cooking spray

1½ cups frozen whole kernel corn

6 6-inch corn tortillas, torn into bite-size pieces

1 cup shredded reduced-fat mozzarella cheese (4 ounces)

½ cup sliced green onion (4)

1 4-ounce can diced green chile peppers, drained

¼ cup finely chopped red sweet pepper

1 cup buttermilk

2 egg whites*

1 egg*

¼ teaspoon garlic salt

⅓ cup salsa

1. Coat a 2-quart square baking dish with cooking spray; set aside. Cook corn according to package directions; drain well. Arrange half of the tortillas in the prepared baking dish. Top with half of the cheese, half of the corn, half of the green onion, half of the chile peppers, and half of the red sweet pepper. Repeat layers.

2. In a medium bowl beat together buttermilk, egg whites, whole egg, and garlic salt. Pour over the tortilla mixture.

3. Bake, uncovered, in a 325° oven about 40 minutes or until a knife inserted near center comes out clean. Let stand for 5 minutes before serving. Serve with salsa.

*Note: You may substitute ½ cup refrigerated or frozen egg product, thawed, for the egg whites and whole egg.

Nutrition Facts per serving: 281 cal., 8 g total fat (4 g sat. fat), 71 mg chol., 653 mg sodium, 36 g carbo., 0 g fiber, 18 g pro.
Exchanges: 1 Vegetable, 2 Starch, 1 Medium-Fat Meat

Garbanzo Beans and Spinach with Ravioli 380 mg calcium

Start to Finish: 20 minutes Makes: 4 servings

1 9-ounce package refrigerated light cheese-filled ravioli

2 teaspoons olive oil

2 cloves garlic, minced

1 15-ounce can garbanzo beans (chickpeas), rinsed and drained

1 medium yellow summer squash, thinly sliced (about 1¼ cups)

4 medium roma tomatoes, quartered

2 teaspoons snipped fresh thyme or ½ teaspoon dried thyme, crushed

¼ teaspoon coarsely ground black pepper

4 cups shredded fresh spinach

1. Cook ravioli according to package directions. Drain; cover and keep warm.

2. Meanwhile, in a large skillet heat oil over medium-high heat. Add garlic; cook and stir for 15 seconds. Add garbanzo beans, squash, tomato, thyme, and pepper; stir to combine. Cook and stir for 4 to 5 minutes or just until squash is tender.

3. Add the cooked ravioli to bean mixture; toss gently to combine. To serve, arrange the shredded spinach on a serving platter. Top with the bean mixture.

Nutrition Facts per serving: 386 cal., 9 g total fat (3 g sat. fat), 26 mg chol., 691 mg sodium, 60 g carbo., 9 g fiber, 19 g pro. **Exchanges:** 2½ Vegetable, 3 Starch, 1 Lean Meat, ½ Fat

Cheese Calzones `480 mg calcium`

Prep: 45 minutes Bake: 20 minutes Oven: 375°F Makes: 8 calzones

Nonstick cooking spray

1 16-ounce loaf frozen bread dough, thawed

$\frac{1}{2}$ cup chopped onion (1 medium)

2 cloves garlic, minced

1 10-ounce package frozen chopped spinach, thawed and well drained

$1\frac{1}{2}$ teaspoons dried Italian seasoning, crushed

1 egg, slightly beaten

1 15-ounce carton low-fat ricotta cheese

$\frac{3}{4}$ cup shredded reduced-fat mozzarella cheese (3 ounces)

$\frac{1}{4}$ cup grated Parmesan cheese

1 8-ounce can low-sodium tomato sauce

1. Lightly coat a very large baking sheet with cooking spray; set aside. Divide bread dough into 8 equal pieces. Place dough on a floured surface and cover with a towel. Let dough rest while preparing filling.

2. For filling, in a small covered saucepan cook onion and garlic in a small amount of boiling water until onion is tender. Drain. Stir in spinach and 1 teaspoon of the Italian seasoning; set aside. In a medium bowl stir together egg, ricotta cheese, mozzarella cheese, and Parmesan cheese.

3. Roll each piece of dough into a 6-inch circle. Spread 2 tablespoons of the spinach mixture over half of each circle to within $\frac{1}{2}$ inch of edge. Top with $\frac{1}{4}$ cup of the cheese mixture. Moisten edges of dough with water. Fold each circle in half, pinching edges or pressing edges together with a fork. Prick tops with a fork. Place calzones on prepared baking sheet.

4. Bake in a 375° oven for 20 to 25 minutes or until golden. Meanwhile, in a small saucepan stir together tomato sauce and the remaining $\frac{1}{2}$ teaspoon Italian seasoning; heat through. Serve with calzones.

Nutrition Facts per calzone: 280 cal., 6 g total fat (3 g sat. fat), 43 mg chol., 542 mg sodium, 35 g carbo., 3 g fiber, 19 g pro.
Exchanges: 1 Vegetable, 2 Starch, 1½ Lean Meat

Tomato Polenta Pizza 340 mg calcium

Prep: 25 minutes   Chill: 2 to 24 hours   Bake: 20 minutes   Oven: 400°F   Makes: 6 servings

3 cups fat-free milk

1½ cups semolina pasta flour or quick-cooking polenta mix

2 eggs, beaten

½ cup finely shredded Asiago or Parmesan cheese (2 ounces)

¼ teaspoon salt

⅛ teaspoon black pepper

Nonstick cooking spray

4 medium roma tomatoes, thinly sliced

1 cup shredded mozzarella cheese (4 ounces)

2 tablespoons snipped fresh basil and/or oregano

1. In a large saucepan bring milk just to boiling over medium heat. Sprinkle the semolina flour over milk, stirring constantly. Cook and stir for 2 minutes (mixture will be very stiff). Remove from heat and cool for 5 minutes. Stir in eggs, Asiago cheese, salt, and pepper.

2. Coat a 12-inch pizza pan with cooking spray. Spread semolina mixture in prepared pizza pan. Cover and chill 2 to 24 hours. Arrange the tomato slices over semolina mixture. Top with mozzarella cheese.

3. Bake in a 400° oven about 20 minutes or until cheese melts and begins to brown. Sprinkle with basil. Serve immediately.

Nutrition Facts per serving: 319 cal., 9 g total fat (5 g sat. fat), 94 mg chol., 376 mg sodium, 39 g carbo., 2 g fiber, 19 g pro.
Exchanges: ½ Milk, ½ Vegetable, 2 Starch, 1 Medium-Fat Meat, ½ Fat

Tortellini-and-Vegetable Chowder 310 mg calcium

Start to Finish: 30 minutes Makes: 6 servings

2 14-ounce cans reduced-sodium chicken broth

1 16-ounce package loose-pack frozen broccoli, cauliflower, and carrots

1 9-ounce package refrigerated cheese-filled tortellini

2 cups reduced-fat or fat-free milk

¼ cup all-purpose flour

1 tablespoon snipped fresh basil or 1 teaspoon dried basil, crushed

1 cup shredded smoked Gouda cheese (4 ounces)

Freshly ground black pepper

Fresh basil leaves (optional)

1. In a large saucepan combine broth and frozen vegetables. Bring to boiling; add tortellini. Return to boiling; reduce heat. Simmer, uncovered, about 4 minutes or just until vegetables are tender.

2. Meanwhile, in a screw-top jar combine about half of the milk and all of the flour; cover and shake well. Add to saucepan along with remaining milk and dried basil (if using). Cook and stir until thickened and bubbly. Cook and stir for 1 minute more. Stir in cheese and fresh basil (if using) until cheese melts. Season to taste with pepper. If desired, top each serving with additional fresh basil.

Nutrition Facts per serving: 302 cal., 10 g total fat (5 g sat. fat), 41 mg chol., 878 mg sodium, 39 g carbo., 3 g fiber, 17 g pro. **Exchanges:** 2 Vegetable, 2 Starch, 1 High-Fat Meat, ½ Fat

Lasagna Roll-Ups with Swiss Cheese Sauce `550 mg calcium`

Prep: 40 minutes Bake: 35 minutes Oven: 350°F Makes: 8 lasagna roll-ups

8 dried lasagna noodles

2 egg whites, slightly beaten

1 15-ounce carton light ricotta
   cheese

1 10-ounce package frozen
   chopped spinach, thawed and
   well drained

6 ounces reduced-fat Swiss
   cheese, finely chopped

½ cup grated Parmesan cheese

¼ teaspoon ground nutmeg
   (optional)

   Nonstick cooking spray

1½ cups sliced fresh mushrooms

½ cup thinly sliced green
   onion (4)

1 12-ounce can (1½ cups)
   evaporated fat-free milk

2 tablespoons all-purpose flour

¼ teaspoon salt

   Paprika

1. Cook lasagna noodles according to package directions. Drain; rinse with cold water. Drain again. Place noodles in a single layer on a sheet of foil; set aside.

2. For filling, in a large bowl combine the egg whites, ricotta cheese, spinach, half of the Swiss cheese, the Parmesan cheese, and, if desired, nutmeg.

3. Lightly coat a 2-quart rectangular baking dish with cooking spray; set aside. Spread about ⅓ cup of the filling on each lasagna noodle. Starting from a short end, roll up each noodle. Place the lasagna rolls, seam sides down, in the prepared baking dish; set aside.

4. For sauce, lightly coat a medium saucepan with cooking spray. Heat saucepan over medium-high heat. Add mushrooms and green onion; cook and stir about 3 minutes or until vegetables are tender. In a medium bowl stir together ¼ cup of the evaporated milk and the flour until smooth; stir in the remaining evaporated milk and the salt. Stir milk mixture into mushroom mixture. Cook and stir until thickened and bubbly. Remove from heat. Stir in remaining Swiss cheese until melted. Pour sauce over lasagna rolls.

5. Bake, covered, in a 350° oven about 35 minutes or until lasagna rolls are heated through. To serve, sprinkle with paprika.

Nutrition Facts per lasagna roll-up: 250 cal., 6 g total fat (3 g sat. fat), 27 mg chol., 383 mg sodium, 27 g carbo., 2 g fiber, 21 g pro.
Exchanges: 1 Vegetable, 1½ Starch, 2 Lean Meat

Classic Monte Cristo Sandwiches 370 mg calcium

Start to Finish: 15 minutes Makes: 2 sandwiches

4 slices firm white bread or sourdough bread

4 teaspoons cranberry or raspberry mustard

2 ounces thinly sliced reduced-sodium cooked ham

2 slices reduced-fat Swiss cheese (2 ounces)

$\frac{1}{4}$ cup reduced-fat milk

1 egg white

Butter-flavor nonstick cooking spray

1 teaspoon butter or margarine

1. Spread 1 side of each bread slice lightly with mustard. Layer ham and cheese between the mustard-spread sides of the bread slices. In a shallow bowl or pie plate beat together milk and egg white.

2. Coat an unheated nonstick griddle or large skillet with cooking spray. Preheat griddle over medium heat. Melt butter on griddle. Dip each sandwich in milk mixture, turning to coat. Place in skillet; cook for 1 to 2 minutes per side or until bread is golden and cheese is melted.

Nutrition Facts per sandwich: 314 cal., 10 g total fat (4 g sat. fat), 41 mg chol., 606 mg sodium, 33 g carbo., 0 g fiber, 21 g pro.
Exchanges: 2 Starch, 2 Medium-Fat Meat, $\frac{1}{2}$ Fat

Chicken Tetrazzini `300 mg calcium`

Prep: 30 minutes Bake: 10 minutes Oven: 400°F Makes: 4 servings

6 ounces dried spaghetti

1½ cups sliced fresh mushrooms

¾ cup chopped red or green
    sweet pepper (1 medium)

½ cup cold water

¼ cup all-purpose flour

1 12-ounce can (1½ cups)
    evaporated low-fat milk

1 teaspoon instant chicken
    bouillon granules

¼ teaspoon black pepper

⅛ teaspoon salt

1 cup chopped cooked chicken or
    turkey (5 ounces)

¼ cup finely shredded Parmesan
    cheese (1 ounce)

2 tablespoons reduced-fat or
    fat-free milk

Nonstick cooking spray

1 tablespoon sliced almonds

1. Cook the spaghetti according to package directions. Drain; set aside.

2. Meanwhile, in a large covered saucepan cook the mushrooms and sweet pepper in a small amount of boiling water about 3 minutes or until the vegetables are tender. Drain well; return to saucepan.

3. In a screw-top jar combine the ½ cup cold water and the flour; cover and shake well. Stir into the vegetable mixture in saucepan. Stir in the evaporated milk, bouillon granules, black pepper, and salt. Cook and stir until thickened and bubbly. Stir in the cooked spaghetti, chicken, Parmesan cheese, and milk.

4. Lightly coat a 2-quart square baking dish with cooking spray. Spoon spaghetti mixture into dish. Sprinkle with almonds.

5. Bake, uncovered, in a 400° oven about 10 minutes or until heated through and nuts are lightly toasted.

Nutrition Facts per serving: 394 cal., 9 g total fat (4 g sat. fat), 44 mg chol., 492 mg sodium, 50 g carbo., 2 g fiber, 26 g pro.
Exchanges: 1 Vegetable, 3 Starch, 2 Lean Meat, ½ Fat

high-
iron recipes

Your iron needs go up during pregnancy to account for your increased blood volume. Although you'll likely take a prenatal vitamin with iron in it, make sure you get iron in your diet as well. This chapter will help you do just that, with recipes for everything from simple salads that are great for lunch to hearty chili that's perfect for a weeknight dinner.

Beefsteak Chili `5 mg iron`

Prep: 25 minutes Cook: 1 hour 5 minutes Makes: 6 servings

1½ pounds boneless beef top round steak

1 tablespoon cooking oil

1 cup chopped onion (1 large)

2 cloves garlic, minced

2 14½-ounce cans diced tomatoes, undrained

1 cup beef broth

1 4-ounce can diced chile peppers, undrained

2 tablespoons chili powder

1 tablespoon packed brown sugar

2 teaspoons dried oregano, crushed

1 teaspoon salt

1 teaspoon ground cumin

2 15-ounce cans pinto beans or red kidney beans, rinsed and drained

1. Partially freeze meat. Trim fat from meat. Cut meat into small, thin strips. In a Dutch oven cook and stir half of meat in hot oil until brown; remove meat and set aside. Add remaining meat, the onion, and garlic to the Dutch oven. Cook and stir until meat is brown and onion is tender, adding more oil if necessary. Drain fat. Return all of the meat to Dutch oven.

2. Stir in undrained tomatoes, broth, undrained chile peppers, chili powder, brown sugar, oregano, salt, and cumin. Bring to boiling; reduce heat. Simmer, covered, for 1 hour. Stir in beans; cook about 5 minutes more or until heated through.

Nutrition Facts per serving: 409 cal., 13 g total fat (4 g sat. fat), 66 mg chol., 1,331 mg sodium, 39 g carbo., 10 g fiber, 36 g pro. **Exchanges:** 1 Vegetable, 2 Starch, 4 Lean Meat

Beefy Italian Skillet `5 mg iron`

Prep: 35 minutes Cook: 1¼ hours Makes: 4 servings

1 pound boneless beef round steak

Nonstick cooking spray

2 cups sliced fresh mushrooms

1 cup chopped onion (1 large)

1 cup coarsely chopped green sweet pepper (1 large)

½ cup chopped celery (1 stalk)

2 cloves garlic, minced

1 14½-ounce can diced tomatoes, undrained

½ teaspoon dried basil, crushed

¼ teaspoon dried oregano, crushed

¼ teaspoon crushed red pepper (optional)

8 ounces dried spaghetti

2 tablespoons grated Parmesan cheese (optional)

1. Trim fat from meat. Cut meat into 4 serving-size pieces. Lightly coat an unheated large skillet with cooking spray. Heat over medium heat. Add meat to skillet; cook each piece on both sides until brown. Remove meat from skillet.

2. Add mushrooms, onion, sweet pepper, celery, and garlic to the skillet. Cook until vegetables are nearly tender. Stir in undrained tomatoes, basil, oregano, and, if desired, crushed red pepper. Add meat to skillet, spooning vegetable mixture over the meat. Simmer, covered, about 1¼ hours or until meat is tender, stirring occasionally. Meanwhile, cook spaghetti according to package directions. Drain; keep warm.

3. Transfer meat to a serving platter. Spoon vegetable mixture over meat. Serve with spaghetti. If desired, sprinkle with Parmesan cheese.

Nutrition Facts per serving: 438 cal., 8 g total fat (3 g sat. fat), 56 mg chol., 273 mg sodium, 55 g carbo., 4 g fiber, 37 g pro.
Exchanges: 2½ Vegetable, 2½ Starch, 3 Lean Meat

Beef-Vegetable Ragout   `6 mg iron`

Start to Finish: 30 minutes   Makes: 4 servings

8 ounces dried wide noodles

12 ounces beef tenderloin, cut into ³/₄-inch pieces

2 tablespoons olive oil or cooking oil

1½ cups sliced fresh cremini or button mushrooms

½ cup chopped onion (1 medium)

2 cloves garlic, minced

3 tablespoons all-purpose flour

½ teaspoon salt

¼ teaspoon black pepper

2 cups reduced-sodium beef broth

2 cups sugar snap peas

1 cup cherry tomatoes, halved

1. In a large saucepan cook noodles according to package directions. Drain; keep warm.

2. Meanwhile, in a large skillet cook and stir the meat in hot oil over medium heat for 2 to 3 minutes or until meat is desired doneness. Remove meat, reserving drippings in skillet. Set meat aside.

3. Cook mushrooms, onion, and garlic in reserved drippings for 4 to 5 minutes or until tender. Sprinkle flour, salt, and pepper over mushroom mixture; stir in. Carefully add broth. Cook and stir until thickened and bubbly.

4. Stir sugar snap peas into the mushroom mixture. Cook for 2 to 3 minutes more or until peas are tender. Stir in meat and tomatoes; heat through.

5. Arrange warm noodles on a serving platter. Spoon the meat and vegetable mixture over noodles.

Nutrition Facts per serving: 511 cal., 16 g total fat (4 g sat. fat), 106 mg chol., 573 mg sodium, 59 g carbo., 5 g fiber, 32 g pro.
Exchanges: 1½ Vegetable, 3 Starch, 3 Lean Meat, 1½ Fat

Paprika Beef Stew [6 mg iron]

Prep: 20 minutes Cook: 8 to 9 hours (low) or 4 to 4½ hours (high) Makes: 6 servings

2 pounds boneless beef chuck pot roast

1½ cups chopped onion (3 medium)

1 14-ounce can reduced-sodium beef broth

1½ cups water

1 6-ounce can tomato paste

3 cloves garlic, minced

1 tablespoon paprika

1 tablespoon caraway seeds

2 teaspoons dried marjoram, crushed

¼ teaspoon black pepper

2 cups coarsely chopped green and/or red sweet pepper (2 large)

½ cup light dairy sour cream

1. Trim fat from meat. Cut meat into ¾-inch pieces. In a 3½- or 4-quart slow cooker combine meat, onion, broth, water, tomato paste, garlic, paprika, caraway seeds, marjoram, and black pepper.

2. Cover and cook on low-heat setting for 8 to 9 hours or on high-heat setting for 4 to 4½ hours. Stir in sweet pepper for the last 45 minutes of cooking. Top each serving with sour cream.

Nutrition Facts per serving: 280 cal., 8 g total fat (3 g sat. fat), 96 mg chol., 259 mg sodium, 15 g carbo., 3 g fiber, 37 g pro.
Exchanges: 2½ Vegetable, 4½ Lean Meat

Home-Style Beef and Vegetables `6 mg iron`

Prep: 20 minutes Cook: 8 to 9 hours (low) or 4 to 4½ hours (high), plus 30 minutes Makes: 8 servings

Nonstick cooking spray

1 3- to 3½-pound boneless beef chuck pot roast

1 0.6-ounce envelope dry Italian salad dressing mix

3 tablespoons quick-cooking tapioca

1 14-ounce can beef broth seasoned with onion

1 16-ounce package loose-pack frozen Italian vegetables (zucchini, carrots, cauliflower, lima beans, Italian beans)

1. Coat a 3½- or 4-quart slow cooker with cooking spray; set aside.

2. Trim fat from meat. Coat a large skillet with cooking spray. Cook meat in hot skillet over medium heat until brown on all sides. Place meat in prepared cooker. Sprinkle with salad dressing mix and tapioca. Add broth.

3. Cover and cook on low-heat setting for 8 to 9 hours or on high-heat setting for 4 to 4½ hours.

4. If using low-heat setting, turn to high-heat setting. Add frozen vegetables to cooker. Cover and cook about 30 minutes more or until vegetables are tender.

Nutrition Facts per serving: 338 cal., 8 g total fat (3 g sat. fat), 134 mg chol., 787 mg sodium, 11 g carbo., 2 g fiber, 50 g pro.
Exchanges: 2½ Other Carbo., 6½ Very Lean Meat, 1 Vegetable, 1 Fat

Roast Beef and Vegetable Soup 5 mg iron

Prep: 15 minutes   Roast: 1 hour Cook: 53 minutes Oven: 350°F Makes: 4 to 5 servings

1 pound boneless beef chuck pot roast

1 tablespoon cooking oil

2 14½-ounce cans diced tomatoes, undrained

1 teaspoon salt

½ teaspoon dried thyme, crushed

1 bay leaf

1 cup water

1½ cups sliced carrot (3 medium)

2 small potatoes, peeled, if desired, and cut into ½-inch cubes

1 cup chopped onion (1 large)

½ cup frozen peas

1. Trim fat from meat. In a large skillet cook meat in hot oil over medium-high heat until brown on all sides. Place meat on a rack in a roasting pan. Roast, uncovered, in a 350° oven for 1 hour. Transfer to a cutting board. Cut into ½-inch cubes.

2. Transfer meat to a 4-quart Dutch oven. Add undrained tomatoes, salt, thyme, and bay leaf. Bring to boiling; reduce heat. Simmer, covered, for 30 minutes. Discard bay leaf.

3. Stir in water, carrot, potato, and onion. Return to boiling; reduce heat. Simmer, covered, about 20 minutes or until vegetables are tender. Stir in peas and cook, covered, for 3 minutes more.

Nutrition Facts per serving: 339 cal., 8 g total fat (2 g sat. fat), 67 mg chol., 1,038 mg sodium, 36 g carbo., 5 g fiber, 29 g pro.
Exchanges: 1½ Starch, 3 Very Lean Meat, 2 Vegetable, 1½ Fat

Gingered Brisket `5 mg iron`

Prep: 20 minutes Cook: 10 to 12 hours (low) or 5 to 6 hours (high) Makes: 6 servings

1 2½- to 3-pound fresh beef brisket

2 4½-ounce jars whole mushrooms, drained

2 tablespoons quick-cooking tapioca

⅓ cup water

¼ cup hoisin sauce

2 tablespoons light soy sauce

1 tablespoon grated fresh ginger

½ teaspoon garlic powder

¼ to ½ teaspoon crushed red pepper

½ cup bias-sliced green onion (4)

3 to 4 cups hot cooked rice

1. Trim fat from meat. If necessary, cut meat to fit into a 3½- or 4-quart slow cooker. Place meat in cooker. Add mushrooms and tapioca.

2. For sauce, in a small bowl combine water, hoisin sauce, soy sauce, ginger, garlic powder, and crushed red pepper. Pour over mixture in cooker.

3. Cover and cook on low-heat setting for 10 to 12 hours or on high-heat setting for 5 to 6 hours.

4. Transfer meat and mushrooms to a serving platter. If necessary, skim fat from sauce. Spoon some of the sauce over meat and mushrooms and sprinkle with sliced green onion. Serve with hot cooked rice. Pass remaining sauce.

Nutrition Facts per serving: 418 cal., 10 g total fat (3 g sat. fat), 109 mg chol., 592 mg sodium, 33 g carbo., 2 g fiber, 44 g pro. **Exchanges:** ½ Vegetable, 1½ Starch, ½ Other Carbo., 5½ Very Lean Meat, ½ Fat

Steak with Onions and Carrots ▸ 6 mg iron

Start to Finish: 1 hour Makes: 4 servings

4 small onions, peeled and cut into wedges

1 tablespoon cooking oil

8 baby carrots with tops

4 small red potatoes, cut up (1 pound)

¾ cup beef broth

1 tablespoon packed brown sugar

1 teaspoon dried thyme, crushed

1 1¼-pound boneless beef top sirloin steak, cut 1½ inches thick

¼ teaspoon salt

¼ teaspoon black pepper

1. In a 12-inch skillet cook onion in hot oil about 5 minutes or until brown, turning occasionally. Remove onion; set aside. Add carrots to skillet; cook about 5 minutes or until light brown, turning occasionally. Remove skillet from heat. Carefully add potato, broth, brown sugar, and ½ teaspoon of the thyme. Return onion to skillet. Return skillet to heat. Bring to boiling; reduce heat. Simmer, covered, for 25 to 30 minutes or until vegetables are tender.

2. Meanwhile, trim fat from meat. Season meat with the remaining ½ teaspoon thyme, the salt, and pepper. Place steak on the unheated rack of a broiler pan. Broil 4 to 5 inches from heat until desired doneness, turning once. (Allow 25 to 27 minutes for medium rare [145°F] or 30 to 32 minutes for medium [160°F].) Cut into 4 pieces.

3. Remove vegetables from skillet with a slotted spoon. Gently boil juices, uncovered, for 1 to 2 minutes or until slightly thickened. Divide steak and vegetables among 4 dinner plates. Spoon juices over.

Nutrition Facts per serving: 358 cal., 9 g total fat (2 g sat. fat), 86 mg chol., 349 mg sodium, 34 g carbo., 5 g fiber, 34 g pro.
Exchanges: 2 Vegetable, 1½ Starch, 3½ Medium-Fat Meat

Spicy Steak and Ranch Salad `5 mg iron`
Start to Finish: 25 minutes Makes: 4 servings

½ cup french-fried onions

1 pound boneless beef top sirloin steak, cut 1 inch thick

1 tablespoon Cajun seasoning

1 tablespoon lime juice

1 clove garlic, minced

Salt (optional)

1 10-ounce package torn European-style salad greens

2 carrots, cut into thin bite-size strips or peeled into thin strips

½ cup thinly sliced radishes

½ cup bottled fat-free ranch salad dressing

1. In a nonstick large skillet cook french-fried onions over medium-high heat about 2 minutes or until brown, stirring occasionally. Remove from skillet; set aside.

2. Trim fat from meat. For rub, in a small bowl combine Cajun seasoning, lime juice, and garlic. Sprinkle evenly over meat; rub in with your fingers. In the same skillet cook meat over medium heat until desired doneness, turning once. (Allow 6 to 8 minutes for medium rare [145°F] or 9 to 12 minutes for medium [160°F].) Cut meat into thin bite-size slices. If desired, season with salt.

3. On a large serving platter toss together the salad greens, carrot strips, and radishes. Arrange meat strips over greens mixture. Drizzle with the ranch dressing. Sprinkle with french-fried onions.

Nutrition Facts per serving: 310 cal., 13 g total fat (4 g sat. fat), 76 mg chol., 557 mg sodium, 16 g carbo., 3 g fiber, 28 g pro.
Exchanges: 2 Vegetable, 2 Lean Meat, 1 Fat

Sizzling Peaches and Steak `6 mg iron`

Start to Finish: 30 minutes Makes: 4 servings

4 slices thick-sliced bacon, cut crosswise into thirds

4 6-ounce boneless beef flat iron, ribeye, or Delmonico steaks, cut ³⁄₄ to 1 inch thick

Salt

Black pepper

Nonstick cooking spray

1 recipe Peach Steak Sauce

2 fresh peaches, pitted and cut into eighths

4 slices Texas toast, toasted

1. In a large skillet cook bacon until crisp and brown. Remove from skillet. Drain on paper towels; set aside. Reserve 1 tablespoon drippings in skillet; set aside.

2. Trim fat from meat; season with salt and pepper. Coat a heavy 12-inch skillet with cooking spray. Preheat skillet over medium-high heat. Add meat. Reduce heat to medium and cook, uncovered, for 8 to 15 minutes for medium rare (145°F) to medium (160°F) doneness, turning occasionally. Brush steaks with ½ cup of the Peach Steak Sauce during the last 5 minutes of cooking.

3. Meanwhile, in the same large skillet cook peaches in the reserved bacon drippings over medium-high heat about 3 minutes or until peaches are brown and heated through, stirring and turning occasionally.

4. To serve, place a toast slice on each of 4 plates. Top with bacon, steak, and peaches. Pass remaining Peach Steak Sauce.

Peach Steak Sauce: Peel, pit, and cut up 2 fresh medium peaches. Place peaches in a blender or food processor. Cover; blend or process until almost smooth. In a small saucepan mix pureed peaches, ¼ cup peach or apricot nectar, 2 tablespoons condensed beef consommé or condensed beef broth, 2 tablespoons balsamic vinegar, 1 tablespoon packed brown sugar, 1 tablespoon minced onion, and ¼ teaspoon ground cinnamon. Bring to boiling; reduce heat. Simmer, uncovered, about 10 minutes or until desired consistency, stirring occasionally.

Nutrition Facts per serving: with sauce: 690 cal., 16 g total fat (6 g sat. fat), 88 mg chol., 840 mg sodium, 87 g carbo., 7 g fiber, 47 g pro. **Exchanges:** 1 Fruit, 2 Starch, 2½ Other Carbo., 6 Lean Meat

Chipotle Pork Chili `6 mg iron`
Start to Finish: 25 minutes Makes: 3 servings

8 ounces lean boneless pork or boneless beef sirloin steak

Nonstick cooking spray

1 teaspoon olive oil

1 cup chopped onion (1 large)

2 cloves garlic, minced

1 14½-ounce can no-salt-added diced tomatoes, undrained

1 8-ounce can no-salt-added tomato sauce

1 cup water

1 canned chipotle pepper in adobo sauce, chopped

1 teaspoon dried basil, crushed

1 teaspoon dried oregano, crushed

1 teaspoon chili powder

¼ teaspoon ground cumin

1½ cups frozen whole kernel corn

1. Trim fat from meat. Cut meat into thin bite-size strips. Lightly coat a large saucepan with cooking spray. Heat over medium-high heat. Add meat. Cook and stir for 2 to 3 minutes or until meat is brown. Remove meat from saucepan and set aside.

2. Carefully add the oil to the hot saucepan. Cook onion and garlic in the hot oil about 4 minutes or until onion is tender. Stir in undrained tomatoes, tomato sauce, water, chipotle pepper, basil, oregano, chili powder, and cumin. Bring to boiling; reduce heat. Simmer, covered, for 15 minutes, stirring occasionally.

3. Stir in frozen corn. Simmer, covered, for 5 minutes more, stirring occasionally. Stir in meat. Heat through.

Nutrition Facts per serving: 355 cal., 12 g total fat (3 g sat. fat), 50 mg chol., 598 mg sodium, 43 g carbo., 4 g fiber, 23 g pro. **Exchanges:** 4 Vegetable, 1½ Starch, 2 Lean Meat, ½ Fat

Tuscan Ham and Bean Soup ◖ 6 mg iron ◗

Prep: 25 minutes Cook: 6 to 8 hours (low) or 3 to 4 hours (high) Makes: 8 servings

3 15-ounce cans small white beans, rinsed and drained

2½ cups cubed cooked ham

1½ cups chopped carrot (3 medium)

1 cup thinly sliced celery (2 stalks)

1 cup chopped onion (1 large)

¼ teaspoon black pepper

2 14½-ounce cans diced tomatoes with garlic and herbs, undrained

2 14-ounce cans reduced-sodium chicken broth

8 cups torn fresh kale or spinach leaves

Freshly shredded Parmesan cheese (optional)

1. In a 5- to 6-quart slow cooker combine beans, ham, carrot, celery, onion, and pepper. Stir in undrained tomatoes and broth.

2. Cover and cook on low-heat setting for 6 to 8 hours or on high-heat setting for 3 to 4 hours. Just before serving, stir in kale. If desired, sprinkle each serving with Parmesan cheese.

Nutrition Facts per serving: 323 cal., 3 g total fat (1 g sat. fat), 21 mg chol., 2,099 mg sodium, 53 g carbo., 12 g fiber, 25 g pro.
Exchanges: 2½ Vegetable, 2½ Starch, 2 Very Lean Meat

Orange and Ginger Chicken [10 mg iron]

Start to Finish: 30 minutes Makes: 4 servings

2 oranges

1 tablespoon cooking oil

2 10-ounce packages fresh
   baby spinach

1 tablespoon light soy sauce

1 teaspoon honey

1 teaspoon grated fresh ginger

½ teaspoon cornstarch

⅛ to ¼ teaspoon crushed
   red pepper

1 pound skinless, boneless
   chicken breast strips

¼ teaspoon salt

¼ teaspoon freshly ground
   black pepper

3 cloves garlic, minced

1. Remove peel and white membrane from 1 orange. Slice orange crosswise; halve slices. Set aside. Squeeze enough juice from the remaining orange to measure ⅓ cup; set aside. In a 4-quart Dutch oven heat 1 teaspoon of the oil over medium heat. Add spinach; cover and cook for 4 to 5 minutes or just until wilted, stirring occasionally. Drain and transfer to a serving platter. Cover and keep warm.

2. Meanwhile, in a small bowl combine the ⅓ cup orange juice, the soy sauce, honey, ginger, cornstarch, and crushed red pepper. Set aside.

3. Sprinkle chicken with salt and black pepper. Wipe out Dutch oven with a paper towel. In Dutch oven heat the remaining 2 teaspoons oil over medium-high heat. Add garlic; cook and stir for 30 seconds. Add chicken; cook and stir for 2 to 3 minutes or until chicken is no longer pink. Stir orange juice mixture; add to chicken in Dutch oven. Cook and stir until thickened and bubbly. Cook and stir for 1 minute more.

4. To serve, arrange orange slices on top of spinach. Spoon chicken mixture over oranges and spinach.

Nutrition Facts per serving: 207 cal., 6 g total fat (1 g sat. fat), 66 mg chol., 521 mg sodium, 8 g carbo., 13 g fiber, 31 g pro.
Exchanges: 2 Vegetable, 4 Very Lean Meat, ½ Fat

Grilled Asian Chicken and Noodles `5 mg iron`

Prep: 20 minutes Grill: 12 minutes Cool: 5 minutes Makes: 4 servings

8 ounces udon or Chinese curly
    noodles

¼ cup light soy sauce

2 tablespoons toasted sesame oil

2 tablespoons rice vinegar

4 cloves garlic, minced

1½ teaspoons grated fresh ginger

¼ teaspoon crushed red pepper

4 medium skinless, boneless
    chicken breast halves (about
    1 pound total)

1 small eggplant, sliced

4 cups packaged shredded
    cabbage with carrot
    (coleslaw mix)

¼ cup chopped cashews
    (optional)

2 to 3 tablespoons snipped
    fresh cilantro

1. Cook noodles according to package directions. Drain; set aside.

2. Meanwhile, combine soy sauce, sesame oil, vinegar, garlic, ginger, and crushed red pepper. Set 2 tablespoons of the soy sauce mixture aside. In a large bowl toss noodles with the remaining soy sauce mixture. Place noodle mixture in freezer to chill quickly.

3. Place chicken on the lightly greased rack of an uncovered grill directly over medium heat. Grill for 12 to 15 minutes or until an instant-read thermometer inserted near the center registers 170°F, turning once and brushing occasionally with the reserved soy sauce mixture. For the last 8 minutes of grilling, place eggplant slices on the rack alongside the chicken; turn once and brush occasionally with reserved soy sauce mixture. Transfer chicken and eggplant to cutting board; cool for 5 minutes and cut into cubes.

4. Toss chicken, eggplant, and cabbage with noodles. Sprinkle with cashews (if desired) and cilantro.

Nutrition Facts per serving: 442 cal., 12 g total fat (2 g sat. fat), 108 mg chol., 646 mg sodium, 51 g carbo., 6 g fiber, 32 g pro.
Exchanges: 2 Vegetable, 2½ Starch, 3 Very Lean Meat, 2 Fat

Southwestern Chicken and Black Bean Salad `5 mg iron`

Start to Finish: 25 minutes Makes: 4 servings

10 cups torn romaine

 1 15-ounce can black beans,
    rinsed and drained

1½ cups chopped cooked chicken
    or turkey (about 8 ounces)

1½ cups red and/or yellow cherry
    tomatoes, halved

 ½ cup bottled reduced-calorie
    Caesar salad dressing

 2 teaspoons chili powder

 ½ teaspoon ground cumin

 2 tablespoons snipped fresh
    cilantro or parsley

 ½ cup broken tortilla chips

1. In a large bowl combine romaine, black beans, chicken, and tomatoes. Set aside.

2. For dressing, in a small bowl whisk together salad dressing, chili powder, and cumin. Pour dressing over salad. Toss lightly to coat. Sprinkle with cilantro and tortilla chips.

Nutrition Facts per serving: 295 cal., 10 g total fat (1 g sat. fat), 55 mg chol., 913 mg sodium, 26 g carbo., 9 g fiber, 27 g pro.
Exchanges: 3 Vegetable, 1 Starch, 2½ Very Lean Meat, 1 Fat

Manhattan Clam Chowder `16 mg iron`

Start to Finish: 40 minutes Makes: 4 servings

1 pint shucked, fresh clams or two 6½-ounce cans minced clams

1 cup chopped celery (2 stalks)

⅓ cup chopped onion (1 small)

¼ cup chopped carrot (1 small)

2 tablespoons olive oil or cooking oil

1 8-ounce bottle clam juice or 1 cup chicken broth

2 cups red potatoes cut into bite-size pieces

1 teaspoon dried thyme, crushed

⅛ teaspoon cayenne pepper

⅛ teaspoon black pepper

1 14½-ounce can diced tomatoes, undrained

2 tablespoons purchased cooked bacon pieces

1. Chop fresh clams (if using), reserving juice; set clams aside. Strain clam juice to remove bits of shell. (Or drain canned clams, reserving juice.) If necessary, add enough water to reserved clam juice to equal 1½ cups liquid. Set juice aside.

2. In a large saucepan cook celery, onion, and carrot in hot oil until tender. Stir in the reserved 1½ cups clam juice and the bottled clam juice. Stir in potato, thyme, cayenne pepper, and black pepper. Bring to boiling; reduce heat. Simmer, covered, for 10 minutes. Stir in tomatoes, clams, and bacon. Return to boiling; reduce heat. Cook for 1 to 2 minutes more or until heated through.

Nutrition Facts per serving: 264 cal., 10 g total fat (2 g sat. fat), 43 mg chol., 375 mg sodium, 23 g carbo., 3 g fiber, 18 g pro.
Exchanges: 1 Vegetable, 1 Starch, 2 Medium-Fat Meat, 1 Fat

Shortcut Shrimp Risotto `6 mg iron`

Prep: 10 minutes Cook: 21 minutes Makes: 4 servings

 2 14-ounce cans reduced-sodium
    chicken broth

1⅓ cups Arborio rice or short grain
    white rice

 ½ cup finely chopped onion
    (1 medium)

 ¾ teaspoon dried basil, crushed,
    or 1 tablespoon fresh snipped
    basil (optional)

 1 12-ounce package frozen
    peeled and cooked shrimp,
    thawed

1½ cups frozen peas, thawed

 ¼ cup grated Parmesan cheese

1. In a large saucepan combine broth, rice, onion, and dried basil (if using). Bring mixture to boiling; reduce heat. Simmer, covered, for 18 minutes.

2. Stir in shrimp and peas. Cover and cook 3 minutes more (do not lift lid). Stir in fresh basil (if using). Sprinkle Parmesan cheese over each serving.

Nutrition Facts per serving: 325 cal., 3 g total fat (1 g sat. fat), 171 mg chol., 842 mg sodium, 45 g carbo., 3 g fiber, 29 g pro. **Exchanges:** 3 Starch, 3 Very Lean Meat

Crispy Tofu and Vegetables `11 mg iron`

Prep: 15 minutes Cook: 9 minutes Stand: 1 hour Makes: 4 servings

1 10½-ounce package light extra-firm tofu (fresh bean curd), well drained

3 tablespoons light soy sauce

8 green onions

8 ounces fresh pea pods (2 cups)

1 tablespoon toasted sesame oil

1 medium red sweet pepper, cut into thin strips

1 medium yellow sweet pepper, cut into thin strips

2 tablespoons cornmeal

1 tablespoon white sesame seeds, toasted* (optional)

1. Cut tofu crosswise into 8 slices. Arrange slices in a single layer in a shallow baking pan. Pour soy sauce over tofu; turn slices to coat. Cover and let stand for 1 hour.

2. Meanwhile, trim ends of green onions, leaving 3 inches of white and light green parts. (Reserve the dark green ends for another use.) Cut green onions in half lengthwise, forming 16 strips. Trim ends of pea pods and remove strings; cut pea pods in half lengthwise.

3. Pour sesame oil into a 12-inch nonstick skillet. Preheat over medium-high heat. Stir-fry sweet peppers in hot oil for 1 minute. Add green onions and pea pods. Stir-fry for 2 to 3 minutes more or until vegetables are crisp-tender. Remove skillet from heat. Drain tofu, reserving soy sauce. Stir the soy sauce into cooked vegetables. Transfer to a serving platter; cover and keep warm.

4. Carefully dip the tofu slices in cornmeal to lightly coat both sides. In the same skillet cook tofu about 6 minutes or until crisp and heated through, gently turning once.

5. To serve, arrange the tofu slices over cooked vegetables. If desired, sprinkle with sesame seeds. Serve immediately.

*Note: To toast sesame seeds, in a nonstick skillet cook and stir sesame seeds over medium heat about 1 minute or just until golden brown. Watch closely so the seeds don't burn. Remove from heat and transfer to a bowl to cool completely.

Nutrition Facts per serving: 198 cal., 10 g total fat (1 g sat. fat), 0 mg chol., 410 mg sodium, 14 g carbo., 3 g fiber, 16 g pro.
Exchanges: 1½ Vegetable, 1 Lean Meat, ½ Fat

Layered Bean and Potato Pie 6 mg iron

Prep: 25 minutes Bake: 45 minutes Oven: 350°F Makes: 5 servings

1 pound small red potatoes, thinly sliced

1 cup chopped onion (1 large)

1 cup sliced celery (2 stalks)

4 cloves garlic, minced

¼ teaspoon cracked black pepper

1 tablespoon cooking oil

1 15-ounce can garbanzo beans (chickpeas), rinsed and drained

1 15-ounce can small red beans, rinsed and drained

1 cup frozen peas

1 cup chopped green sweet pepper

1 10¾-ounce can condensed cream of potato soup

¼ cup fat-free milk

½ teaspoon ground cumin

½ teaspoon ground coriander

½ cup shredded reduced-fat Monterey Jack cheese (2 ounces)

1. In a large saucepan cook potato slices, covered, in enough boiling water to cover for 4 to 5 minutes or until nearly tender. Drain. Run cold water over potato slices in colander. Drain; set aside.

2. Wash and dry pan. In the saucepan cook onion, celery, garlic, and black pepper in hot oil about 5 minutes or until vegetables are tender. Mash ½ cup of the garbanzo beans; add to vegetable mixture along with remaining garbanzo beans, red beans, peas, sweet pepper, soup, milk, cumin, and coriander. Gently stir to combine.

3. Grease a 2-quart casserole. Place a single layer of potato slices in casserole. Spoon bean mixture on top and cover with remaining potato slices in layers, overlapping if necessary.

4. Bake, covered, in a 350° oven for 35 minutes. Uncover and sprinkle with cheese. Bake about 10 minutes more or until the cheese melts.

To Make Ahead: Prepare as directed through step 3. Cover tightly and chill overnight. To serve, cover and bake in a 350°F oven about 1 hour or until heated through. Uncover and sprinkle with cheese. Bake, uncovered, about 5 minutes more or until the cheese melts.

Nutrition Facts per serving: 376 cal., 8 g total fat (2 g sat. fat), 11 mg chol., 1,073 mg sodium, 63 g carbo., 12 g fiber, 19 g pro.
Exchanges: ½ Vegetable, 3½ Starch, 1 Very Lean Meat, 1 Fat

high-fiber recipes

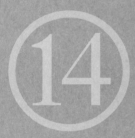

Fiber is key to healthy digestion, but sometimes it's hard to get enough. This is especially true if you eat a lot of processed or packaged foods, which tend to be low in fiber. This chapter is full of recipes that can help you get the fiber you need.

Fruit Granola 5 g fiber

Prep: 20 minutes Bake: 25 minutes Oven: 325°F Makes: 10 servings

Nonstick cooking spray

3 cups regular rolled oats

⅓ cup toasted wheat germ

⅓ cup unsalted, shelled sunflower seeds

⅓ cup sliced almonds

3 tablespoons nonfat dry milk powder

1½ teaspoons ground cinnamon

⅓ cup orange juice

⅓ cup honey

1 tablespoon cooking oil

1 cup mixed dried fruit bits

Milk (optional)

1. Lightly coat a 15×10×1-inch baking pan with cooking spray; set aside. In a large bowl stir together oats, wheat germ, sunflower seeds, almonds, milk powder, and cinnamon.

2. In a small bowl stir together orange juice, honey, and oil. Pour juice mixture over oat mixture; toss to coat. Spread in the prepared baking pan.

3. Bake in a 325° oven about 25 minutes or until oats are light brown, stirring twice. Immediately turn out onto a large piece of foil. Stir in fruit bits. Cool completely. If desired, serve the granola with milk.

4. To store, spoon granola into food storage bags or containers and store at room temperature up to 2 weeks. For longer storage, spoon granola into freezer bags or containers. Seal, label, and freeze up to 3 months.

Nutrition Facts per serving: 272 cal., 8 g total fat (1 g sat. fat), 0 mg chol., 18 mg sodium, 44 g carbo., 5 g fiber, 8 g pro.
Exchanges: 1 Fruit, 2 Starch, 1 Fat

Breakfast Couscous with Fruit `5 g fiber`

Start to Finish: 15 minutes Makes: 4 servings

1   cup fat-free milk

¼ teaspoon ground cinnamon

     Dash ground nutmeg

1   cup couscous

⅓ cup orange juice

1   cup fresh cranberries

2   tablespoons water

2   tablespoons honey

1   11-ounce can mandarin orange
     sections, drained

2   tablespoons slivered almonds,
     toasted

1. In a medium saucepan combine milk, cinnamon, and nutmeg. Bring to boiling over medium heat. Stir in couscous. Cover and remove from heat; let stand for 5 minutes. Stir in orange juice. Fluff with a fork.

2. Meanwhile, in a small saucepan combine cranberries, water, and honey. Cook over low heat for 4 to 5 minutes or until cranberry skins begin to pop. Remove from heat. Gently stir in mandarin oranges.

3. To serve, spoon the couscous mixture into serving bowls. Top with warm cranberry-orange mixture. Sprinkle with almonds.

Nutrition Facts per serving: 298 cal., 3 g total fat (0 g sat. fat), 1 mg chol., 35 mg sodium, 60 g carbo., 5 g fiber, 10 g pro.
Exchanges: 1 Fruit, 3 Starch

Granola French Toast `6 g fiber`

Start to Finish: 40 minutes Makes: 4 servings

3 eggs, slightly beaten

¾ cup reduced-fat or fat-free milk

1 tablespoon sugar

1 tablespoon finely shredded orange peel

½ teaspoon vanilla

¼ teaspoon ground cinnamon

12 ½-inch bias-cut slices baguette-style French bread

2 tablespoons butter

1 cup granola, coarsely crushed

1 recipe Cinnamon Yogurt Sauce

Maple syrup (optional)

1. In a shallow bowl whisk together eggs, milk, sugar, 1½ teaspoons of the orange peel, the vanilla, and cinnamon. Dip bread slices into egg mixture, coating both sides.

2. In a large skillet or on a griddle melt 1 tablespoon of the butter over medium heat; add half of the bread slices. Sprinkle some of the granola on top of each slice of bread in the skillet, pressing in gently with spatula so granola sticks. Cook for 2 to 3 minutes or until bottoms are golden brown. Flip slices, pressing lightly with the spatula. Cook about 2 minutes more or until golden brown. When removing from pan, flip slices so granola side is on top. Repeat with remaining butter, bread slices, and granola. Serve immediately with Cinnamon Yogurt Sauce, remaining orange peel, and, if desired, maple syrup.

Cinnamon Yogurt Sauce: In a small bowl combine 1 cup plain low-fat yogurt, 1 tablespoon honey, ¼ teaspoon ground cinnamon (if desired), and ¼ teaspoon vanilla. Makes about 1 cup.

Nutrition Facts per serving: 501 cal., 16 g total fat (7 g sat. fat), 183 mg chol., 516 mg sodium, 70 g carbo., 6 g fiber, 20 g pro.
Exchanges: ½ Milk, 3 Starch, 1 Other Carbo., 1 Medium-Fat Meat, 1½ Fat

Chicken Salad with Berry Dressing [6 g fiber]

Prep: 20 minutes Broil: 12 minutes Makes: 4 servings

1 10-ounce package frozen red raspberries, thawed

2 tablespoons olive oil or salad oil

2 tablespoons lemon juice

1 clove garlic, minced

4 skinless, boneless chicken breast halves

2 tablespoons honey-mustard

7 cups torn mixed salad greens

2 medium oranges, peeled and sectioned

1 pink grapefruit, peeled and sectioned

1 avocado, halved, pitted, peeled, and sliced lengthwise

2 green onions, thinly bias-sliced

1. For raspberry vinaigrette, in a blender or food processor combine raspberries, oil, lemon juice, and garlic. Cover and blend or process until smooth. Strain dressing through a sieve; discard seeds. Cover and refrigerate dressing until serving time.

2. Place chicken on the unheated rack of a broiler pan; broil 4 to 5 inches from the heat for 12 to 15 minutes or until chicken is tender and no longer pink (170°F), turning once and brushing with honey-mustard during the last 2 minutes of broiling. Cool chicken slightly; cut into $\frac{1}{4}$-inch strips.

3. In a large bowl toss together chicken strips, salad greens, orange sections, grapefruit sections, and avocado slices. Divide salad mixture among 4 dinner plates. Sprinkle with green onion. Drizzle each salad with 2 tablespoons of the raspberry vinaigrette. (Store remaining dressing in refrigerator up to 1 week; use on tossed salads.)

Nutrition Facts per serving: 340 cal., 11 g total fat (2 g sat. fat), 66 mg chol., 145 mg sodium, 32 g carbo., 6 g fiber, 29 g pro.
Exchanges: 2 Vegetable, 1½ Fruit, 3½ Medium-Fat Meat, 1½ Fat

Apple-Glazed Chicken and Spinach Salad 5 g fiber

Start to Finish: 30 minutes Makes: 2 servings

¼ cup apple jelly

1 tablespoon light soy sauce

½ teaspoon dried thyme, crushed

½ teaspoon finely shredded
 lemon peel

½ teaspoon grated fresh ginger

2 medium skinless, boneless
 chicken breast halves

 Salt (optional)

 Black pepper (optional)

 Nonstick cooking spray

1 cup chopped, peeled apple
 (1 large)

¼ cup sliced onion

1 clove garlic, minced

6 cups packaged prewashed
 spinach, stems removed

1. For glaze, in a small saucepan stir together apple jelly, soy sauce, thyme, lemon peel, and ginger. Cook over low heat just until jelly melts, stirring once. Reserve 2 tablespoons of the glaze.

2. If desired, lightly sprinkle chicken with salt and pepper. Place chicken on the unheated rack of a broiler pan. Broil 4 to 5 inches from the heat for 12 to 15 minutes or until chicken is tender and no longer pink (170°F), turning once and brushing with the remaining glaze the last 5 minutes of broiling.

3. Meanwhile, lightly coat a large saucepan with cooking spray. Add apple, onion, and garlic; cook and stir for 3 minutes over medium heat. Stir in the reserved 2 tablespoons glaze; bring to boiling. Add spinach; toss just until wilted. Remove from heat.

4. To serve, slice each chicken breast half crosswise into 6 to 8 pieces. Divide spinach mixture between 2 dinner plates. Top with the sliced chicken.

Nutrition Facts per serving: 302 cal., 2 g total fat (1 g sat. fat), 66 mg chol., 433 mg sodium, 42 g carbo., 5 g fiber, 30 g pro.
Exchanges: 3 Vegetable, ½ Fruit, 1 Other Carbo., 3 Very Lean Meat

Kale, Lentil, and Chicken Soup ▐ 5 g fiber ▌

Prep: 25 minutes Cook: 25 minutes Makes: 6 servings

1 tablespoon olive oil

1 cup chopped onion (1 large)

1 cup coarsely chopped carrot (2 medium)

2 cloves garlic, minced

6 cups reduced-sodium chicken broth

1 tablespoon snipped fresh basil or 1 teaspoon dried basil, crushed

4 cups coarsely chopped kale (about 8 ounces)

$\frac{1}{2}$ teaspoon salt

$\frac{1}{8}$ teaspoon black pepper

$1\frac{1}{2}$ cups cubed cooked chicken or turkey

1 medium tomato, seeded and chopped

$\frac{1}{2}$ cup red lentils, rinsed and drained

1. In a large saucepan heat oil over medium-low heat. Add onion, carrot, and garlic. Cover and cook for 5 to 7 minutes or until vegetables are nearly tender, stirring occasionally.

2. Add broth and dried basil (if using) to vegetable mixture. Bring to boiling; reduce heat. Simmer, covered, for 10 minutes. Stir in kale, salt, and pepper. Return to boiling; reduce heat. Simmer, covered, for 10 minutes.

3. Stir in chicken, tomato, lentils, and fresh basil (if using). Simmer, covered, for 5 to 10 minutes more or until kale and lentils are tender.

Nutrition Facts per serving: 199 cal., 5 g total fat (1 g sat. fat), 31 mg chol., 833 mg sodium, 20 g carbo., 5 g fiber, 19 g pro.
Exchanges: 1 Vegetable, 1 Starch, 1½ Lean Meat, ½ Fat

Turkey Sausage and Bean Soup `11 g fiber`

Start to Finish: 25 minutes Makes: 4 servings

4 cups reduced-sodium
  chicken broth

2 15-ounce cans cannellini (white
  kidney), Great Northern, or
  red kidney beans, rinsed and
  drained

½ pound cooked turkey kielbasa,
  halved lengthwise and cut
  into ½-inch pieces

½ cup chopped onion (1 medium)

1 teaspoon dried basil, crushed

¼ teaspoon coarsely ground black
  pepper

1 clove garlic, minced

3 cups packaged prewashed
  spinach

1. In a large saucepan or Dutch oven combine broth, beans, kielbasa, onion, basil, pepper, and garlic. Bring to boiling; reduce heat. Simmer, covered, for 10 to 15 minutes or until onion is tender.

2. Meanwhile, remove stems from spinach. Stack the leaves one on top of the other and cut into 1-inch-wide strips. Just before serving, stir spinach into soup.

Nutrition Facts per serving: 236 cal., 5 g total fat (0 g sat. fat), 0 mg chol., 1,445 mg sodium, 34 g carbo., 11 g fiber, 26 g pro.
Exchanges: 1 Vegetable, 1½ Starch, 1½ Very Lean Meat, 1 Lean Meat

Curried Beef with Apple Couscous `8 g fiber`
Prep: 20 minutes Broil: 15 minutes Makes: 4 servings

10 ounces boneless beef top
   sirloin steak, cut 1 inch thick

Salt

Black pepper

1 tablespoon apple jelly

½ teaspoon curry powder

2 medium tart green apples,
  chopped

1 medium red and/or green
  sweet pepper, cut into thin
  strips

½ cup coarsely chopped onion
  (1 medium)

1 teaspoon cooking oil

1 tablespoon curry powder

2 cups apple juice or water

1 tablespoon instant beef
  bouillon granules

1 10-ounce package couscous

⅓ cup chopped peanuts

1. Trim fat from meat. Lightly sprinkle meat with salt and black pepper. For glaze, in a small saucepan combine apple jelly and the ½ teaspoon curry powder. Cook and stir over medium heat until jelly melts.

2. Place meat on the unheated rack of a broiler pan. Broil 3 to 4 inches from the heat until desired doneness, turning meat over after half of the broiling time and brushing occasionally with glaze during the last 2 to 3 minutes of broiling. Allow 15 to 17 minutes for medium rare (145°F) or 20 to 22 minutes for medium (160°F).

3. Meanwhile, in a large skillet cook apple, sweet pepper, and onion in hot oil over medium heat for 5 minutes. Stir in the 1 tablespoon curry powder. Cook and stir for 1 minute. Add juice and bouillon granules. Bring to boiling. Stir in couscous; remove from heat. Cover and let stand about 5 minutes or until liquid is absorbed.

4. To serve, fluff the couscous with a fork. Thinly slice the meat across the grain. Serve the sliced meat on top of the couscous. Sprinkle with peanuts.

Nutrition Facts per serving: 506 cal., 11 g total fat (2 g sat. fat), 43 mg chol., 818 mg sodium, 74 g carbo., 8 g fiber, 29 g pro.
Exchanges: ½ Vegetable, 1 Fruit, 3½ Starch, 1 Medium-Fat Meat

Taco Soup `13 g fiber`

Prep: 15 minutes Cook: 1 hour Makes: 8 servings

1 pound lean ground beef

1 15-ounce can black-eyed peas, undrained

1 15-ounce can black beans, undrained

1 15-ounce can chili beans in chili gravy, undrained

1 15-ounce can garbanzo beans (chickpeas), undrained

1 14½-ounce can Mexican-style stewed tomatoes, undrained

1 11-ounce can whole kernel corn with sweet peppers, undrained

1 1.25-ounce package taco seasoning mix

   Light dairy sour cream

   Salsa

   Tortilla chips

1. In a 4-quart Dutch oven cook ground beef until brown; drain off fat. Stir in undrained black-eyed peas, undrained black beans, undrained chili beans, undrained garbanzo beans, undrained tomatoes, and undrained corn. Stir in taco seasoning mix until well combined.

2. Bring mixture to boiling; reduce heat. Simmer, covered, for 1 to 2 hours, stirring occasionally. Serve with sour cream, salsa, and tortilla chips.

Slow Cooker Directions: In a large skillet cook ground beef until brown. Drain off fat. Place meat in a 3½- or 4-quart slow cooker. Stir in undrained black-eyed peas, undrained black beans, undrained chili beans, undrained garbanzo beans, undrained tomatoes, and undrained corn. Stir in taco seasoning mix until well combined. Cover and cook on low-heat setting for 6 to 8 hours or on high-heat setting for 3 to 4 hours. Serve as above.

Nutrition Facts per serving: 443 cal., 13 g total fat (4 g sat. fat), 41 mg chol., 1,496 mg sodium, 60 g carbo., 13 g fiber, 27 g pro.
Exchanges: 1 Vegetable, 3½ Starch, 1½ Very Lean Meat, 1 Medium-Fat Meat, ½ Fat

Fajita Chops 7 g fiber

Prep: 20 minutes Broil: 9 minutes Stand: 30 minutes Makes: 4 servings

1 lime

1 15-ounce can Great Northern beans, rinsed and drained

1 large mango, pitted, peeled, and chopped, or 2 medium nectarines or peaches, peeled, pitted, and chopped

1 small roma tomato, seeded and chopped

1/4 cup sliced green onion (2)

2 tablespoons cider vinegar

1 tablespoon finely chopped, seeded fresh jalapeño chile pepper* (optional)

1 teaspoon sugar

1 1/2 teaspoons fajita seasoning

2 cloves garlic, minced

4 boneless pork loin chops, cut 3/4 inch thick (about 1 1/2 pounds)

Lime wedges (optional)

1. Finely shred 1/2 teaspoon peel from lime. Squeeze juice from lime. Reserve 2 teaspoons lime juice for pork chops.

2. For salad, in a medium bowl combine finely shredded lime peel, remaining lime juice, beans, mango, tomato, green onion, vinegar, jalapeño pepper (if desired), sugar, 1/2 teaspoon of the fajita seasoning, and the garlic. Let stand at room temperature for 30 minutes, stirring occasionally. (Or cover and refrigerate up to 24 hours.)

3. Trim fat from chops. Brush the reserved 2 teaspoons lime juice onto both sides of each chop. Sprinkle chops with the remaining 1 teaspoon fajita seasoning; pat into meat with your fingers.

4. Preheat broiler. Place chops on the unheated rack of a broiler pan. Broil 3 to 4 inches from the heat for 9 to 11 minutes or until juices run clear (160°F), turning once. Slice chops and serve with salad. If desired, serve with lime wedges.

*Note: When working with chile peppers, wear plastic or rubber gloves. If your bare hands do touch the peppers, wash your hands well with soap and water.

Grilling Directions: Prepare as above through step 3. Place chops on the rack of an uncovered grill directly over medium coals. Grill for 12 to 15 minutes or until juices run clear (160°F), turning once. Slice chops and serve with salad.

Nutrition Facts per serving: 385 cal., 9 g total fat (3 g sat. fat), 93 mg chol., 402 mg sodium, 32 g carbo., 7 g fiber, 43 g pro.
Exchanges: 1/2 Fruit, 1 1/2 Starch, 5 Medium-Fat Meat

Caribbean-Style Pork Stew 7 g fiber

Start to Finish: 30 minutes Makes: 6 servings

1 15-ounce can black beans,
   rinsed and drained

1 14-ounce can beef broth

1³/₄ cups water

12 ounces cooked pork, cut into
    bite-size strips

3 plantains, peeled and sliced

1 cup chopped tomato
   (2 medium)

¹/₂ of a 16-ounce package (2 cups)
   frozen pepper stir-fry
   vegetables (yellow, green, and
   red sweet peppers and onion)

1 tablespoon grated fresh ginger

1 teaspoon ground cumin

¹/₄ teaspoon salt

¹/₄ teaspoon crushed red pepper

3 cups hot cooked brown or
   white rice

1. In a Dutch oven combine black beans, broth, and water; heat to boiling.

2. Add the pork, plantain, and tomato to the bean mixture. Stir in the frozen vegetables, ginger, cumin, salt, and crushed red pepper. Return mixture to boiling; reduce heat. Simmer, covered, about 10 minutes or until the plantain is tender. Serve with hot cooked rice.

Nutrition Facts per serving: 401 cal., 7 g total fat (2 g sat. fat), 46 mg chol., 543 mg sodium, 64 g carbo., 7 g fiber, 25 g pro.
Exchanges: 1 Vegetable, 2 Fruit, 2 Starch, 2¹/₂ Medium-Fat Meat

Mediterranean Shrimp Packets `7 g fiber`

Prep: 25 minutes Bake: 25 minutes Oven: 425°F Makes: 4 servings

8 ounces fresh or frozen medium shrimp, peeled and deveined, with tails

1 cup quick-cooking couscous

1 cup boiling water

2 small zucchini and/or yellow summer squash, halved lengthwise and thinly sliced

1 small red, yellow, or green sweet pepper, cut into bite-size strips

1 9-ounce package frozen artichoke hearts, thawed

1/4 teaspoon coarsely ground black pepper

1/8 teaspoon salt

1/2 cup bottled reduced-calorie Italian salad dressing

1/4 cup thinly sliced fresh basil or fresh spinach

1. Thaw shrimp, if frozen. Rinse shrimp; pat dry with paper towels. Set aside. Cut four 16×12-inch pieces of parchment or use precut sheets. (Or tear off four 24×18-inch pieces of heavy foil. Fold each piece in half to make four 18×12-inch pieces.)

2. In a small saucepan combine couscous and boiling water; cover and let stand for 5 minutes. Divide couscous mixture, shrimp, squash, sweet pepper, and artichokes evenly among the 4 pieces of parchment. Sprinkle with black pepper and salt. Drizzle with salad dressing.

3. Bring together 2 opposite edges of parchment or foil; seal with a double fold. Fold remaining ends to completely enclose the food, allowing space for steam to build. Place the packets in a single layer on a baking pan.

4. Bake in a 425° oven about 25 minutes or until shrimp turn opaque (carefully open a packet to check). Carefully open packets and sprinkle with basil.

Nutrition Facts per serving: 292 cal., 3 g total fat (0 g sat. fat), 88 mg chol., 696 mg sodium, 46 g carbo., 7 g fiber, 20 g pro.
Exchanges: 2 Vegetable, 2 Starch, 1½ Medium-Fat Meat

Slow Cooker Stuffed Peppers `11 g fiber`

Prep: 15 minutes Cook: 6 to 6½ hours (low) or 3 to 3½ hours (high) Makes: 4 servings

4 medium green, red, or yellow
   sweet peppers

1 cup converted rice, cooked
   according to package
   directions

1 12-ounce package frozen
   cooked and crumbled ground
   meat substitute (soy protein)

1 cup shredded reduced-fat
   mozzarella cheese (4 ounces)

1 teaspoon fennel seeds, crushed

½ teaspoon crushed red pepper

½ teaspoon dried thyme, crushed

½ teaspoon paprika

½ teaspoon black pepper

2 cups light spaghetti sauce

¼ cup water

1. Remove tops, membranes, and seeds from sweet peppers. In a medium bowl stir together rice, ground meat substitute, ½ cup of the cheese, the fennel seeds, crushed red pepper, thyme, paprika, and black pepper. Spoon rice mixture into peppers. Pour spaghetti sauce and water into a 5- to 6-quart slow cooker. Place peppers, filled sides up, in cooker.

2. Cover and cook on low-heat setting for 6 to 6½ hours or on high-heat setting for 3 to 3½ hours. Transfer peppers to a serving platter. Spoon sauce over peppers and sprinkle with remaining cheese.

Nutrition Facts per serving: 434 cal., 5 g total fat (3 g sat. fat), 10 mg chol., 568 mg sodium, 69 g carbo., 11 g fiber, 32 g pro.
Exchanges: 1 Vegetable, 2½ Starch, 1½ Other Carbo., 2½ Very Lean Meat

Vegetable Two-Grain Casserole `17 g fiber`

Prep: 15 minutes Bake: 1¼ hours Stand: 5 minutes Oven: 350°F Makes: 4 servings

1 cup fresh small mushrooms, quartered

1 cup sliced carrot (2 medium)

1 18.8-ounce can ready-to-serve lentil soup

1 15-ounce can black beans, rinsed and drained

1 cup frozen whole kernel corn

½ cup regular barley

⅓ cup bulgur

¼ cup chopped onion

½ teaspoon black pepper

¼ teaspoon salt

½ cup water

½ cup shredded cheddar cheese (2 ounces)

1. In a 2-quart casserole combine mushrooms, carrot, lentil soup, black beans, corn, barley, bulgur, onion, pepper, and salt; stir in the water.

2. Bake, covered, in a 350° oven about 1¼ hours or until barley and bulgur are tender, stirring twice. Stir again; sprinkle with cheese. Cover and let stand about 5 minutes or until cheese melts.

Nutrition Facts per serving: 384 cal., 8 g total fat (3 g sat. fat), 15 mg chol., 929 mg sodium, 66 g carbo., 17 g fiber, 22 g pro. **Exchanges:** 1 Vegetable, 4 Starch, 1 Fat

Vegetable Stew `10 g fiber`

Prep: 15 minutes Cook: 9 to 11 hours (low) or 4½ to 5½ hours (high) Makes: 5 servings

1 pound potatoes, cut into
  1-inch cubes

1 cup chopped onion (1 large)

1 cup sliced carrot (2 medium)

1 15-ounce can red kidney beans,
  rinsed and drained

1 15-ounce can tomato sauce

1 14½-ounce can diced tomatoes
  with basil, garlic, and oregano,
  undrained

1 10-ounce package frozen
  whole kernel corn

2 teaspoons steak sauce

⅔ cup shredded cheddar cheese

1. In a 3½- or 4-quart slow cooker combine potato, onion, carrot, beans, tomato sauce, undrained tomatoes, corn, and steak sauce.

2. Cover and cook on low-heat setting for 9 to 11 hours or on high-heat setting for 4½ to 5½ hours. Serve stew in bowls; sprinkle with cheese.

Nutrition Facts per serving: 325 cal., 6 g total fat (3 g sat. fat), 16 mg chol., 1,219 mg sodium, 60 g carbo., 10 g fiber, 16 g pro.
Exchanges: 1½ Vegetable, 3 Starch, ½ High-Fat Meat

Tomato and Lentil Medley `21 g fiber`

Prep: 25 minutes Cook: 30 minutes Makes: 4 servings

1 cup chopped green sweet pepper (1 large)

1 cup chopped yellow sweet pepper (1 large)

1 cup sliced celery (2 stalks)

1 cup chopped onion (1 large)

4 cloves garlic, minced

2 tablespoons olive oil or cooking oil

1½ cups water

1 10-ounce can condensed vegetarian vegetable soup

1 cup brown lentils, rinsed and drained

½ teaspoon salt

½ teaspoon ground turmeric

1 cup chopped, seeded tomato (2 medium)

1 cup frozen peas, thawed

¼ cup snipped fresh parsley (optional)

Salt

Black pepper

1. In a large saucepan cook green and yellow sweet peppers, celery, onion, and garlic in hot oil until vegetables are tender. Stir in the water, soup, lentils, the ½ teaspoon salt, and the turmeric.

2. Bring to boiling; reduce heat. Simmer, covered, about 30 minutes or until lentils are tender and liquid is absorbed, stirring twice during cooking. Stir in tomato, peas, and, if desired, parsley. Heat through. Season to taste with additional salt and black pepper.

Nutrition Facts per serving: 353 cal., 8 g total fat (1 g sat. fat), 0 mg chol., 831 mg sodium, 56 g carbo., 21 g fiber, 19 g pro.
Exchanges: 1½ Vegetable, 3 Starch, 1 Very Lean Meat, 1 Fat

Southwestern Black Bean Cakes with Guacamole

Prep: 20 minutes Grill: 8 minutes Makes: 4 servings   9 g fiber

½ of a medium avocado, peeled

1 tablespoon lime juice

Salt

Black pepper

2 slices whole wheat bread, torn

3 tablespoons fresh cilantro leaves

2 cloves garlic

1 15-ounce can black beans, rinsed and drained

1 canned chipotle pepper in adobo sauce

1 to 2 teaspoons adobo sauce

1 teaspoon ground cumin

1 egg, slightly beaten

1 small roma tomato, chopped

1. For guacamole, in a small bowl mash avocado. Stir in lime juice; season to taste with salt and black pepper. Cover surface with plastic wrap and set aside until ready to serve.

2. Place torn bread in a food processor or blender. Cover and process or blend until bread resembles coarse crumbs. Transfer bread crumbs to a large bowl; set aside.

3. Place cilantro and garlic in the food processor or blender. Cover and process or blend until finely chopped. Add the beans, chipotle pepper, adobo sauce, and cumin. Cover and process or blend using on/off pulses until beans are coarsely chopped and mixture begins to pull away from side of container. Add mixture to bread crumbs in bowl. Add egg; mix well. Shape into four ½-inch-thick patties.

4. Lightly grease a grill rack. For a charcoal grill, grill patties on the lightly greased rack of an uncovered grill directly over medium coals for 8 to 10 minutes or until patties are heated through, turning once halfway through grilling. (For a gas grill, preheat grill. Reduce heat to medium. Place patties on lightly greased rack. Cover; grill as above.) Serve the patties with guacamole and tomato.

Nutrition Facts per serving: 178 cal., 7 g total fat (1 g sat. fat), 53 mg chol., 487 mg sodium, 25 g carbo., 9 g fiber, 11 g pro.
Exchanges: ½ Vegetable, ½ Starch, ½ Lean Meat

Farmer's Market Vegetable Soup `8 g fiber`

Prep: 30 minutes Cook: 8 to 9 hours (low) or 4 to 4½ hours (high), plus 20 minutes (high)
Makes: 4 servings

½ of a small rutabaga, peeled and chopped (2 cups)

2 large roma tomatoes, chopped

2 medium carrots or parsnips, chopped

1 large red-skinned potato, chopped

2 medium leeks, chopped

3 14-ounce cans vegetable broth

1 teaspoon fennel seeds, crushed

½ teaspoon dried sage, crushed

½ to ¼ teaspoon black pepper

½ cup dried tiny bow tie pasta

3 cups torn fresh spinach

1. In a 3½- or 4-quart slow cooker combine rutabaga, tomato, carrot, potato, and leek. Add broth, fennel seeds, sage, and pepper.

2. Cover and cook on low-heat setting for 8 to 9 hours or on high-heat setting for 4 to 4½ hours. If using low-heat setting, turn to high-heat setting. Stir in pasta. Cover and cook for 20 to 30 minutes more or until pasta is tender. Just before serving, stir in spinach.

Nutrition Facts per serving: 198 cal., 2 g total fat (0 g sat. fat), 0 mg chol., 1,313 mg sodium, 41 g carbo., 8 g fiber, 8 g pro.
Exchanges: 2 Vegetable, 2 Starch

Herb and Pepper Lentil Stew   `10 g fiber`

Start to Finish: 35 minutes   Makes: 4 servings

1 tablespoon cooking oil

2 medium onions, quartered

1 medium green sweet pepper, cut into ½-inch rings

1 tablespoon snipped fresh thyme or 1 teaspoon dried thyme, crushed

¼ teaspoon crushed red pepper

5 cups water

1¼ cups red lentils, rinsed and drained*

1 teaspoon salt

1. In a Dutch oven heat oil over medium-high heat. Add onion; cook about 8 minutes or until brown, stirring occasionally. Add sweet pepper, thyme, and crushed red pepper. Cook and stir for 2 minutes.

2. Add the water, 1 cup of the lentils, and the salt. Bring to boiling; reduce heat. Simmer, uncovered, for 15 minutes.

3. Stir in the remaining ¼ cup lentils. Simmer, uncovered, for 4 minutes more.

*Note: Brown or green lentils may be substituted for the red lentils. Prepare as directed above, except add all of the lentils with water. Bring to boiling; reduce heat. Simmer, covered, for 25 minutes. Simmer, uncovered, for 5 minutes more.

Nutrition Facts per serving: 241 cal., 4 g total fat (1 g sat. fat), 0 mg chol., 609 mg sodium, 39 g carbo., 10 g fiber, 15 g pro.
Exchanges: 1 Vegetable, 1 Starch, 1 Lean Meat

Bean-and-Barley Tostadas 11 g fiber

Start to Finish: 20 minutes Makes: 4 servings

1½ cups water

¾ cup quick-cooking barley

1 15-ounce can chili beans in chili gravy, undrained

½ cup salsa

4 cups low-fat tortilla chips

4 cups shredded iceberg lettuce

¾ cup shredded reduced-fat cheddar cheese (3 ounces)

Light dairy sour cream (optional)

Salsa (optional)

1. In a medium saucepan bring the water to boiling; add barley. Reduce heat. Simmer, covered, for 10 to 12 minutes or until tender. Drain off any excess liquid. Stir undrained chili beans in gravy and the ½ cup salsa into barley; heat through.

2. Place 1 cup tortilla chips on each of 4 plates. Top with lettuce and barley mixture; sprinkle with cheese. If desired, top each serving with sour cream and additional salsa.

Nutrition Facts per serving: 454 cal., 7 g total fat (3 g sat. fat), 15 mg chol., 778 mg sodium, 76 g carbo., 11 g fiber, 18 g pro.
Exchanges: 1 Vegetable, 4 Starch, 1 Very Lean Meat, 1 Lean Meat, ½ Fat

Orzo with Root Vegetables   9 g fiber

Start to Finish: 30 minutes   Makes: 4 servings

1 large onion, halved and thinly sliced

2 cloves garlic, minced

1 tablespoon olive oil

1 14-ounce can chicken or vegetable broth

¼ cup water

½ teaspoon dried thyme, crushed

⅛ teaspoon cayenne pepper

¾ cup dried orzo (rosamarina)

2 medium carrot, cut into thin bite-size strips

1 15-ounce can red beans, rinsed and drained

1 medium turnip, cut into thin bite-size strips

1 medium red sweet pepper, cut into thin bite-size strips

1. In a large saucepan cook onion and garlic in hot oil just until tender. Stir in broth, the water, thyme, and cayenne pepper. Bring to boiling. Add orzo and carrot. Simmer, covered, for 10 minutes.

2. Stir in red beans, turnip, and sweet pepper. Return to boiling; reduce heat. Simmer, covered, for 2 to 3 minutes more or until orzo is tender.

Nutrition Facts per serving: 250 cal., 5 g total fat (1 g sat. fat), 0 mg chol., 524 mg sodium, 43 g carbo., 9 g fiber, 13 g pro.
Exchanges: 2 Vegetable, 2½ Starch, ½ Fat

Savory Bean and Spinach Soup   8 g fiber

Prep: 15 minutes Cook: 5 to 7 hours (low) or 2½ to 3½ hours (high) Makes: 6 servings

3 14-ounce cans vegetable broth

1 15-ounce can tomato puree

1 15-ounce can cannellini (white kidney) or Great Northern beans, rinsed and drained

½ cup converted rice

½ cup finely chopped onion (1 medium)

2 cloves garlic, minced

1 teaspoon dried basil, crushed

¼ teaspoon salt

¼ teaspoon black pepper

8 cups coarsely chopped fresh spinach or kale leaves

Finely shredded Parmesan cheese

1. In a 3½- or 4-quart slow cooker combine broth, tomato puree, beans, rice, onion, garlic, basil, salt, and pepper.

2. Cover and cook on low-heat setting for 5 to 7 hours or on high-heat setting for 2½ to 3½ hours.

3. Stir spinach into soup. Ladle soup into bowls; sprinkle with Parmesan cheese.

Nutrition Facts per serving: 150 cal., 3 g total fat (1 g sat. fat), 4 mg chol., 1,137 mg sodium, 31 g carbo., 8 g fiber, 9 g pro.
Exchanges: 2 Vegetable, 1½ Starch

Risotto with Beans and Vegetables 7 g fiber

Start to Finish: 40 minutes Makes: 4 servings

3 cups vegetable or
  chicken broth

2 cups sliced fresh mushrooms
  (such as shiitake or button
  mushrooms)

½ cup chopped onion (1 medium)

2 cloves garlic, minced

2 tablespoons olive oil

1 cup Arborio rice

1 cup finely chopped zucchini
  (1 small)

1 cup finely chopped carrot
  (2 medium)

1 15-ounce can cannellini (white
  kidney) or pinto beans, rinsed
  and drained

½ cup grated Parmesan cheese

1. In a medium saucepan bring broth to boiling; reduce heat and simmer until needed. Meanwhile, in a large saucepan cook mushrooms, onion, and garlic in hot oil over medium heat about 5 minutes or until the onion is tender. Add uncooked rice. Cook and stir about 5 minutes more or until rice is golden brown.

2. Slowly add 1 cup of the broth to the rice mixture, stirring constantly. Continue to cook and stir until liquid is absorbed. Add another ½ cup of the broth, the zucchini, and carrot to rice mixture, stirring constantly. Continue to cook and stir until liquid is absorbed. Add another 1 cup of the broth, ½ cup at a time, stirring constantly until the broth is absorbed. (This should take about 20 minutes.)

3. Stir the remaining ½ cup broth into rice mixture. Cook and stir until rice is slightly creamy and just tender. Stir in beans and Parmesan cheese; heat through.

Nutrition Facts per serving: 328 cal., 11 g total fat (3 g sat. fat), 9 mg chol., 1,050 mg sodium, 51 g carbo., 7 g fiber, 15 g pro.
Exchanges: 1 Vegetable, 3 Starch, ½ Very Lean Meat, 1½ Fat

light
mini meals

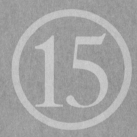

During pregnancy, you may not always feel like eating a big meal; perhaps you're not feeling well or are just short on time. But you need to eat something to keep your energy up and get the nutrients you require. Mini meals are the answer. They give you good nutrition in a smaller amount. Eat them as a snack or a light meal. Some are lighter than others, so let your appetite guide you.

Fruit and Caramel Oatmeal

Start to Finish: 10 minutes Makes: 2 servings

2 1-ounce envelopes instant
   oatmeal (plain)

1 ripe medium banana, peeled
   and sliced

   Desired fresh fruit (such
   as blueberries, sliced
   strawberries, and/or sliced
   peaches)

2 tablespoons chopped pecans,
   toasted

2 teaspoons caramel-flavored
   ice cream topping

   Milk, reduced-fat or fat-free
   (optional)

1. In 2 microwave-safe bowls prepare oatmeal according to package directions. Top each serving with banana slices, desired fresh fruit, and pecans. Drizzle with ice cream topping. If desired, heat in microwave on 100 percent power (high) for 30 seconds. If desired, serve with milk.

Nutrition Facts per serving: 231 cal., 7 g total fat (1 g sat. fat), 0 mg chol., 302 mg sodium, 39 g carbo., 6 g fiber, 6 g pro.
Exchanges: 1½ Fruit, 1 Starch, 1 Fat

Fruit and Cheese Pitas

Start to Finish: 20 minutes Makes: 2 servings

½ cup low-fat cottage cheese

½ cup shredded reduced-fat
  cheddar cheese (2 ounces)

2 kiwifruits, peeled and chopped,
  or ½ cup small strawberries,
  hulled and chopped

¼ cup drained pineapple tidbits

1 large pita bread round, halved
  crosswise

2 tablespoons sliced almonds,
  pecan pieces, or walnut pieces,
  toasted if desired (optional)

1. In a small bowl combine cottage cheese,
cheddar cheese, kiwifruits, and pineapple.
Stir gently to mix. Set aside.

2. Fill pita bread halves with the fruit and
cheese mixture. If desired, sprinkle with
almonds. Serve immediately.

Nutrition Facts per serving: 273 cal., 6 g total fat (3 g sat. fat),
22 mg chol., 604 mg sodium, 35 g carbo., 44 g fiber, 19 g pro.
Exchanges: 1 Fruit, 1 Starch, 2½ Very Lean Meat, 1 Fat

Egg Salad Pitas

Start to Finish: 15 minutes Makes: 4 servings

4 hard-cooked eggs, chopped

4 ounces low-fat cooked ham, cut into thin strips

2 tablespoons light mayonnaise or salad dressing

1 tablespoon yellow or Dijon-style mustard

2 large whole wheat pita bread rounds, halved crosswise

1. In a medium bowl combine eggs, ham, mayonnaise, and mustard. Stir gently to mix.

2. Spoon ⅓ cup of the egg salad into each pita half.

Nutrition Facts per serving: 216 cal., 9 g total fat (2 g sat. fat), 227 mg chol., 629 mg sodium, 20 g carbo., 2 g fiber, 15 g pro. **Exchanges:** 1 Starch, 2 Lean Meat, ½ Fat

Egg Salad Bagels: Prepare egg salad as directed in step 1. Split 2 whole wheat bagels. If desired, toast halves. Top each bagel half with ⅓ cup of the egg salad.

Nutrition Facts per serving: 228 cal., 9 g total fat (2 g sat. fat), 227 mg chol., 649 mg sodium, 21 g carbo., 1 g fiber, 15 g protein. **Exchanges:** 1 Starch, 2 lean Meat, ½ Fat

Egg Salad Wraps: Prepare egg salad as directed in step 1. Spoon ⅓ cup of the egg salad onto each of two 6-inch whole wheat tortillas; roll tortillas around filling.

Nutrition Facts per serving: 204 cal., 10 g total fat (3 g sat. fat), 227 mg chol., 639 mg sodium, 10 g carbo., 6 g fiber, 16 g protein. **Exchanges:** 1 Starch, 2 Lean Meat, ½ Fat

Curried Apple Spread

Start to Finish: 10 minutes Makes: ³/₄ cup spread

½ of an 8-ounce package
   reduced-fat cream cheese
   (Neufchâtel), softened

1 teaspoon finely shredded
   orange peel

1 tablespoon orange juice

½ teaspoon curry powder

¼ of a medium apple (such as
   Delicious, Gala, or Braeburn),
   finely chopped

6 mini bagels, halved, or
   12 melba toast rounds

1. In a small bowl combine cream cheese, orange peel, orange juice, and curry powder. Gently stir in apple.

2. Serve the spread with mini bagels.

Per 1 tablespoon spread with half of a mini bagel: 51 cal.,
2 g total fat (1 g sat. fat), 7 mg chol., 85 mg sodium, 6 g carbo.,
0 g fiber, 2 g pro.
Exchanges: ½ Starch, ½ High-Fat Meat

Chicken and Pear Salad

Start to Finish: 25 minutes Makes: 4 servings

½ cup buttermilk

2 tablespoons low-fat mayonnaise dressing

1 tablespoon frozen apple juice concentrate or frozen orange juice concentrate, thawed

1 teaspoon Dijon-style mustard

6 cups torn mixed salad greens

2 medium pears and/or apples, thinly sliced

8 ounces cooked chicken or turkey, cut into bite-size strips (1½ cups)

¼ cup broken walnuts, toasted (optional)

1. For dressing, in a small bowl stir together buttermilk, mayonnaise dressing, apple juice concentrate, and mustard.

2. In a salad bowl combine salad greens, pear slices, and chicken. Drizzle with dressing; toss to coat. If desired, sprinkle with walnuts.

Nutrition Facts per serving: 188 cal., 4 g total fat (1 g sat. fat), 46 mg chol., 179 mg sodium, 20 g carbo., 3 g fiber, 19 g pro.
Exchanges: 1 Vegetable, 1 Fruit, 2 Medium-Fat Meat

Asian Spring Rolls

Start to Finish: 30 minutes Makes: 4 servings (8 rolls)

8 8-inch round spring roll
 wrappers

8 ounces fresh or frozen cooked
 peeled and deveined shrimp,
 coarsely chopped (1⅓ cups)

1 small head Bibb lettuce, cored
 and shredded (2 cups)

1 cup shredded carrot
 (2 medium)

¼ cup sliced green onion (2)

2 tablespoons snipped fresh
 cilantro

1 recipe Peanut Sauce

1 tablespoon seasoned rice
 vinegar

 Hot water

1. Place some warm water in a shallow dish. Dip each spring roll wrapper in warm water; place between damp paper towels for 10 minutes.

2. Meanwhile, for filling, in a large bowl combine shrimp, lettuce, carrot, green onion, and cilantro. Add 2 tablespoons of the Peanut Sauce and the vinegar. Toss to coat.

3. For the dipping sauce, in a small bowl whisk together the remaining Peanut Sauce and enough hot water to make dipping consistency; set aside.

4. Place about ½ cup of the filling about ½ inch from the bottom edge of one of the moistened spring roll wrappers. Fold the bottom edge of the wrapper over the filling. Fold in sides. Roll up. Repeat with remaining filling and spring roll wrappers. Cut rolls in half; serve with dipping sauce.

Peanut Sauce: In a small saucepan combine 3 tablespoons creamy peanut butter; 2 tablespoons water; 1 tablespoon light soy sauce; 1 clove garlic, minced; and ¼ teaspoon ground ginger. Heat over very low heat until smooth, whisking constantly.

Nutrition Facts per serving: 232 cal., 7 g total fat (1 g sat. fat), 111 mg chol., 397 mg sodium, 26 g carbo., 3 g fiber, 17 g pro.
Exchanges: 1 Vegetable, 1 Starch, 1½ Very Lean Meat, 1 Fat

Chef Salad

Start to Finish: 30 minutes Makes: 4 servings

6 cups packaged torn mixed
  salad greens

4 ounces low-fat cooked ham or
  turkey, cut into bite-size pieces

1/2 cup shredded reduced-fat
  cheddar cheese (2 ounces)

1 hard-cooked egg, sliced

8 cherry tomatoes, halved

1 small yellow or red sweet
  pepper, cut into bite-size strips

1/2 cup purchased croutons

1/2 cup bottled reduced-calorie
  ranch salad dressing

1. Divide salad greens among 4 large salad plates. Arrange ham, cheese, egg, tomato, and sweet pepper on top of the greens. Sprinkle with croutons. Drizzle with dressing.

Nutrition Facts per serving: 194 cal., 11 g total fat (2 g sat. fat), 85 mg chol., 782 mg sodium, 11 g carbo., 2 g fiber, 12 g pro.
Exchanges: 2 Vegetable, 1 Lean Meat, 2 Fat

Turkey and Spinach Salad

Start to Finish: 25 minutes Makes: 4 servings

8 cups fresh baby spinach or torn fresh spinach

8 ounces cooked turkey, cubed

2 grapefruit, peeled and sectioned

2 oranges, peeled and sectioned

¼ cup orange juice

2 tablespoons olive oil

1 teaspoon honey

½ teaspoon poppy seeds

¼ teaspoon salt

¼ teaspoon dry mustard

2 tablespoons sliced almonds, toasted (optional)

1. Place spinach in a large bowl. Add turkey, grapefruit sections, and orange sections.

2. For dressing, in a screw-top jar combine orange juice, oil, honey, poppy seeds, salt, and dry mustard. Cover and shake well. Pour the dressing over salad; toss gently. If desired, sprinkle with almonds.

Nutrition Facts per serving: 228 cal., 10 g total fat (2 g sat. fat), 43 mg chol., 261 mg sodium, 16 g carbo., 8 g fiber, 20 g pro.
Exchanges: 1 Vegetable, 1 Fruit, 2 Medium-Fat Meat, 1½ Fat

Banana Crunch Pops

Prep: 15 minutes Freeze: 2 hours Stand: 10 minutes Makes: 4 servings

²/₃ cup fat-free yogurt (any flavor)

¼ teaspoon ground cinnamon

1 cup crisp rice cereal

2 ripe medium bananas, cut in half crosswise

4 wooden sticks

1. Place yogurt in a small shallow dish; stir in cinnamon. Place cereal in another small shallow dish. Insert a wooden stick into each banana piece. Roll banana pieces in yogurt mixture, covering the entire piece of banana. Roll in cereal to coat. Place on a baking sheet lined with waxed paper. Freeze about 2 hours or until firm.

2. When frozen, wrap each banana pop in freezer wrap. Store pops in the freezer. Before serving, let stand at room temperature for 10 to 15 minutes.

Nutrition Facts per serving: 99 cal., 0 g total fat (0 g sat. fat), 1 mg chol., 94 mg sodium, 23 g carbo., 2 g fiber, 3 g pro.
Exchanges: 1 Fruit, ½ Starch

Honey Granola with Yogurt

Prep: 15 minutes Bake: 30 minutes Oven: 325°F Makes: 12 servings

Nonstick cooking spray

2½ cups regular rolled oats

1 cup wheat flakes

⅓ cup toasted wheat germ

⅓ cup sliced almonds or pecan pieces

⅓ cup unsweetened pineapple juice or apple juice

⅓ cup honey

¼ teaspoon ground allspice

¼ teaspoon ground cinnamon

6 cups fat-free yogurt (any flavor)

4 cups fresh fruit (such as blueberries, seedless green grapes, raspberries, sliced strawberries, and/or chopped peaches)

1. Coat a 15×10×1-inch baking pan with cooking spray; set aside. In a large bowl stir together oats, wheat flakes, wheat germ, and nuts. In a small saucepan stir together pineapple juice, honey, allspice, and cinnamon. Cook and stir just until boiling. Remove from heat. Pour over oat mixture, tossing just until coated. Spread the oat mixture evenly in prepared pan.

2. Bake in a 325° oven for 30 to 35 minutes or until oats are light brown, stirring twice. Remove from oven. Immediately turn out onto a large piece of foil; cool completely.

3. For each serving, spoon ½ cup of the yogurt into a bowl. Top with ⅓ cup of the oat mixture and ⅓ cup fresh fruit.

To Make Ahead: Prepare as above through step 2. Cover and chill up to 2 weeks. For longer storage, seal in freezer bags and freeze up to 3 months.

Nutrition Facts per serving: 244 cal., 4 g total fat (1 g sat. fat), 2 mg chol., 96 mg sodium, 44 g carbo., 5 g fiber, 11 g pro.
Exchanges: 1 Milk, ½ Fruit, 1½ Starch, ½ Fat

Fresh Fruit with Minted Yogurt

Start to Finish: 15 minutes Makes: 6 servings

2 cups carton plain low-fat yogurt

3 tablespoons honey

2 tablespoons snipped fresh mint

4 medium plums, pitted and thinly sliced (about 3 cups)

3 cups blueberries, raspberries, and/or sliced strawberries

1. In a small bowl stir together yogurt, honey, and mint. Cover and chill until ready to serve.

2. In a medium bowl combine plums and berries. Spoon the fruit mixture into serving bowls. Top with the yogurt mixture. If desired, garnish with additional fresh mint.

Nutrition Facts per serving: 135 cal., 2 g total fat (1 g sat. fat), 5 mg chol., 55 mg sodium, 27 g carbo., 3 g fiber, 5 g pro.
Exchanges: ½ Milk, 1½ Fruit

Tropical Fruit Pops

Prep: 15 minutes Freeze: 6 hours Makes: 8 or 12 pops

½ cup boiling water

1 4-serving-size package sugar-free lemon-, mixed fruit-, or strawberry-flavored gelatin

1 15¼-ounce can crushed pineapple (juice pack)

2 ripe medium bananas, cut into chunks

1. In a 1- or 2-cup glass measuring cup stir together boiling water and gelatin until gelatin dissolves. Pour into a blender. Add undrained pineapple and banana chunks. Cover and blend until smooth.

2. Pour a scant ½ cup of the fruit mixture into each of eight 5- to 6-ounce paper or plastic drink cups. (Or pour a scant ⅓ cup into each of twelve 3-ounce cups.) Cover each cup with foil. Using the tip of a knife, make a small hole in the foil over each cup. Insert a wooden stick into the cup through the hole. Freeze about 6 hours or until firm.

3. To serve, quickly dip the cups in warm water to slightly soften fruit mixture. Remove foil and loosen sides of pops from drink cups.

Nutrition Facts per pop: 65 cal., 0 g total fat (0 g sat. fat), 0 mg chol., 29 mg sodium, 15 g carbo., 1 g fiber, 1 g pro.
Exchanges: 1 Fruit

Banana-Berry Smoothies

Start to Finish: 10 minutes   Makes: 3 (about 12-ounce) servings

2 cups plain fat-free yogurt

2 ripe medium bananas, peeled and frozen

1 cup sliced fresh strawberries or unsweetened frozen strawberries

1 cup mixed fresh berries (raspberries, blueberries, and/ or blackberries) or unsweet- ened frozen mixed berries

1 tablespoon honey (optional)

Additional fresh berries (optional)

1. In a blender combine yogurt, fruit, and, if desired, honey. Cover and blend until pureed. If desired, top each serving with a few fresh berries.

Nutrition Facts per serving: 199 cal., 1 g total fat (0 g sat. fat), 3 mg chol., 126 mg sodium, 39 g carbo., 3 g fiber, 11 g pro. **Exchanges:** 1 Milk, 1½ Fruit

Tango Mango Smoothies

Start to Finish: 10 minutes Makes: 6 servings

2 ripe medium bananas, chilled

²/₃ cup peeled mango slices

1 12-ounce can mango, peach, apricot, or other fruit nectar, chilled

1 cup plain fat-free yogurt

1 tablespoon honey (optional)

Cut-up fresh fruit (such as bananas, peeled kiwifruit, and/ or peeled mango) (optional)

1. Cut bananas into chunks. In a blender combine banana, mango, fruit nectar, yogurt, and, if desired, honey.

2. Cover and blend until smooth. Pour into chilled glasses. If desired, garnish each serving with cut-up fresh fruit.

Nutrition Facts per serving: 108 cal., 0 g total fat (0 g sat. fat), 1 mg chol., 33 mg sodium, 24 g carbo., 1 g fiber, 3 g pro.
Exchanges: ½ Milk, 1 Fruit

Nectarine-Soy Smoothies

Start to Finish: 15 minutes Makes: 2 (10-ounce) servings

1½ cups cut-up, peeled nectarines
    or peaches (2 medium)

1 cup soymilk,* chilled

⅓ cup orange juice

1 tablespoon sugar

   Ice cubes

   Fresh mint sprigs (optional)

1. In a blender or food processor combine nectarines, soymilk, orange juice, and sugar. Cover and blend or process until mixture is thick and smooth.

2. Serve the fruit mixture over ice cubes. If desired, garnish with mint.

*Note: Make sure you purchase calcium-fortified soymilk to get the benefit of this important nutrient.

Nutrition Facts per serving: 132 cal., 3 g total fat (0 g sat. fat), 0 mg chol., 15 mg sodium, 25 g carbo., 3 g fiber, 5 g pro.
Exchanges: 1½ Fruit, ½ Medium-Fat Meat

Orange-Melon Smoothies

Start to Finish: 10 minutes Makes: 4 (about 8-ounce) servings

2 cups orange or orange-
  tangerine juice, chilled

1 cup cubed cantaloupe

1 cup plain low-fat yogurt

2 to 4 tablespoons sugar or
  honey

1/2 teaspoon vanilla

  Toasted wheat germ (optional)

  Peeled cantaloupe wedges
  (optional)

1. In a blender combine orange juice, cubed cantaloupe, yogurt, sugar, and vanilla. Cover and blend until nearly smooth.

2. Divide among 4 glasses. If desired, sprinkle with wheat germ and garnish with cantaloupe wedges.

Nutrition Facts per serving: 130 cal., 1 g total fat (1 g sat. fat),
3 mg chol., 45 mg sodium, 26 g carbo., 1 g fiber, 4 g pro.
Exchanges: 1/2 Milk, 1 1/2 Fruit

Peach Shakes

Start to Finish: 10 minutes Makes: 3 (about 8-ounce) servings

2 cups frozen unsweetened
    peach slices

1¾ cups milk

1 to 2 tablespoons honey

1 teaspoon vanilla

1. In a blender combine frozen peach slices, milk, honey, and vanilla. Cover and blend until smooth. Pour into glasses.

Nutrition Facts per serving: 145 cal., 3 g total fat (2 g sat. fat), 11 mg chol., 72 mg sodium, 25 g carbo., 2 g fiber, 5 g pro.
Exchanges: ½ Milk, 1 Fruit

Fresh Fruit Floats

Start to Finish: 10 minutes Makes: 4 servings

2 cups cut-up fresh fruit (such as strawberries, seedless grapes, peeled oranges or bananas, and/or apples)

4 cups low-calorie lemon-lime carbonated beverage or low-calorie ginger ale

2 cups fruit-flavored sherbet

1. Divide fruit evenly among 4 tall glasses. Slowly pour 1 cup carbonated beverage over fruit in each glass. Top each serving with ½ cup sherbet.

Nutrition Facts per serving: 155 cal., 2 g total fat (1 g sat. fat), 5 mg chol., 80 mg sodium, 34 g carbo., 2 g fiber, 2 g pro. **Exchanges:** 2 Fruit, ½ Fat

Icy Melon-Berry Smoothies

Start to Finish: 15 minutes Makes: 4 (about 6-ounce) servings

1 cup frozen unsweetened whole strawberries

1 cup cut-up cantaloupe

1/3 cup orange juice

1/4 cup fat-free milk

1 tablespoon honey or sugar

1 cup ice cubes

1. In a blender combine strawberries, cantaloupe, orange juice, milk, and honey. Cover and blend until smooth. Add ice cubes; cover and blend until smooth. Immediately pour into glasses and serve.

Nutrition Facts per serving: 57 cal., 0 g total fat (0 g sat. fat), 0 mg chol., 14 mg sodium, 14 g carbo., 1 g fiber, 1 g pro. **Exchanges:** 1/2 Fruit, 1/2 Other Carbo.

on-the-go
foods

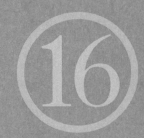

Moms both new and experienced often spend their days on the go. There's so much to do and so little time! But that doesn't mean your diet should suffer. If eating on the go means heading for the nearest vending machine or fast-food place, these recipes are for you. They offer healthy alternatives to the usual, often unhealthy, get-and-go foods.

Chicken Pockets

Start to Finish: 15 minutes Makes: 4 sandwiches

¼ cup plain low-fat yogurt

¼ cup bottled reduced-calorie
  ranch salad dressing

1½ cups chopped cooked chicken
  or turkey

½ cup chopped broccoli

¼ cup shredded carrot

¼ cup chopped pecans or walnuts
  (optional)

2 6- to 7-inch whole wheat
  pita bread rounds, halved
  crosswise

1. In a small bowl stir together yogurt and
ranch salad dressing.

2. In a medium bowl combine chicken,
broccoli, carrot, and, if desired, nuts. Pour
yogurt mixture over chicken; toss to coat.
Spoon chicken mixture into pita halves.
Wrap tightly in plastic wrap and chill up to
24 hours.

3. To tote, pack sandwiches in insulated
containers with ice packs.

Nutrition Facts per sandwich: 231 cal., 8 g total fat (1 g sat. fat),
53 mg chol., 392 mg sodium, 21 g carbo., 3 g fiber, 20 g pro.
Exchanges: ½ Vegetable, 1 Starch, 2 Lean Meat, ½ Fat

Chicken Waldorf Salad
Start to Finish: 20 minutes Makes: 4 servings

1/3 cup fat-free mayonnaise
dressing or salad dressing

1/3 cup fat-free dairy sour cream

1 tablespoon lemon juice

1 tablespoon honey

1 teaspoon dried rosemary,
crushed

2 cups shredded or cubed cooked
chicken breast

2 cups coarsely chopped red and/
or green apple (2 medium)

1/4 cup thinly sliced celery

1/3 cup dried tart cherries

1/3 cup coarsely chopped pecans
or peanuts

Lettuce leaves (optional)

1. For dressing, in a small bowl stir together mayonnaise dressing, sour cream, lemon juice, honey, and rosemary; set aside.

2. In a medium bowl combine chicken, apple, celery, cherries, and nuts. Stir dressing into chicken mixture just until evenly coated. Divide salad among 4 individual containers. Cover and refrigerate up to 24 hours.

3. To tote, pack in insulated containers with ice packs. If desired, place lettuce leaves in plastic bags, seal, and add to the insulated containers; serve salad on lettuce leaves.

Nutrition Facts per serving: 272 cal., 9 g total fat (1 g sat. fat), 314 mg sodium, 30 g carbo., 2 g fiber, 19 g pro.
Exchanges: 2 Fruit, 3 Lean Meat, 1 Fat

Chicken-Zucchini Salad

Start to Finish: 25 minutes Makes: 3 to 4 servings

1½ cups shredded cooked chicken

¾ cup chopped zucchini or yellow summer squash (1 medium)

½ cup chopped fennel (½ of a small bulb)

¼ cup sliced green onion (2)

¼ cup chopped celery

¼ cup chopped carrot

1 tablespoon snipped dried apricots (optional)

1 recipe Herbed Mustard Mayonnaise

Salt

Black pepper

Lettuce leaves (optional)

1. In a large bowl combine chicken, zucchini, fennel, green onion, celery, carrot, and, if desired, dried apricots. Pour Herbed Mustard Mayonnaise over chicken mixture; toss gently to coat. Season to taste with salt and pepper. Cover and refrigerate up to 24 hours.

2. To tote, pack individual servings in containers. Pack in insulated containers with ice packs. If desired, place lettuce leaves in plastic bags, seal, and add to insulated containers; serve salad on lettuce leaves.

Herbed Mustard Mayonnaise: In a small bowl stir together ⅓ cup fat-free mayonnaise dressing or salad dressing, 2 teaspoons Dijon-style mustard, 2 teaspoons snipped fresh dill or tarragon, ½ teaspoon finely shredded lemon peel, 1 teaspoon lemon juice, 1 tablespoon frozen orange juice concentrate, and ⅛ teaspoon black pepper. Makes about ⅓ cup.

Nutrition Facts per serving: 193 cal., 6 g total fat (2 g sat. fat), 68 mg chol., 514 mg sodium, 11 g carbo., 6 g fiber, 23 g pro.
Exchanges: 1 Vegetable, 1½ Lean Meat, ½ Fat

Chicken and Egg Salad Sandwiches

Start to Finish: 20 minutes Makes: 4 servings

1 cup chopped cooked chicken

1/3 cup chopped apple or finely chopped celery

1 hard-cooked egg, peeled and chopped

2 tablespoons plain low-fat yogurt

2 tablespoons light mayonnaise or salad dressing

Salt

Black pepper

8 slices whole wheat bread

1. In a medium bowl stir together chicken, apple, and egg. Add yogurt and mayonnaise; stir to combine. Season to taste with salt and pepper. If desired, cover and refrigerate overnight.

2. Spread chicken mixture on half of the bread slices. Top with remaining bread slices. Cut sandwiches in half. Pack sandwiches in sandwich containers or plastic sandwich bags.

3. To tote, place sandwiches in insulated containers with ice packs.

Nutrition Facts per serving: 248 cal., 8 g total fat (2 g sat. fat), 87 mg chol., 434 mg sodium, 27 g carbo., 2 g fiber, 17 g pro.
Exchanges: 2 Starch, 1 1/2 Lean Meat, 1/2 Fat

Shake-It-Up Turkey Salad
Start to Finish: 15 minutes Makes: 1 serving

¼ cup coarsely chopped cucumber

1 ounce cooked turkey or ham, cut into ½-inch pieces

1 cup packaged torn mixed salad greens

¼ cup grape or cherry tomatoes

2 tablespoons shredded part-skim mozzarella cheese

1 tablespoon sliced almonds or walnut pieces (optional)

2 tablespoons bottled reduced-fat or reduced-calorie salad dressing (any flavor)

1. In a 4-cup plastic container or 1-quart self-sealing plastic bag place cucumber, turkey, salad greens, tomatoes, cheese, and, if desired, nuts. Cover the container or seal the bag.

2. To tote, pack in an insulated container with an ice pack. Place salad dressing in another small plastic container; cover the container and add to insulated container.

3. To serve, uncover the salad and dressing; pour dressing over the salad in the container or bag. Put the lid on the container or seal the bag and shake to mix.

Nutrition Facts per serving: 166 cal., 10 g total fat (3 g sat. fat), 31 mg chol., 530 mg sodium, 7 g carbo., 1 g fiber, 13 g pro.
Exchanges: 1½ Vegetable, 1½ Very Lean Meat, 2 Fat

Ranch-Style Turkey Pockets

Start to Finish: 15 minutes Makes: 2 servings

¾ cup packaged shredded broccoli (broccoli slaw mix) or shredded cabbage with carrot (coleslaw mix)

2 ounces cooked turkey or chicken breast, cut into bite-size pieces

½ of a small tomato, chopped

1 large wheat pita bread round, halved crosswise

2 tablespoons bottled reduced-calorie ranch salad dressing

1. For filling, in a medium bowl combine shredded broccoli, turkey, and tomato. Spoon half of the broccoli mixture into each pita pocket. Wrap each pita half in plastic wrap or place in plastic bags. Refrigerate up to 6 hours.

2. To tote, pack in insulated containers with ice packs. Divide the salad dressing between two small containers and add to insulated containers.

3. To serve, drizzle dressing over broccoli mixture in pita pockets.

Nutrition Facts per serving: 174 cal., 5 g total fat (1 g sat. fat), 20 mg chol., 406 mg sodium, 21 g carbo., 3 g fiber, 13 g pro.
Exchanges: 1 Vegetable, 1 Starch, 1 Very Lean Meat, 1 Fat

Dip-and-Eat Lunch

Prep: 15 minutes　Chill: 1 hour　Makes: 1 serving

½ of a small zucchini, 1 carrot,
　½ of a medium green sweet
　pepper, ½ cup broccoli florets,
　and/or ½ cup grape or cherry
　tomatoes

1 ounce smoked turkey sausage,
　sliced

1 ounce mozzarella or
　provolone cheese, cut into
　bite-size cubes

1 ounce Italian bread, cut into
　bite-size pieces

¼ cup tomato sauce

⅛ teaspoon dried Italian
　seasoning

　Dash garlic powder

1. Cut the zucchini, carrot, and/or sweet pepper (if using) into bite-size pieces.

2. Pack vegetables, sausage, cheese, and bread into a 2-cup plastic container or a plastic bag. Seal and chill for 1 to 6 hours.

3. In a small container stir together tomato sauce, Italian seasoning, and garlic powder. Cover and chill for 1 to 6 hours.

4. To tote, pack dipper and tomato mixture containers in an insulated container with an ice pack.

5. To eat, dip the vegetables, sausage, cheese, and bread in the tomato mixture.

Nutrition Facts per serving with zucchini: 217 cal., 8 g total fat (4 g sat. fat), 37 mg chol., 876 mg sodium, 21 g carbo., 2 g fiber, 15 g pro.
Exchanges: 1 Vegetable, 1 Starch, 2 Lean Meat

Turkey-Tomato Wraps
Prep: 20 minutes Chill: 2 hours Makes: 6 wraps

1 7-ounce container prepared hummus

3 8- to 10-inch tomato-basil flour tortillas or plain flour tortillas

8 ounces thinly sliced cooked turkey breast

6 romaine lettuce leaves, ribs removed

3 small tomatoes, thinly sliced

3 thin slices red onion, separated into rings

1. Spread hummus evenly over tortillas. Layer turkey breast, romaine, tomato, and onion on top of each tortilla. Roll up each tortilla into a spiral. Cut each roll in half and wrap with plastic wrap. Refrigerate for 2 to 4 hours.

2. To tote, pack in insulated containers with ice packs.

Per wrap: 236 cal., 6 g total fat (1 g sat. fat), 32 mg chol., 458 mg sodium, 29 g carbo., 4 g fiber, 19 g pro.
Exchanges: 1 Vegetable, 1½ Starch, 2 Lean Meat

Turkey-and-Chutney Pitas

Prep: 25 minutes   Chill: 2 to 24 hours   Makes: 4 servings

¼ cup chutney

3 tablespoons light mayonnaise
  or salad dressing

2 large pita bread rounds, halved
  crosswise

4 small romaine lettuce leaves

4 ounces thinly sliced cooked
  turkey or chicken

3 ounces thinly sliced smoked
  Gouda cheese

½ cup coarsely shredded carrot
  (1 medium)

¼ cup shredded fresh basil leaves

1. Cut up any large pieces of chutney. In a small bowl stir together the chutney and mayonnaise; cover and refrigerate.

2. Line the pita halves with lettuce leaves. Fill with turkey, cheese, carrot, and basil. Wrap each sandwich in plastic wrap. Refrigerate for 2 to 24 hours.

3. To tote, pack wrapped pita halves and mayonnaise mixture in insulated containers with ice packs.

4. To serve, top each sandwich with some of the mayonnaise mixture.

Nutrition Facts per serving: 265 cal., 10 g total fat (5 g sat. fat), 42 mg chol., 632 mg sodium, 28 g carbo., 2 g fiber, 16 g pro.
Exchanges: 1 Vegetable, 1 Starch, ½ Other Carbo., 1½ Very Lean Meat, 1½ Fat

Gazpacho to Go

Prep: 30 minutes Chill: 2 hours Makes: 6 servings

1 15-ounce can chunky Italian- or salsa-style tomatoes, undrained

2 cups quartered yellow pear-shape and/or halved cherry tomatoes

1 15-ounce can garbanzo beans (chickpeas), rinsed and drained

1¼ cups vegetable juice

1 cup beef broth

½ cup coarsely chopped seeded cucumber

½ cup coarsely chopped yellow and/or red sweet pepper

¼ cup coarsely chopped red onion

¼ cup snipped fresh cilantro

3 tablespoons lime juice or lemon juice

2 cloves garlic, minced

¼ to ½ teaspoon bottled hot pepper sauce (optional)

1. In a large bowl combine undrained canned tomatoes, fresh tomatoes, garbanzo beans, vegetable juice, broth, cucumber, sweet pepper, onion, cilantro, lime juice, garlic, and, if desired, hot pepper sauce. Cover and refrigerate for 2 to 24 hours.

2. To tote, transfer individual servings to individual containers; seal tightly. Pack in insulated containers with ice packs.

Nutrition Facts per serving: 136 cal., 3 g total fat (0 g sat. fat), 0 mg chol., 1,145 mg sodium, 23 g carbo., 6 g fiber, 6 g pro.
Exchanges: 1 Vegetable, ½ Starch, ½ Other Carbo., ½ Very Lean Meat

Easy Spiral Sandwich

Start to Finish: 15 minutes   Makes: 1 serving

1   slice reduced-fat American cheese

1   ounce thinly sliced cooked chicken, turkey, or lean beef

1   7- to 8-inch flour tortilla

2   teaspoons honey mustard or yellow mustard

¼   cup shredded carrot

2   teaspoons dried tart cherries or raisins

1. Layer cheese and chicken on tortilla. Spread the mustard on chicken. Top with carrot and cherries. Tightly roll up tortilla. Cut in half. Wrap tightly in plastic wrap.

3. To tote, pack in an insulated container with an ice pack.

Nutrition Facts per serving: 227 cal., 7 g total fat (3 g sat. fat), 35 mg chol., 495 mg sodium, 25 g carbo., 2 g fiber, 15 g pro. **Exchanges:** ½ Vegetable, 1½ Starch, 1½ Lean Meat

Chilly Pizza Rolls

Prep: 25 minutes Bake: 13 minutes Cool: 1 hour Chill: 4 to 24 hours Oven: 400°F Makes: 6 rolls

Nonstick cooking spray

Cornmeal (optional)

1 10-ounce package refrigerated pizza dough

1 3½-ounce package pizza-style Canadian-style bacon (1½-inch diameter)

⅓ cup pizza sauce

3 1-ounce pieces string cheese, cut in half crosswise

1. Lightly coat a baking sheet with cooking spray. If desired, lightly sprinkle cornmeal over baking sheet. Set aside.

2. On a lightly floured surface, unroll pizza dough. Press dough to form a 13½×9-inch rectangle. Cut into six 4½×4½-inch squares. Place Canadian bacon in the center of each square. Top with pizza sauce and string cheese. Bring up 2 opposite edges and pinch to seal. Pinch ends to seal. Place rolls, seam sides down, on prepared baking sheet.

3. Bake in a 400° oven for 13 to 18 minutes or until golden brown. Remove to a wire rack; cool. Wrap each roll in plastic wrap; refrigerate for 4 to 24 hours.

4. To tote, pack in insulated containers with ice packs.

Nutrition Facts per roll: 187 cal., 6 g total fat (2 g sat. fat), 16 mg chol., 613 mg sodium, 23 g carbo., 1 g fiber, 11 g pro.
Exchanges: 1½ Starch, 1 Medium-Fat Meat

Mexican Fiesta Salad

Start to Finish: 30 minutes Makes: 4 servings

2 cups dried penne (mostaccioli) or rotini pasta (about 6 ounces)

½ cup frozen whole kernel corn

½ cup light dairy sour cream

⅓ cup bottled chunky salsa

1 tablespoon snipped fresh cilantro

1 tablespoon lime juice

1 15-ounce can black beans, rinsed and drained

3 medium roma tomatoes, chopped

1¼ cups chopped zucchini (1 medium)

½ cup shredded sharp cheddar cheese (2 ounces)

1. Cook pasta according to package directions, adding corn for the last 5 minutes of cooking. Drain in colander. Rinse with cold water; drain again.

2. Meanwhile, for dressing, in a small bowl stir together sour cream, salsa, snipped cilantro, and lime juice. Set dressing aside.

3. In a large bowl combine the pasta-corn mixture, black beans, tomato, zucchini, and cheese. Pour dressing over pasta mixture. Toss lightly to coat. (If desired, pack in individual serving containers; cover.) Refrigerate up to 24 hours.

4. To tote, pack in insulated containers with ice packs.

Nutrition Facts per serving: 330 cal., 8 g total fat (5 g sat. fat), 25 mg chol., 470 mg sodium, 50 g carbo., 7 g fiber, 18 g pro.
Exchanges: ½ Vegetable, 3 Starch, 1 Medium-Fat Meat

Lunch Box Sub Sandwiches

Start to Finish: 15 minutes Makes: 4 sandwiches

¼ cup low-fat mayonnaise or salad dressing

1 teaspoon Dijon-style mustard

¼ cup finely snipped dried tart cherries or raisins

4 hamburger buns, split

4 ¾-ounce slices mozzarella cheese

6 ounces thinly sliced cooked turkey breast

1 medium tomato, thinly sliced

1. In a small bowl stir together the mayonnaise dressing, mustard, and cherries. Spread the bottoms of the buns with the mayonnaise mixture. Top with cheese, turkey, and tomato. Add bun tops.

2. Wrap each sandwich in plastic wrap. Refrigerate up to 24 hours.

3. To tote, place in insulated containers with ice packs.

Nutrition Facts per sandwich: 301 cal., 8 g total fat (3 g sat. fat), 45 mg chol., 515 mg sodium, 34 g carbo., 2 g fiber, 22 g pro. **Exchanges:** 2 Starch, 2½ Medium-Fat Meat

Gazpacho Sandwiches to Go

Prep: 20 minutes Chill: 4 hours Makes: 2 sandwiches

½ of an 8-ounce loaf baguette-
  style French bread

¾ cup yellow pear-shaped, cherry,
  and/or grape tomatoes,
  quartered

¼ cup coarsely chopped
  cucumber

2 thin slices red onion, separated
  into rings

2 ounces mozzarella cheese,
  cubed

1 tablespoon snipped fresh mint

1 tablespoon red wine vinegar

1 teaspoon olive oil

¼ teaspoon salt

⅛ teaspoon white pepper

½ cup fresh basil leaves

1. Cut the bread in half crosswise. Cut a thin horizontal slice from the top of each portion and reserve. Use a knife to carefully remove bread from the centers, leaving ¼-inch shells. (Reserve the bread from centers for another use.) Set bread shells aside.

2. In a medium bowl combine tomatoes, cucumber, onion, mozzarella cheese, mint, vinegar, oil, salt, and white pepper. Line the bottoms of the bread shells with basil leaves. Fill the shells with tomato mixture. Replace tops of bread. Wrap each sandwich in plastic wrap. Refrigerate for at least 4 hours or overnight.

3. To tote, pack sandwiches in insulated containers with ice packs.

Nutrition Facts per sandwich: 237 cal., 8 g total fat (3 g sat. fat), 16 mg chol., 691 mg sodium, 29 g carbo., 3 g fiber, 12 g pro. **Exchanges:** 1 Vegetable, 1½ Starch, 1 Lean Meat

Egg and Vegetable Wraps

Start to Finish: 30 minutes Makes: 6 servings

4 hard-cooked eggs, chopped

1 cup chopped cucumber

1 cup chopped zucchini or yellow summer squash (1 small)

½ cup finely chopped red onion (1 medium)

½ cup shredded carrot (1 medium)

¼ cup fat-free or light mayonnaise or salad dressing

2 tablespoons Dijon-style mustard

1 tablespoon fat-free milk

1 teaspoon snipped fresh tarragon or basil

⅛ teaspoon paprika

6 10-inch whole wheat, spinach, or vegetable flour tortillas

6 leaf lettuce leaves

2 roma tomatoes, thinly sliced

1. In a large bowl combine eggs, cucumber, zucchini, red onion, and carrot. For dressing, in a small bowl stir together mayonnaise dressing, mustard, milk, tarragon, and paprika. Pour dressing over the egg mixture; toss gently to coat.

2. For each sandwich, place a lettuce leaf on a tortilla. Place 3 or 4 tomato slices on top of the lettuce, slightly off center. Spoon about ⅔ cup of the egg mixture on top of the tomato slices. Fold in 2 opposite sides of the tortilla; roll up from the bottom. Cut the rolls in half diagonally. Wrap each tightly in plastic wrap.

3. To tote, pack wraps in insulated lunch bags with ice packs.

Nutrition Facts per serving: 265 cal., 7 g total fat (2 g sat. fat), 141 mg chol., 723 mg sodium, 40 g carbo., 4 g fiber, 11 g pro.
Exchanges: 1 Vegetable, 2½ Starch, 1 Fat

Shake-It-Up Black Bean Salad

Prep: 15 minutes Makes: 1 serving

1 cup packaged torn mixed
   salad greens

⅓ cup chopped yellow or green
   sweet pepper

¼ cup grape or cherry tomatoes

¼ cup rinsed, drained canned
   black beans

2 tablespoons crushed purchased
   baked tortilla chips

2 tablespoons shredded reduced-
   fat cheddar cheese

2 tablespoons bottled salsa

1. In a 4-cup plastic container or 1-quart self-sealing plastic bag combine salad greens, sweet pepper, tomatoes, black beans, crushed chips, and cheese. Cover the container or seal the bag. Put the salsa in a small covered container.

2. To tote, pack the salad and salsa in an insulated lunch bag with ice packs.

3. To serve, uncover the salad and salsa; pour the salsa over the salad in the container or bag. Put the lid on the container or seal the bag and shake to mix.

Nutrition Facts per serving: 149 cal., 4 g total fat (2 g sat. fat), 10 mg chol., 411 mg sodium, 23 g carbo., 5 g fiber, 10 g pro.
Exchanges: 2 Vegetable, 1 Starch, ½ Lean Meat

Citrus Tuna Pasta Salad

Prep: 30 minutes Chill: 1 hour Makes: 4 servings

6 ounces dried mafalda pasta or medium shell macaroni

1 9-ounce package frozen artichoke hearts, thawed

1 9¼-ounce can chunk light tuna (water pack), drained and broken into chunks

1 cup sliced fresh mushrooms

1 cup chopped yellow sweet pepper (1 large)

¼ cup sliced pitted ripe olives

1 recipe Lemon Dressing

1 cup cherry tomatoes, halved

2 tablespoons finely shredded Parmesan cheese

1. Cook pasta according to package directions, adding artichoke hearts for the last 5 minutes of cooking. Drain in colander. Rinse with cold water; drain again. Halve any large artichoke hearts.

2. Transfer pasta mixture to a large bowl. Gently stir in tuna, mushrooms, sweet pepper, and olives. Pour Lemon Dressing over pasta mixture; toss to coat. Pack salad in individual containers. Put ¼ cup of cherry tomatoes into each of 4 small plastic bags. Divide Parmesan cheese into 4 portions; wrap each portion tightly in plastic wrap.

3. To tote, for each serving, pack a portion of salad, tomatoes, and cheese into an insulated lunch bag with ice packs. To serve, stir tomatoes into salad; sprinkle with cheese.

Lemon Dressing: In a small bowl whisk together 1 teaspoon finely shredded lemon peel; 3 tablespoons lemon juice; 3 tablespoons rice vinegar or white wine vinegar; 2 tablespoons salad oil; 1 tablespoon snipped fresh thyme or basil or 1 teaspoon dried thyme or basil, crushed; 1 clove garlic, minced; ½ teaspoon sugar; and ¼ teaspoon black pepper.

Nutrition Facts per serving: 389 cal., 11 g total fat (1 g sat. fat), 22 mg chol., 369 mg sodium, 49 g carbo., 5 g fiber, 27 g pro.
Exchanges: 1½ Vegetable, 2½ Starch, 2½ Very Lean Meat, 1½ Fat

Traveling Tuna Subs

Prep: 20 minutes Chill: 2 to 24 hours Makes: 4 sandwiches

1/3 cup low-fat mayonnaise
   dressing or salad dressing

1 1/2 teaspoons yellow mustard

1/4 teaspoon dried dill

   Dash black pepper

1 12-ounce can light tuna (water
   pack), drained and flaked

1/2 cup chopped carrot, celery, or
   red sweet pepper

4 frankfurter buns, split

1/2 cup shredded reduced-fat
   cheddar cheese (2 ounces)

1. In a medium bowl stir together mayonnaise dressing, mustard, dill, and black pepper. Stir in tuna and carrot; set aside.

2. Use a fork to hollow out the tops and bottoms of frankfurter buns, leaving 1/4-inch shells. Sprinkle cheese over the bottom shells. Spoon tuna mixture over cheese. Add bun tops. Wrap tightly in plastic wrap. Refrigerate for 2 to 24 hours.

3. To tote, pack in insulated containers with ice packs.

Nutrition Facts per sandwich: 307 cal., 7 g total fat (3 g sat. fat), 39 mg chol., 858 mg sodium, 29 g carbo., 2 g fiber, 29 g pro.
Exchanges: 2 Starch, 3 Very Lean Meat, 1 Fat

quick &
easy foods

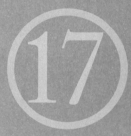

When juggling all the events of your hectic life has you pressed for time, start your search for the perfect meal right here. Each recipe in this chapter takes a mere 30 minutes or less from start to finish. So even when you're in a hurry to get to prenatal classes, doctor's appointments, work, and home, you have plenty of time to savor a healthful, delicious meal that provides you and your baby with necessary nutrients.

Sweet-and-Sour Chicken

Start to Finish: 30 minutes Makes: 6 servings

¾ cup reduced-sodium chicken broth

3 tablespoons red wine vinegar

2 tablespoons light soy sauce

4 teaspoons sugar

1 tablespoon cornstarch

1 clove garlic, minced

2 medium carrots, thinly sliced

1 medium red sweet pepper, cut into bite-size strips

4 teaspoons cooking oil

1 cup fresh pea pods, tips and stems removed

12 ounces skinless, boneless chicken breast halves, cut into 1-inch pieces

1 8-ounce can pineapple chunks (juice pack), drained

3 cups hot cooked rice

1. For sauce, in a small bowl stir together broth, vinegar, soy sauce, sugar, cornstarch, and garlic; set aside.

2. In a large nonstick skillet cook and stir carrot and sweet pepper in 3 teaspoons of the hot oil over medium-high heat for 3 minutes. Add pea pods. Cook and stir about 1 minute more or until vegetables are crisp-tender. Remove from skillet; set aside.

3. Add remaining 1 teaspoon oil to skillet. Add chicken to skillet. Cook and stir for 3 to 4 minutes or until chicken is no longer pink. Push chicken from center of skillet. Stir sauce; add to center of skillet. Cook and stir until thickened and bubbly. Add vegetable mixture and pineapple chunks; heat through. Serve with hot cooked rice.

Nutrition Facts per serving: 259 cal., 4 g total fat (1 g sat. fat), 33 mg chol., 311 mg sodium, 37 g carbo., 2 g fiber, 17 g pro.
Exchanges: ½ Vegetable, 2 Starch, 1½ Very Lean Meat, 1 Fat

Chicken and Rice Salad

Start to Finish: 30 minutes Makes: 4 servings

1 recipe Thyme Vinaigrette

3 medium skinless, boneless chicken breast halves (about 12 ounces)

1 cup frozen French-cut green beans

2 cups cooked brown rice, chilled

1 14-ounce can artichoke hearts, drained and quartered

1 cup shredded red cabbage

½ cup shredded carrot (1 medium)

2 tablespoons sliced green onion (1)

Lettuce leaves (optional)

1. Pour 2 tablespoons of the Thyme Vinaigrette into a small bowl; brush onto chicken. Set aside the remaining vinaigrette.

2. Place chicken on the unheated rack of a broiler pan; broil 4 to 5 inches from heat for 12 to 15 minutes or until chicken is tender and no longer pink (170°F), turning once halfway through broiling time. Cut chicken into slices.

3. Meanwhile, rinse green beans with cool water for 30 seconds; drain. In a large bowl toss together beans, chilled rice, artichoke hearts, cabbage, carrot, and green onion. Pour the remaining vinaigrette over rice mixture; toss gently to coat.

4. If desired, arrange lettuce leaves on 4 dinner plates. Top with the rice mixture and chicken slices.

Thyme Vinaigrette: In a screw-top jar combine ¼ cup white wine vinegar; 2 tablespoons olive oil; 2 tablespoons water; 1 tablespoon grated Parmesan cheese; 2 teaspoons snipped fresh thyme; 1 clove garlic, minced; ¼ teaspoon salt; and ¼ teaspoon black pepper. Cover and shake well.

Nutrition Facts per serving: 325 cal., 9 g total fat (2 g sat. fat), 50 mg chol., 545 mg sodium, 32 g carbo., 6 g fiber, 25 g pro.
Exchanges: 2 Vegetable, 1½ Starch, 2½ Medium-Fat Meat

Honey-Crusted Chicken

Prep: 10 minutes Bake: 18 minutes Oven: 350°F Makes: 4 servings

Nonstick cooking spray

4 small skinless, boneless
  chicken breast halves (about
  12 ounces)

1 tablespoon honey

1 tablespoon orange juice

1/4 teaspoon ground ginger

1/4 teaspoon black pepper

  Dash cayenne pepper
  (optional)

3/4 cup cornflakes, crushed (about
  1/3 cup)

1/2 teaspoon dried parsley flakes

1. Lightly coat a shallow baking pan with cooking spray. Place chicken in baking pan.

2. In a small bowl combine honey, orange juice, ginger, black pepper, and, if desired, cayenne pepper. Brush the honey mixture over chicken.

3. Combine the cornflakes and parsley flakes. Sprinkle cornflake mixture over chicken.

4. Bake, uncovered, in a 350° oven for 18 to 20 minutes or until chicken is tender and no longer pink (170°F).

Nutrition Facts per serving: 130 cal., 1 g total fat (0 g sat. fat), 49 mg chol., 79 mg sodium, 9 g carbo., 0 g fiber, 20 g pro.
Exchanges: 1/2 Starch, 3 Very Lean Meat

Mediterranean Chicken and Pasta

Start to Finish: 30 minutes Makes: 4 servings

1 6-ounce jar marinated artichoke hearts

1 tablespoon olive oil

12 ounces skinless, boneless
   chicken breast halves, cut into
   ¾-inch pieces

3 cloves garlic, thinly sliced

½ cup chicken broth

1 tablespoon small fresh oregano
   leaves or 1 teaspoon dried
   oregano, crushed

1 cup roasted red sweet peppers,
   drained and cut into strips

¼ cup pitted kalamata olives

3 cups hot cooked whole wheat
   penne or rotini pasta

1. Drain artichokes, reserving marinade. Set aside. In a large skillet heat oil over medium-high heat. Add chicken and garlic; cook and stir until chicken is no longer pink. Add the reserved artichoke marinade, chicken broth, and dried oregano (if using).

2. Bring to boiling; reduce heat. Simmer, covered, for 10 minutes. Stir in artichokes, roasted pepper, olives, and fresh oregano (if using). Heat through.

3. To serve, spoon the chicken mixture over hot cooked pasta.

Nutrition Facts per serving: 320 cal., 9 g total fat (1 g sat. fat), 50 mg chol., 396 mg sodium, 36 g carbo., 4 g fiber, 27 g pro. **Exchanges:** ½ Vegetable, 2 Starch, 2½ Very Lean Meat, 1 Fat

Summer Chicken and Mushroom Pasta

Start to Finish: 30 minutes Makes: 6 servings

8 ounces dried penne pasta

12 ounces skinless, boneless chicken breast halves, cut into bite-size strips

1/4 teaspoon salt

1/8 teaspoon black pepper

2 tablespoons olive oil or cooking oil

3 large cloves garlic, minced

3 cups sliced fresh mushrooms

1 medium onion, thinly sliced

3/4 cup chicken broth

1 cup cherry tomatoes, halved

1/4 cup shredded fresh basil

3 tablespoons snipped fresh oregano

1/4 cup finely shredded Parmesan cheese

1/8 teaspoon black pepper

1. Cook pasta according to package directions; drain. Return pasta to saucepan; cover and keep warm.

2. Meanwhile, sprinkle chicken with salt and 1/8 teaspoon of the pepper. In a large skillet heat 1 tablespoon of the oil over medium-high heat. Add chicken and garlic. Cook and stir for 3 to 4 minutes or until chicken is no longer pink. Remove from skillet; cover and keep warm.

3. Add the remaining 1 tablespoon oil to skillet. Add mushrooms and onion; cook just until tender, stirring occasionally. Carefully add broth. Bring to boiling; reduce heat. Boil gently, uncovered, about 2 minutes or until liquid is reduced by half. Remove skillet from heat.

4. Add cooked pasta, chicken, cherry tomatoes, basil, and oregano to mushroom mixture; toss gently to coat. Transfer chicken mixture to a serving dish; sprinkle with Parmesan cheese and 1/8 teaspoon pepper. Serve immediately.

Nutrition Facts per serving: 299 cal., 8 g total fat (2 g sat. fat), 37 mg chol., 249 mg sodium, 33 g carbo., 2 g fiber, 22 g pro.
Exchanges: 1 1/2 Vegetable, 1 Starch, 1 Lean Meat, 1/2 Fat

Lemon-Tarragon Chicken Toss

Start to Finish: 20 minutes Makes: 4 servings

6 ounces dried fettuccine
   or linguine

2 cups broccoli or cauliflower
   florets

½ cup reduced-sodium
   chicken broth

3 tablespoons lemon juice

1 tablespoon honey

2 teaspoons cornstarch

¼ teaspoon ground white pepper

12 ounces skinless, boneless
   chicken breast halves, cut into
   bite-size strips

2 teaspoons olive oil or
   cooking oil

½ cup shredded carrot
   (1 medium)

1 tablespoon snipped fresh
   tarragon or ½ teaspoon dried
   tarragon, crushed

   Lemon slices, halved (optional)

1. Cook pasta according to package directions, adding the broccoli for the last 4 minutes of cooking. Drain.

2. Meanwhile, in a small bowl combine broth, lemon juice, honey, cornstarch, and white pepper; set aside.

3. In a large nonstick skillet cook and stir chicken in hot oil for 3 to 4 minutes or until no longer pink. Stir broth mixture; add to skillet. Cook and stir until thickened and bubbly. Add carrot and tarragon; cook 1 minute more.

4. To serve, spoon chicken mixture over pasta. If desired, garnish with lemon slices. Serve immediately.

Nutrition Facts per serving: 320 cal., 4 g total fat (1 g sat. fat), 49 mg chol., 143 mg sodium, 43 g carbo., 3 g fiber, 27 g pro.
Exchanges: 1 Vegetable, 2½ Starch, 2½ Very Lean Meat

Sweet and Spicy Turkey Skillet

Start to Finish: 30 minutes Makes: 4 servings

½ cup apple juice

¼ cup hoisin sauce

1 teaspoon grated fresh ginger

¼ teaspoon salt

⅛ teaspoon cayenne pepper

2 small red, green, and/or yellow sweet peppers, cut into bite-size strips

1 medium onion, cut into thin wedges

2 tablespoons cooking oil

4 turkey breast tenderloin steaks, cut ½ inch thick (about 1 pound)

1 tablespoon cold water

2 teaspoons cornstarch

1 small apple or pear, cored and cut into wedges

1. In a small bowl combine apple juice, hoisin sauce, ginger, salt, and cayenne pepper; set aside.

2. In a large skillet cook sweet pepper and onion in hot oil over medium-high heat for 4 to 5 minutes or until nearly tender. Remove vegetables, reserving oil in skillet. Add turkey to skillet; cook about 4 minutes or until light brown, turning once.

3. Return vegetables to skillet; add apple juice mixture. Bring to boiling; reduce heat. Cover and simmer for 8 to 10 minutes or until turkey is no longer pink (170°F).

4. Using a slotted spoon, transfer turkey and vegetables to a serving platter; cover and keep warm.

5. In a small bowl combine water and cornstarch; stir into liquid in skillet. Cook and stir over medium heat until thickened and bubbly. Stir in apple. Cover and cook about 3 minutes more or just until apple is slightly softened. Serve over turkey and vegetables.

Nutrition Facts per serving: 267 cal., 8 g total fat (1 g sat. fat), 70 mg chol., 395 mg sodium, 18 g carbo., 2 g fiber, 29 g pro.
Exchanges: ½ Fruit, 1 Other Carbo., 1 Very Lean Meat, 1½ Fat

Turkey Burgers with Cranberry Sauce

Prep: 12 minutes Broil: 11 minutes Makes: 4 servings

⅓ cup herb-seasoned stuffing mix, crushed

2 tablespoons reduced-fat milk

1 tablespoon snipped fresh sage or ½ teaspoon dried sage, crushed

¼ teaspoon salt

1 pound uncooked ground turkey

1 cup torn mixed salad greens, watercress leaves, or shredded fresh spinach

4 whole wheat hamburger buns, split and toasted

½ cup whole cranberry sauce

1. In a large bowl combine stuffing mix, milk, sage, and salt. Add ground turkey; mix well. Shape into four ½-inch-thick patties.

2. Place patties on the unheated rack of a broiler pan. Broil 4 to 5 inches from the heat for 11 to 13 minutes or until internal temperature registers 170°F on an instant-read meat thermometer; turn once.

3. Divide salad greens among buns; top with patties and cranberry sauce.

Nutrition Facts per serving: 350 cal., 11 g total fat (3 g sat. fat), 71 mg chol., 503 mg sodium, 37 g carbo., 3 g fiber, 28 g pro. **Exchanges:** 2 Starch, ½ Other Carbo., 3 Lean Meat

Tall Turkey Sandwiches

Start to Finish: 15 minutes Makes: 4 sandwiches

¼ cup fat-free plain yogurt

3 tablespoons horseradish mustard

8 slices multigrain bread, toasted

12 lettuce leaves

8 ounces thinly sliced cooked turkey or chicken breast

1 tomato, sliced

1 yellow sweet pepper, sliced

1 cup fresh pea pods

1. In a small bowl stir together yogurt and horseradish mustard. Spread yogurt mixture on 4 of the toasted bread slices.

2. Top the remaining bread slices with lettuce leaves, turkey, tomato, sweet pepper, and pea pods. Top with remaining bread slices, spread sides down.

Per sandwich: 260 cal., 3 g total fat (1 g sat. fat), 47 mg chol., 403 mg sodium, 32 g carbo., 5 g fiber, 25 g pro.
Exchanges: 1 Vegetable, 2 Starch, 2 Very Lean Meat

Fast Fajita Roll-Ups

Start to Finish: 20 minutes Oven: 350°F Makes: 4 servings

12 ounces beef flank steak or sirloin steak or skinless, boneless chicken breast halves

4 8-inch spinach or flour tortillas

1 tablespoon cooking oil

1/3 cup finely chopped onion (1 small)

1/3 cup finely chopped green sweet pepper

1/2 cup chopped tomato (1 medium)

2 tablespoons bottled reduced-calorie Italian salad dressing

1/2 cup shredded reduced-fat cheddar cheese (2 ounces)

1/4 cup salsa or taco sauce

1/4 cup light dairy sour cream (optional)

1. If desired, partially freeze beef for easier slicing. If using steak, trim fat from meat. Cut beef or chicken into bite-size strips.

2. Wrap tortillas tightly in foil. Heat in a 350° oven about 10 minutes or until heated through.

3. Meanwhile, heat oil in a 12-inch skillet over medium-high heat. Add meat, onion, and sweet pepper; cook and stir for 2 to 3 minutes or until desired doneness for steak or chicken is no longer pink. Remove from heat. Drain well. Stir in tomato and salad dressing.

4. To serve, fill warm tortillas with meat mixture. Roll up tortillas. Serve with cheese, salsa, and, if desired, sour cream.

Nutrition Facts per serving: 324 cal., 15 g total fat (6 g sat. fat), 43 mg chol., 462 mg sodium, 21 g carbo., 2 g fiber, 24 g pro.
Exchanges: 1 Vegetable, 1 Starch, 3 Lean Meat, 1 Fat

Ginger Beef Stir-Fry

Start to Finish: 30 minutes Makes: 4 servings

8 ounces beef top round steak

½ cup reduced-sodium beef broth

3 tablespoons light soy sauce

2½ teaspoons cornstarch

1 teaspoon sugar

1 teaspoon grated fresh ginger

Nonstick cooking spray

1¼ pounds fresh asparagus spears, trimmed and cut into 2-inch pieces (3 cups), or 3 cups small broccoli florets

1½ cups sliced fresh mushrooms

4 green onions, bias-sliced into 2-inch lengths (½ cup)

1 tablespoon cooking oil

2 cups hot cooked rice

1. If desired, partially freeze meat for easier slicing. Trim fat from meat. Thinly slice meat across the grain into bite-size strips. Set aside. For the sauce, in a small bowl stir together broth, soy sauce, cornstarch, sugar, and ginger; set aside.

2. Lightly coat an unheated wok or large skillet with cooking spray. Preheat over medium-high heat. Add asparagus, mushrooms, and green onion. Stir-fry for 3 to 4 minutes or until vegetables are crisp-tender. Remove vegetables from wok or skillet.

3. Carefully add the oil to wok or skillet. Add meat; stir-fry for 2 to 3 minutes or until brown. Push the meat from center of the wok or skillet. Stir sauce. Add sauce to center of wok or skillet. Cook and stir until thickened and bubbly.

4. Return vegetables to wok or skillet. Stir all ingredients together to coat with sauce; heat through. Serve immediately over hot cooked rice.

Nutrition Facts per serving: 258 cal., 7 g total fat (2 g sat. fat), 25 mg chol., 523 mg sodium, 31 g carbo., 3 g fiber, 19 g pro.
Exchanges: 1½ Vegetable, 1½ Starch, 1½ Lean Meat, ½ Fat

Greek Beef and Pasta Skillet

Start to Finish: 25 minutes Makes: 4 servings

12 ounces boneless beef sirloin steak or top round steak

2 cups dried rotini

1 10-ounce package frozen chopped spinach, thawed

1 tablespoon cooking oil

2 cups ripe olive and mushroom pasta sauce, ripe olive and green olive pasta sauce, or marinara pasta sauce

1/4 teaspoon ground cinnamon

1. If desired, partially freeze meat for easier slicing. Trim fat from meat. Thinly slice across the grain into bite-size pieces. Cook pasta according to package directions; drain.

2. Meanwhile, place spinach in a colander. Using the back of a spoon, press spinach to remove excess liquid.

3. In a large skillet cook and stir beef in hot oil for 2 to 3 minutes or until it reaches desired doneness. Add pasta sauce and cinnamon. Cook and stir until sauce is bubbly. Add cooked pasta and spinach. Cook and stir until heated through.

Nutrition Facts per serving: 445 cal., 12 g total fat (4 g sat. fat), 58 mg chol., 683 mg sodium, 53 g carbo., 5 g fiber, 29 g pro.
Exchanges: 1 1/2 Vegetable, 3 Starch, 2 1/2 Lean Meat, 1/2 Fat

Saucy Strip Steak

Prep: 10 minutes Cook: 3 minutes Grill: 11 minutes Makes: 4 servings

²/₃ cup orange marmalade

2 tablespoons butter or margarine

1 teaspoon snipped fresh rosemary or ¼ teaspoon dried rosemary, crushed

4 8-ounce boneless beef top loin steaks, cut about 1 inch thick

Salt

Black pepper

1. In a small saucepan combine the marmalade, butter, and rosemary. Cook and stir over low heat until butter is melted and mixture is heated through. Set aside.

2. Trim fat from meat. Sprinkle both sides of steaks with salt and pepper. For a charcoal grill, grill steaks on the rack of an uncovered grill directly over medium coals to desired doneness, turning once halfway through cooking and brushing with marmalade mixture during the last 5 minutes of cooking time. (Allow 11 to 15 minutes for medium rare [145°] or 14 to 18 minutes for medium [160°F].) (For a gas grill, preheat grill. Reduce heat to medium. Place steaks on grill rack over heat. Cover; grill as above.)

3. Transfer steaks to a serving platter. Spoon any remaining marmalade mixture over steaks.

Nutrition Facts per serving: 464 cal., 14 g total fat (7 g sat. fat), 123 mg chol., 357 mg sodium, 35 g carbo., 0 g fiber, 49 g pro.
Exchanges: ½ Other Carbo., 6 Lean Meat, 1½ Fat

Pork Medallions with Pear-Maple Sauce

Start to Finish: 25 minutes Makes: 4 servings

1 12- to 16-ounce pork tenderloin

2 teaspoons snipped fresh rosemary or $\frac{1}{2}$ teaspoon dried rosemary, crushed

1 teaspoon snipped fresh thyme or $\frac{1}{4}$ teaspoon dried thyme, crushed

$\frac{1}{4}$ teaspoon salt

$\frac{1}{4}$ teaspoon black pepper

1 tablespoon olive oil or cooking oil

2 medium pears, peeled and coarsely chopped

$\frac{1}{4}$ cup pure maple syrup or maple-flavored syrup

2 tablespoons dried tart red cherries, halved

2 tablespoons apple juice

1. Trim fat from meat. Cut meat into $\frac{1}{4}$-inch slices. In a medium bowl combine rosemary, thyme, salt, and pepper. Add meat slices; toss to coat.

2. In a large skillet cook meat, half at a time, in hot oil for 2 to 3 minutes or until meat is slightly pink in center, turning once. Remove meat from skillet; set aside.

3. In the same skillet combine pear, maple syrup, dried cherries, and apple juice. Bring to boiling; reduce heat. Boil gently, uncovered, about 3 minutes or just until pear is tender. Return meat to skillet with pear; heat through.

4. To serve, use a slotted spoon to transfer meat to a warm serving platter. Spoon the pear mixture over meat.

Nutrition Facts per serving: 255 cal., 7 g total fat (2 g sat. fat), 60 mg chol., 179 mg sodium, 29 g carbo., 3 g fiber, 19 g pro. **Exchanges:** 1 Fruit, 1½ Lean Meat

Squirt-of-Orange Chops

Prep: 10 minutes Broil: 9 minutes Makes: 4 servings

1 large orange

4 boneless pork top loin chops,
   cut 1 inch thick (about
   1¼ pounds)

½ teaspoon garlic-pepper
   seasoning

¼ teaspoon salt

¼ cup orange marmalade

2 teaspoons snipped fresh
   rosemary

1. Cut orange in half. Cut one half of the orange into 4 wedges; set wedges aside. Squeeze juice from remaining orange half. Remove 1 tablespoon of the juice and brush on both sides of each chop. Sprinkle chops with garlic-pepper seasoning and salt. In a small bowl combine remaining orange juice, orange marmalade, and rosemary; set aside.

2. Preheat broiler. Place chops on the unheated rack of a broiler pan. Broil 3 to 4 inches from the heat for 9 to 12 minutes or until juices run clear (160°F), turning once and brushing with orange marmalade mixture for the last 2 to 3 minutes of broiling.

3. Serve orange wedges with chops. If desired, squeeze juice from orange wedges over chops.

Nutrition Facts per serving: 262 cal., 7 g total fat (3 g sat. fat), 83 mg chol., 343 mg sodium, 17 g carbo., 1 g fiber, 31 g pro.
Exchanges: 1 Fruit, 4½ Medium-Fat Meat

Hoisin and Citrus Shrimp Saute

Start to Finish: 25 minutes Makes: 4 servings

12 ounces fresh or frozen large
   shrimp in shells

2 tablespoons cooking oil

2 cloves garlic, minced

1 medium red sweet pepper, cut
   into thin strips

1/3 cup orange juice

3 tablespoons bottled hoisin
   sauce

1 1/2 cups shredded fresh spinach

2 cups hot cooked rice

1. Thaw shrimp, if frozen. Peel and devein shrimp. Rinse shrimp; pat dry with paper towels. Set aside.

2. In a large skillet heat 1 tablespoon of the oil over medium-high heat. Add garlic; cook and stir for 15 seconds. Add sweet pepper; cook and stir about 3 minutes or until pepper is crisp-tender. Remove from skillet.

3. Add the remaining 1 tablespoon oil to skillet. Add the shrimp. Cook and stir about 3 minutes or until shrimp are opaque. Remove from skillet. Add the orange juice and hoisin sauce. Bring to boiling; reduce heat. Simmer, uncovered, about 1 minute or until slightly thickened. Return shrimp and sweet pepper to skillet. Add the spinach; toss just until combined. To serve, spoon the shrimp mixture over hot cooked rice.

Nutrition Facts per serving: 306 cal., 9 g total fat (1 g sat. fat), 129 mg chol., 372 mg sodium, 34 g carbo., 1 g fiber, 20 g pro.
Exchanges: 1 Vegetable, 1 Starch, 1 Lean Meat, 1/2 Fat

Snapper Veracruz

Start to Finish: 30 minutes   Makes: 6 servings

1½ pounds fresh or frozen skinless red snapper or other fish fillets, ½ to ¾ inch thick

⅛ teaspoon salt

⅛ teaspoon black pepper

1 large onion, sliced and separated into rings

2 cloves garlic, minced

1 tablespoon cooking oil

2 cups chopped, seeded tomato (2 large)

¼ cup sliced pimiento-stuffed green olives

¼ cup chicken broth

2 tablespoons capers, drained

½ teaspoon sugar

1 bay leaf

Snipped fresh parsley

1. Thaw fish, if frozen. Rinse fish; pat dry with paper towels. Cut fish into 6 serving-size pieces. Sprinkle with salt and pepper.

2. For sauce, in a large skillet cook onion and garlic in hot oil until onion is tender. Stir in tomato, olives, broth, capers, sugar, and bay leaf. Bring to boiling. Add fish to skillet. Return to boiling; reduce heat. Simmer, covered, for 6 to 10 minutes or until fish flakes easily when tested with a fork. Use a slotted spatula to carefully transfer fish from skillet to a serving platter. Cover and keep warm.

3. Bring sauce in skillet to boiling. Boil sauce for 5 to 6 minutes or until reduced to about 2 cups, stirring occasionally. Discard bay leaf. Spoon sauce over fish. Sprinkle with parsley.

Nutrition Facts per serving: 166 cal., 5 g total fat (1 g sat. fat), 41 mg chol., 332 mg sodium, 6 g carbo., 1 g fiber, 24 g pro.
Exchanges: ½ Vegetable, 3 Very Lean Meat, ½ Fat

Fish Fillets with Roasted Red Pepper Sauce

Start to Finish: 25 minutes Makes: 4 servings

1 12-ounce jar roasted red sweet peppers, drained

2 cloves garlic, minced

1 cup water

2 tablespoons tomato paste

1 tablespoon red wine vinegar

2 teaspoons dried basil, crushed

½ teaspoon sugar

⅛ teaspoon salt

   Dash cayenne pepper

1 pound cod, orange roughy, or other fish fillets

1 lemon, sliced

¼ teaspoon salt

¼ teaspoon lemon-pepper seasoning

1. For sauce, in a blender or food processor combine roasted sweet peppers and garlic. Cover and blend or process until nearly smooth. Add ½ cup of the water, the tomato paste, vinegar, basil, sugar, the ⅛ teaspoon salt, and cayenne pepper. Cover; blend or process with several on-off pulses until mixture is nearly smooth. Transfer to a small saucepan; cook over medium heat until heated through, stirring frequently.

2. Meanwhile, rinse fish; pat dry with paper towels. Measure thickness of fish. Cut fish into 4 serving-size pieces. In a large skillet bring the remaining ½ cup water and half of the lemon slices just to boiling. Carefully add fish. Return just to boiling; reduce heat. Simmer, covered, for 4 to 6 minutes per ½-inch thickness of fish or until fish flakes easily when tested with a fork. Gently pat tops of fish dry with paper towels. Sprinkle fish lightly with the ¼ teaspoon salt and the lemon-pepper seasoning.

3. To serve, spoon the sauce onto dinner plates. Place the fish on top of sauce. Garnish with remaining lemon slices.

Nutrition Facts per serving: 119 cal., 1 g total fat (0 g sat. fat), 49 mg chol., 343 mg sodium, 6 g carbo., 1 g fiber, 21 g pro.
Exchanges: ½ Other Carbo., 3 Very Lean Meat

Soft Fish Tacos with Mango Salsa

Prep: 20 minutes Broil: 8 minutes Makes: 4 servings

1 pound fresh or frozen
    swordfish or halibut steaks,
    1 inch thick

½ teaspoon Jamaican jerk
    seasoning

4 8- to 10-inch whole wheat or
    flour tortillas

2 cups fresh small spinach leaves
    or shredded lettuce

1 recipe Mango Salsa

   Lime wedges (optional)

1. Thaw fish, if frozen. Rinse fish; pat dry with paper towels. Cut fish into ¾-inch slices; sprinkle with Jamaican jerk seasoning.

2. Place seasoned fish slices on the greased, unheated rack of a broiler pan. Broil fish 4 inches from the heat for 5 minutes; turn fish. Broil for 3 to 7 minutes more or until fish flakes easily when tested with a fork. Meanwhile, wrap tortillas in foil. Heat package on lower rack of oven for 5 to 7 minutes.

3. Fill each warm tortilla with spinach, fish, and Mango Salsa. If desired, serve with lime wedges.

Mango Salsa: In a large bowl combine 1 thinly sliced green onion; 1 large mango, peeled, seeded, and chopped; 1 large tomato, seeded and chopped; 1 small cucumber, seeded and chopped; 2 to 4 tablespoons snipped, fresh cilantro; 1 fresh jalapeño chile pepper, seeded and chopped*; and 1 tablespoon lime juice. Cover and chill until serving time. Serve with a slotted spoon. Makes about 3 cups.

*Note: When working with chile peppers, wear plastic or rubber gloves. If your bare hands do touch the chile peppers, wash your hands well with soap and water.

Nutrition Facts per serving: 261 cal., 5 g total fat (1 g sat. fat), 43 mg chol., 346 mg sodium, 28 g carbo., 13 g fiber, 26 g pro.
Exchanges: 1 Vegetable, ½ Fruit, 1 Starch, 3 Medium-Fat Meat

Deli-Style Pasta Salad

Start to Finish: 30 minutes Makes: 4 servings

½ of a 16-ounce package frozen cheese-filled tortellini or one 9-ounce package refrigerated cheese-filled tortellini (about 2 cups)

1½ cups broccoli florets

¾ cup thinly sliced carrot (1 large)

¾ cup chopped yellow and/or red sweet pepper (1 medium)

¼ cup white wine vinegar

2 tablespoons olive oil

1 teaspoon dried Italian seasoning, crushed

1 teaspoon Dijon-style mustard

¼ teaspoon black pepper

⅛ teaspoon garlic powder

Kale leaves (optional)

1. Cook pasta in a large saucepan according to package directions, except omit any oil and salt and add the broccoli, carrot, and sweet pepper for the last 3 minutes of cooking time. Return to boiling; reduce heat. Simmer, uncovered, about 3 minutes or until pasta is just tender and vegetables are crisp-tender. Drain. Rinse with cold water; drain again.

2. For dressing, in a screw-top jar combine the vinegar, oil, Italian seasoning, mustard, pepper, and garlic powder. Cover and shake well. Pour over pasta mixture; toss to coat. If desired, serve in kale-lined salad bowls.

Nutrition Facts per serving: 262 cal., 10 g total fat (1 g sat. fat), 31 mg chol., 300 mg sodium, 33 g carbo., 2 g fiber, 11 g pro.
Exchanges: 2 Vegetable, 1½ Starch, ½ Medium-Fat Meat, 1 Fat

Lentil and Veggie Tostadas

Start to Finish: 25 minutes Makes: 4 servings

1¾ cups water

¾ cup dry red lentils, rinsed
   and drained

¼ cup chopped onion

1 to 2 tablespoons snipped
   fresh cilantro

1 clove garlic, minced

½ teaspoon salt

½ teaspoon ground cumin

4 tostada shells

2 cups chopped fresh vegetables
   (such as broccoli, tomato, zucchini, and/or yellow summer
   squash)

¾ cup shredded Monterey Jack
   cheese (3 ounces)

1. In a medium saucepan stir together water, lentils, onion, cilantro, garlic, salt, and cumin. Bring to boiling; reduce heat. Simmer, covered, for 12 to 15 minutes or until lentils are tender and most of the liquid is absorbed. Use a fork to mash the cooked lentils.

2. Spread the lentil mixture on tostada shells; top with the vegetables and cheese. Place on a large baking sheet. Broil tostadas 3 to 4 inches from the heat about 2 minutes or until cheese is melted.

Nutrition Facts per serving: 288 cal., 11 g total fat (5 g sat. fat), 20 mg chol., 497 mg sodium, 34 g carbo., 7 g fiber, 16 g pro. **Exchanges:** ½ Milk, 1 Vegetable, 1 Starch, ½ Lean Meat

Ravioli Skillet

Prep: 6 minutes Cook: 7 minutes Makes: 4 servings

1 14-ounce can vegetable or
  chicken broth

1 14½-ounce can Italian-style
  stewed tomatoes, undrained

2 medium zucchini, halved
  lengthwise and cut into
  ½-inch slices (about 2½ cups)

1 9-ounce package refrigerated
  cheese ravioli

1 15- to 16-ounce can cannellini
  (white kidney) or navy beans,
  rinsed and drained

2 tablespoons snipped fresh basil
  or parsley

2 tablespoons grated
  Parmesan cheese

1. In a large saucepan combine broth and undrained tomatoes; bring to boiling. Add zucchini and ravioli. Return to boiling; reduce heat. Boil gently, uncovered, for 6 to 7 minutes or until ravioli is tender and sauce has thickened slightly, gently stirring once or twice.

2. Add beans to ravioli mixture; heat through. Sprinkle each serving with basil and Parmesan cheese.

Nutrition Facts per serving: 335 cal., 11 g total fat (5 g sat. fat), 58 mg chol., 1,131 mg sodium, 47 g carbo., 7 g fiber, 19 g pro.
Exchanges: 2 Vegetable, 2½ Starch, 1½ Fat

Sweet Bean Pilaf

Prep: 15 minutes Cook: 10 minutes Makes: 4 servings

½ cup chopped onion (1 medium)

2 cloves garlic, minced

1 tablespoon olive oil

1 cup bulgur

1 cup frozen green or sweet soy-beans (edamame)

1 cup orange juice

1 cup chicken broth

1 medium carrot, cut into thin bite-size strips

½ cup bias-sliced celery (1 stalk)

2 oranges, peeled and sectioned

⅓ cup dried tart cherries or raisins

1. In a large saucepan cook onion and garlic in hot oil until onion is tender. Stir in bulgur, soybeans, orange juice, broth, carrot, and celery.

2. Bring to boiling; reduce heat. Simmer, covered, for 10 to 12 minutes or until soybeans are tender and liquid is absorbed. Stir in oranges and dried cherries.

Nutrition Facts per serving: 348 cal., 9 g total fat (1 g sat. fat), 0 mg chol., 227 mg sodium, 56 g carbo., 19 g fiber, 16 g pro. **Exchanges:** 2 Vegetable, 1 Fruit, 2½ Starch, ½ Fat

Triple-Decker Tortilla

Start to Finish: 20 minutes Oven: 450°F Makes: 4 servings

Nonstick cooking spray

1 cup canned pinto beans, rinsed and drained

1 cup salsa

4 6-inch corn tortillas

½ cup frozen whole kernel corn

½ cup shredded reduced-fat Monterey Jack or cheddar cheese (2 ounces)

½ cup shredded lettuce

1. Lightly coat a 9-inch pie plate with cooking spray; set aside. Place beans in a small bowl; mash the beans slightly. In a small saucepan or skillet cook and stir beans over medium heat for 2 to 3 minutes. Set aside.

2. Spoon ¼ cup of the salsa into bottom of prepared pie plate. Top with 1 of the tortillas. Layer half of the mashed beans, 1 tortilla, corn, ¼ cup of the cheese, ¼ cup salsa, 1 tortilla, remaining bean mixture, remaining tortilla, and remaining ½ cup salsa.

3. Cover with foil; bake for 12 minutes in a 450° oven. (Or cover with microwave-safe plastic wrap; microwave at 100 percent power [high] for 4 minutes, rotating once.) Remove foil. Sprinkle with remaining ¼ cup cheese.

4. Bake, uncovered, 3 minutes more. (Or microwave, uncovered, on high for 30 seconds more.) Top with lettuce.

Nutrition Facts per serving: 219 cal., 5 g total fat (2 g sat. fat), 10 mg chol., 813 mg sodium, 38 g carbo., 6 g fiber, 10 g pro.
Exchanges: ½ Vegetable, 2 Starch, ½ Lean Meat, ½ Fat

Tortellini and Tomato Soup

Start to Finish: 20 minutes Makes: 4 servings

1 9-ounce package refrigerated
    cheese tortellini

1 14-ounce can reduced-sodium
    chicken broth

1 14½-ounce can diced tomatoes
    with basil, garlic, and oregano,
    undrained

1 cup water

2 tablespoons tomato paste

1 cup finely chopped zucchini
    (1 small)

1 tablespoon snipped fresh sage
    or 1 teaspoon dried sage,
    crushed

¼ cup shredded Asiago or
    Parmesan cheese (1 ounce)

1. Cook tortellini according to package directions; drain.

2. Meanwhile, in a large saucepan combine chicken broth, undrained tomatoes, water, and tomato paste. Bring to boiling. Stir in drained tortellini, zucchini, and sage; heat through.

3. To serve, ladle soup into serving bowls; top each serving with cheese.

Nutrition Facts per serving: 287 cal., 7 g total fat (3 g sat. fat), 38 mg chol., 1,113 mg sodium, 41 g carbo., 1 g fiber, 15 g pro. **Exchanges:** 1 Vegetable, 2 Starch, 1 Medium-Fat Meat

Penne with Fennel

Start to Finish: 30 minutes Makes: 4 servings

2 cups dried penne pasta
   (6 ounces)

2 medium bulbs fennel (about
   2 pounds)

3 cloves garlic, minced

¼ teaspoon crushed red pepper

1 tablespoon olive oil

2 small yellow, green, and/or red
   sweet peppers, cut into thin
   bite-size strips (about 1 cup)

1 15-ounce can Great Northern
   beans, rinsed and drained

2 teaspoons snipped fresh thyme
   or ¼ teaspoon dried thyme,
   crushed

   Freshly ground black pepper
   (optional)

1. In a large saucepan cook pasta according to package directions. Drain; return pasta to saucepan and keep warm.

2. Meanwhile, cut off feathery leaves and upper stalks of fennel bulbs. If desired, reserve some of the feathery leaves for garnish; discard upper stalks. Remove any wilted outer layers of stalks. Wash fennel and cut lengthwise into quarters. Remove core and discard; cut fennel into thin strips.

3. In a large skillet cook garlic and crushed red pepper in hot oil for 30 seconds. Add fennel to skillet; cook and stir for 5 minutes. Add sweet pepper strips; cook for 3 minutes more. Add beans and thyme; cook about 2 minutes or until heated through.

4. To serve, add fennel mixture to pasta; toss gently to combine. If desired, season to taste with freshly ground black pepper. If desired, garnish with reserved fennel leaves.

Nutrition Facts per serving: 370 cal., 5 g total fat (1 g sat. fat), 0 mg chol., 93 mg sodium, 69 g carbo., 12 g fiber, 16 g pro.
Exchanges: ½ Vegetable, 3½ Starch, 1 Very Lean Meat, 1 Fat

Vegetable and Tofu Stir-Fry

Start to Finish: 30 minutes Makes: 4 servings

1½ cups quick-cooking brown rice

¼ cup vegetable broth or chicken broth

¼ cup water

1 tablespoon cornstarch

1 tablespoon light soy sauce

1 teaspoon sugar

1 teaspoon grated fresh ginger

½ teaspoon crushed red pepper (optional)

Nonstick cooking spray

1 cup thinly bias-sliced carrot (2 medium)

3 cloves garlic, minced

3 cups broccoli florets

6 ounces firm tofu (fresh bean curd), cut into ½-inch cubes

1. Cook rice according to package directions; keep warm.

2. For sauce, in a small bowl stir together broth, water, cornstarch, soy sauce, sugar, ginger, and, if desired, crushed red pepper. Set sauce aside.

3. Coat an unheated wok or large skillet with cooking spray. Preheat over medium-high heat. Add carrot and garlic; stir-fry for 2 minutes. Add broccoli; stir-fry for 3 to 4 minutes more or until vegetables are crisp-tender. Push vegetables from center of wok.

4. Stir sauce; add to center of wok. Cook and stir until thickened and bubbly. Add tofu; stir together all ingredients to coat. Cook and stir for 1 minute more.

5. To serve, spoon vegetable mixture over hot cooked rice.

Nutrition Facts per serving: 211 cal., 3 g total fat (0 g sat. fat), 0 mg chol., 248 mg sodium, 38 g carbo., 5 g fiber, 9 g pro.
Exchanges: 1 Vegetable, 2 Starch, ½ Medium-Fat Meat

Pasta Salad with Italian Beans and Parmesan

Start to Finish: 25 minutes Makes: 4 servings

6 ounces dried ziti, elbow macaroni, or penne pasta

1 9-ounce package frozen Italian green beans, thawed

1/3 cup bottled fat-free Italian salad dressing

1 tablespoon snipped fresh tarragon or 1/2 teaspoon dried tarragon, crushed

1/2 teaspoon freshly ground pepper

2 cups torn radicchio or 1 cup finely shredded red cabbage

4 cups fresh spinach leaves

1/4 cup finely shredded Parmesan cheese (1 ounce)

1. Cook pasta according to package directions, adding green beans for the last 3 to 4 minutes of cooking; drain. Rinse pasta and beans with cold water; drain again.

2. In a large bowl combine Italian salad dressing, tarragon, and pepper. Add pasta mixture and radicchio; toss gently to coat.

3. To serve, divide spinach leaves among individual plates. Top with pasta mixture. Sprinkle each serving with Parmesan cheese.

Nutrition Facts per serving: 218 cal., 2 g total fat (1 g sat. fat), 4 mg chol., 301 mg sodium, 40 g carbo., 4 g fiber, 10 g pro. **Exchanges:** 2 Vegetable, 2 Starch, 1/2 Lean Meat

Eggplant Panini

Start to Finish: 25 minutes Makes: 6 servings

1 cup torn arugula

2 teaspoons red wine vinegar

1 teaspoon olive oil

1/3 cup seasoned fine dry
    bread crumbs

2 tablespoons grated Romano or
    Parmesan cheese

1 egg

1 tablespoon reduced-fat or fat-
    free milk

2 tablespoons all-purpose flour

1/2 teaspoon salt

1 medium eggplant, cut cross-
    wise into 1/2-inch slices

1 tablespoon olive oil

3 ounces mozzarella cheese,
    thinly sliced

6 individual focaccia rolls or one
    12-inch plain or seasoned
    Italian flatbread (focaccia),*
    halved horizontally

1 large tomato, thinly sliced

1. In a small bowl toss together arugula, red wine vinegar, and the 1 teaspoon oil; set aside. In a shallow dish stir together the bread crumbs and Romano cheese. In another shallow dish beat together egg and milk. In a third shallow dish stir together flour and salt. Dip the eggplant slices into flour mixture to coat. Dip the slices into egg mixture; coat both sides with bread crumb mixture.

2. In a 12-inch nonstick skillet heat the 1 tablespoon oil over medium heat. Add eggplant slices; cook for 6 to 8 minutes or until light brown, turning once. (Add more oil as necessary during cooking.) Top the eggplant with mozzarella cheese; reduce heat to low. Cook, covered, just until cheese begins to melt.

3. To serve, place the tomato slices on bottom halves of rolls. Top with eggplant slices, cheese sides up, and the arugula mixture. Add top halves of rolls.

*Note: For easier slicing, purchase focaccia that is at least 2 1/2 inches thick.

Nutrition Facts per serving: 271 cal., 10 g total fat (3 g sat. fat), 53 mg chol., 687 mg sodium, 37 g carbo., 3 g fiber, 12 g pro.
Exchanges: 1 Vegetable, 2 Starch, 1 Medium-Fat Meat, 1/2 Fat

one-dish meals

Cleanup is one of the things people dread the most about cooking. So make it easy on yourself with a one-dish meal! The recipes combine steps so you can cook everything using fewer dishes. Plus, most of these are complete meals—no need to cook any additional sides. Give these recipes a try. You'll have more time to enjoy the many things on your to-do list before your baby arrives.

Garden Pot Roast

Prep: 25 minutes Bake: 2½ hours Oven: 325°F Makes: 8 servings

1 3-pound boneless beef bottom
   round roast

   Salt

   Black pepper

1 tablespoon cooking oil

1 14-ounce can beef broth

½ cup coarsely chopped onion
   (1 medium)

½ teaspoon dried marjoram,
   crushed

½ teaspoon dried thyme, crushed

2 cloves garlic, minced

4 cups cut-up vegetables (such
   as 2-inch pieces of peeled
   winter squash, carrots,
   parsnips, and/or green beans)

2 tablespoons cold water

1 tablespoon cornstarch

1. Trim fat from meat. Sprinkle meat lightly with salt and pepper. In a 4- to 6-quart Dutch oven brown meat on all sides in hot oil for 5 minutes, turning to brown evenly. Drain off fat. Carefully pour broth over meat. Add onion, marjoram, thyme, and garlic. Bake, covered, in a 325° oven for 2 hours.

2. Add vegetables. Cover and bake for 30 to 40 minutes more or until tender. Transfer meat and vegetables to a serving platter; reserve cooking liquid in Dutch oven. Cover platter with foil to keep warm.

3. For gravy, strain juices into a glass measuring cup. Skim fat from juices; return 1¼ cups of the juices to Dutch oven (discard remaining juices). In a small bowl stir together the cold water and cornstarch. Stir into juices in Dutch oven. Cook and stir until thickened and bubbly. Cook and stir for 2 minutes more. Season to taste with salt and pepper. Slice meat. Spoon some of the gravy over meat and vegetables. Pass remaining gravy.

Nutrition Facts per serving: 250 cal., 8 g total fat (2 g sat. fat), 83 mg chol., 337 mg sodium, 9 g carbo., 2 g fiber, 33 g pro.
Exchanges: 1½ Vegetable, 4 Lean Meat

Maple Harvest Pot Roast

Prep: 25 minutes Cook: 1¾ hours Makes: 6 to 8 servings

1 2-pound boneless beef chuck pot roast

Salt

Black pepper

1 tablespoon cooking oil

1 teaspoon finely shredded orange peel

1½ cups orange juice

1 cup water

¼ cup maple syrup or maple-flavor syrup

½ teaspoon salt

¼ teaspoon ground ginger

⅛ teaspoon ground allspice

1½ pounds sweet potatoes (about 2 medium), peeled and cut into bite-size chunks

1 medium onion, cut into thin wedges

1 tablespoon cornstarch

1 tablespoon cold water

1. Trim fat from pot roast. Sprinkle pot roast with salt and pepper. In a 4-quart Dutch oven brown roast on all sides in hot oil. Drain off fat.

2. In a medium bowl combine orange peel, orange juice, the 1 cup water, the syrup, the ½ teaspoon salt, the ginger, and allspice. Pour over pot roast. Bring to boiling; reduce heat. Simmer, covered, for 1¼ hours. Add sweet potato and onion to meat. Return to boiling; reduce heat. Simmer, covered, about 30 minutes more or until meat and vegetables are tender, adding additional water if necessary.

3. Transfer meat and vegetables to a serving platter, reserving juices in Dutch oven. If desired, cut meat into bite-size pieces. Keep warm.

4. For sauce, measure juices; skim off fat. If necessary, add enough water to make 2 cups total liquid. Return to Dutch oven. In a small bowl stir together cornstarch and the 1 tablespoon cold water. Stir into juices in Dutch oven. Cook and stir over medium heat until thickened and bubbly. Cook and stir for 2 minutes more. If desired, season to taste with additional pepper. Serve sauce over meat and vegetables.

Nutrition Facts per serving: 399 cal., 8 g total fat (2 g sat. fat), 89 mg chol., 362 mg sodium, 46 g carbo., 4 g fiber, 35 g pro.
Exchanges: 1 Starch, 2 Other Carbo., 4 Medium-Fat Meat

Beef and Rutabaga Stew

Prep: 25 minutes Cook: 1 ½ hours Makes: 4 or 5 servings

12 ounces boneless beef chuck
   roast

2 tablespoons all-purpose flour

12 peeled pearl onions or 1 cup
   chopped onion (1 large)

2 tablespoons olive oil or
   cooking oil

2¼ cups reduced-sodium
   beef broth

1 cup water

1 tablespoon Worcestershire
   sauce

½ teaspoon dried thyme, crushed

¼ teaspoon black pepper

2 cloves garlic, minced

1 bay leaf

1 pound rutabaga, peeled and
   cut into ¾-inch cubes

6 ounces green beans, trimmed
   and cut into 2½-inch pieces,
   or 1 cup loose-pack frozen cut
   green beans

1 tablespoon tomato paste or
   ketchup

   Salt

   Black pepper

1. Trim fat from roast. Cut roast into ¾-inch cubes. Place flour in a plastic bag. Add meat cubes, a few at a time, shaking to coat.

2. In a large saucepan or Dutch oven cook meat and onions in hot oil over medium heat for 4 to 5 minutes or until meat is brown. Drain off fat. Stir in broth, water, Worcestershire sauce, thyme, pepper, garlic, and bay leaf. Bring to boiling; reduce heat. Simmer, covered, for 30 minutes.

3. Stir in rutabaga. Bring to boiling; reduce heat. Simmer, covered, about 1 hour more or until meat and rutabaga are tender, adding fresh green beans for the last 20 minutes or frozen green beans for the last 10 minutes of cooking. Discard bay leaf. Stir in tomato paste. Season to taste with salt and additional black pepper.

Nutrition Facts per serving: 265 cal., 10 g total fat (2 g sat. fat), 50 mg chol., 382 mg sodium, 21 g carbo., 5 g fiber, 22 g pro.
Exchanges: 1 Vegetable, 1 Starch, 2 Medium-Fat Meat, ½ Fat

Mushroom Beef Stew

Prep: 25 minutes Cook: 9 to 10 hours (low) or 4½ to 5 hours (high), plus 15 minutes (high)
Makes: 8 servings (8 cups)

2 pounds boneless beef chuck
   pot roast

8 ounces portobello mushrooms,
   cut into 1-inch pieces

8 ounces shiitake mushrooms or
   button mushrooms, stemmed
   and halved

1 cup chopped onion (1 large)

2 tablespoons Dijon-style
   mustard

2 cloves garlic, minced

½ teaspoon salt

½ teaspoon black pepper

2¼ cups reduced-sodium
   beef broth

1 8-ounce carton light dairy
   sour cream

2 tablespoons cornstarch

1 tablespoon snipped
   fresh chives

1. Trim fat from meat. Cut meat into 1-inch pieces. In a 4½- to 5½-quart slow cooker combine beef, mushrooms, onion, mustard, garlic, salt, and pepper. Stir in broth.

2. Cover and cook on low-heat setting for 9 to 10 hours or on high-heat setting for 4½ to 5 hours.

3. If using low-heat setting, turn to high-heat setting. In a small bowl combine sour cream and cornstarch. Stir ½ cup of the hot cooking liquid into the sour cream mixture. Return all of the sour cream mixture to the slow cooker; stir well. Cover and cook about 15 minutes more or until thickened. Top each serving with chives.

Nutrition Facts per serving: 224 cal., 7 g total fat (3 g sat. fat), 76 mg chol., 457 mg sodium, 12 g carbo., 1 g fiber, 29 g pro.
Exchanges: ½ Vegetable, ½ Other Carbo., 3 Lean Meat, 1 Fat

Country Italian Beef Stew

Prep: 25 minutes Cook: 8 to 10 hours (low) or 4 to 5 hours (high), plus 15 minutes (high)
Makes: 6 servings

2 pounds boneless beef chuck
   pot roast

3 medium parsnips, cut into
   1-inch pieces

2 cups chopped onions (2 large)

1 medium fennel bulb, trimmed
   and coarsely chopped (1 cup)

1 teaspoon dried rosemary,
   crushed

1¾ cups reduced-sodium beef
   broth

1 6-ounce can tomato paste

1 teaspoon salt

1 teaspoon finely shredded
   orange peel

½ teaspoon black pepper

2 cloves garlic, minced

2 tablespoons cornstarch

2 tablespoons cold water

3 cups torn fresh spinach

1. Trim fat from meat. Cut meat into 2-inch pieces. Set aside. In a 3½- or 4-quart slow cooker place parsnip, onion, and fennel. Add meat; sprinkle with rosemary. In a medium bowl combine broth, tomato paste, salt, orange peel, pepper, and garlic. Pour over mixture in cooker.

2. Cover and cook on low-heat setting for 8 to 10 hours or on high-heat setting for 4 to 5 hours.

3. If using low-heat setting, turn to high-heat setting. In a small bowl combine cornstarch and water. Stir into meat mixture. Cover and cook 15 minutes more or until thickened. Just before serving, stir in spinach.

Nutrition Facts per serving: 284 cal., 6 g total fat (2 g sat. fat), 89 mg chol., 659 mg sodium, 21 g carbo., 4 g fiber, 36 g pro.
Exchanges: 2 Vegetable, ½ Starch, 4 Lean Meat

Southwest Steak and Potato Soup

Prep: 25 minutes Cook: 8 to 10 hours (low) or 4 to 5 hours (high) Makes: 6 servings

1½ pounds boneless beef sirloin steak, cut 1 inch thick

2 medium potatoes, cut into 1-inch pieces

2 cups frozen cut green beans

1 small onion, sliced and separated into rings

1 16-ounce jar thick and chunky salsa

1 14-ounce can beef broth

1 teaspoon dried basil, crushed

2 cloves garlic, minced

Shredded Monterey Jack or Mexican blend cheese (optional)

1. Trim fat from meat. Cut meat into 1-inch pieces. Set aside.

2. In a 3½- or 4-quart slow cooker place potato, green beans, and onion. Add meat. In a medium bowl stir together salsa, broth, basil, and garlic. Pour over mixture in cooker.

3. Cover and cook on low-heat setting for 8 to 10 hours or on high-heat setting for 4 to 5 hours. If desired, sprinkle each serving with cheese.

Nutrition Facts per serving: 206 cal., 4 g total fat (1 g sat. fat), 68 mg chol., 624 mg sodium, 16 g carbo., 3 g fiber, 27 g pro.
Exchanges: ½ Vegetable, ½ Starch, 2½ Lean Meat

Teriyaki Beef Soup

Start to Finish: 40 minutes Makes: 5 servings

8 ounces boneless beef sirloin
   steak

2 teaspoons olive oil

1 large shallot, thinly sliced

4 cups water

1 cup apple juice or apple cider

2 carrots, cut into thin
   bite-size strips

1/3 cup uncooked long grain rice

1 tablespoon grated fresh ginger

1 clove garlic, minced

1 teaspoon instant beef bouillon
   granules

2 cups coarsely chopped broccoli

1 to 2 tablespoons light teriyaki
   sauce

1. Trim fat from meat. Cut meat into thin bite-size strips. In a large saucepan heat olive oil over medium-high heat. Add meat and shallot. Cook and stir for 2 to 3 minutes or until meat is brown. Use a slotted spoon to remove meat mixture; set aside.

2. In the same saucepan combine water, apple juice, carrot, rice, ginger, garlic, and bouillon granules. Bring to boiling; reduce heat. Simmer, covered, about 15 minutes or until carrot is tender.

3. Stir in broccoli and the meat mixture. Simmer, covered, for 3 minutes more. Stir in the teriyaki sauce.

Nutrition Facts per serving: 197 cal., 6 g total fat (2 g sat. fat), 30 mg chol., 382 mg sodium, 22 g carbo., 2 g fiber, 13 g pro.
Exchanges: 2 Vegetable, 1/2 Starch, 1 Lean Meat

Pineapple Beef

Prep: 15 minutes Marinate: 15 minutes Cook: 5 minutes Makes: 4 servings

12 ounces beef top round steak

1 8-ounce can pineapple slices
(juice pack)

2 tablespoons light soy sauce

1/2 teaspoon grated fresh ginger
or 1/8 teaspoon ground ginger

1/4 teaspoon crushed red pepper

1 tablespoon cornstarch

Nonstick cooking spray

4 green onions, cut into 1/2-inch
pieces

1 6-ounce package frozen pea
pods

1 medium tomato, cut into
wedges

2 cups hot cooked rice

1. If desired, partially freeze meat for easier slicing. Trim fat from meat. Thinly slice meat across the grain into bite-size strips. Drain pineapple, reserving juice. Cut pineapple slices into quarters. Set aside.

2. In a bowl stir together reserved pineapple juice, soy sauce, ginger, and crushed red pepper. Add the meat; stir until coated. Cover and marinate meat in refrigerator for 15 minutes. Drain, reserving marinade. For sauce, stir cornstarch into reserved marinade. Set aside.

3. Lightly coat an unheated large nonstick skillet or wok with cooking spray. Heat over medium heat. Add meat and green onion. Cook and stir for 2 to 3 minutes or until meat is desired doneness. Push from center of skillet.

4. Stir sauce; add to center of skillet. Cook and stir over medium heat until thickened and bubbly. Add pineapple, pea pods, and tomato. Cook and stir for 2 minutes more. Serve immediately over hot cooked rice.

Nutrition Facts per serving: 284 cal., 2 g total fat (1 g sat. fat), 37 mg chol., 340 mg sodium, 39 g carbo., 3 g fiber, 24 g pro.
Exchanges: 1 Vegetable, 1/2 Fruit, 1 1/2 Starch, 2 1/2 Very Lean Meat

Creamy Tomato-Sauced Round Steak

Prep: 20 minutes Cook: 8 to 10 hours (low) or 4 to 5 hours (high), plus 15 minutes (high)
Makes: 6 servings

2 pounds boneless beef top
   round steak, cut 1 inch thick

Black pepper

1 tablespoon cooking oil

1 large onion, sliced and
   separated into rings

1 14½-ounce can diced
   tomatoes, undrained

1 10¾-ounce can reduced-fat
   and reduced-salt condensed
   cream of mushroom soup

1 teaspoon dried thyme, crushed

1 teaspoon Worcestershire sauce

⅛ teaspoon garlic powder

2 tablespoons cornstarch

2 tablespoons cold water

9 ounces dried whole wheat
   pasta, cooked and drained

1. Cut meat into 6 serving-size pieces.
Sprinkle pepper over meat. In a large skillet
cook meat, half at a time, in hot oil over
medium heat until brown on both sides.
Drain off fat.

2. Place onion in a 3½- to 5-quart slow
cooker. Add meat. In a bowl combine
undrained tomatoes, mushroom soup, thyme,
Worcestershire sauce, and garlic powder.
Pour over mixture in cooker.

3. Cover and cook on low-heat setting for
8 to 10 hours or on high-heat setting for 4 to
5 hours.

4. Transfer meat to a serving platter,
reserving cooking liquid. Cover meat with
foil to keep warm.

5. If using low-heat setting, turn to high-heat
setting. For sauce, in a small bowl combine
cornstarch and water. Stir into liquid in
cooker. Cover and cook about 15 minutes
more or until thickened. Serve meat and
sauce over hot cooked pasta.

Nutrition Facts per serving: 277 cal., 8 g total fat (2 g sat. fat),
87 mg chol., 506 mg sodium, 13 g carbo., 1 g fiber, 35 g pro.
Exchanges: 1 Vegetable, ½ Starch, 4 Lean Meat

Mashed Potato Chicken Potpie

Prep: 30 minutes Bake: 30 minutes Stand: 5 minutes Oven: 375°F Makes: 6 servings

3 tablespoons butter or margarine

$\frac{1}{3}$ cup all-purpose flour

$\frac{1}{2}$ teaspoon seasoned pepper

$\frac{1}{4}$ teaspoon salt

1 14-ounce can reduced-sodium chicken broth

$\frac{3}{4}$ cup reduced-fat or fat-free milk

2 cups frozen peas and carrots, thawed

2 cups frozen cut green beans, thawed

$2\frac{1}{2}$ cups chopped cooked chicken or turkey (about 12 ounces)

1 20-ounce package refrigerated mashed potatoes (about $2\frac{2}{3}$ cups)

2 tablespoons grated Parmesan cheese

1 clove garlic, minced, or $\frac{1}{2}$ teaspoon bottled minced garlic

1. In a large saucepan melt butter over medium heat. Stir in flour, $\frac{1}{4}$ teaspoon of the seasoned pepper, and the salt. Add broth and milk all at once. Cook and stir over medium heat until thickened and bubbly. Stir in thawed vegetables and cooked chicken. Pour into an ungreased 3-quart rectangular baking dish.

2. In a medium bowl combine mashed potatoes, Parmesan cheese, garlic, and the remaining $\frac{1}{4}$ teaspoon seasoned pepper. Using a spoon, drop potato mixture in large mounds over chicken mixture in baking dish.

3. Bake, uncovered, in a 375° oven for 30 to 40 minutes or until heated through. Let stand for 5 minutes before serving.

Nutrition Facts per serving: 330 cal., 13 g total fat (6 g sat. fat), 72 mg chol., 616 mg sodium, 29 g carbo., 4 g fiber, 25 g pro. **Exchanges:** 1$\frac{1}{2}$ Vegetable, 1 Starch, $\frac{1}{2}$ Other Carbo., 3 Very Lean Meat, 1$\frac{1}{2}$ Fat

Chicken and Dumplings

Prep: 20 minutes Cook: 50 minutes Makes: 4 servings

4 chicken breast halves or thighs (about 1½ pounds)

2½ cups water

1 medium onion, sliced and separated into rings

1 teaspoon instant chicken bouillon granules

1 teaspoon snipped fresh thyme or ¼ teaspoon dried thyme, crushed

¼ teaspoon black pepper

2 cups sliced carrot (4 medium)

1 medium bulb fennel, cut into bite-size strips (1½ cups)

¼ cup cold water

2 tablespoons cornstarch

1 recipe Dumplings

Fresh herb sprigs (optional)

1. Remove the skin from the chicken. In a large saucepan combine the chicken pieces, the 2½ cups water, the onion, bouillon granules, dried thyme (if using), and pepper. Bring to boiling; reduce heat. Simmer, covered, for 25 minutes. Add the carrot and fennel. Return to boiling; reduce heat. Simmer, covered, for 10 minutes more.

2. Remove chicken pieces from saucepan; set aside. Skim fat from broth in pan. In a small bowl stir together the ¼ cup cold water and the cornstarch; stir into broth in saucepan. Cook and stir until thickened and bubbly. Return chicken to pan; add fresh thyme (if using).

3. Drop Dumplings batter from a tablespoon into 8 mounds onto the hot chicken mixture. Cover; simmer about 10 minutes or until a wooden toothpick inserted into a dumpling comes out clean. If desired, garnish with herb sprigs.

Dumplings: In a small bowl stir together 1 cup all-purpose flour, 1½ teaspoons baking powder, ⅛ teaspoon salt, and ⅛ teaspoon coarsely ground black pepper. In another small bowl stir together 1 beaten egg, ¼ cup fat-free milk, and 1 tablespoon cooking oil. Pour into flour mixture; stir with a fork until combined.

Nutrition Facts per serving: 327 cal., 6 g total fat (1 g sat. fat), 110 mg chol., 558 mg sodium, 37 g carbo., 12 g fiber, 29 g pro.
Exchanges: 1½ Vegetable, 2 Starch, 3 Very Lean Meat, ½ Fat

Chicken and Tortellini Stew

Start to Finish: 45 minutes Makes: 6 servings

2 cups water

1 14-ounce can chicken broth

6 cups torn fresh spinach

1½ cups sliced carrot (3 medium)

1 medium zucchini or yellow summer squash, halved lengthwise and cut into ½-inch slices

1 cup dried cheese-filled tortellini

1 red or green sweet pepper, coarsely chopped

1 medium onion, cut into bite-size wedges

1 teaspoon dried basil, crushed

½ teaspoon dried oregano, crushed

¼ teaspoon black pepper

2 cups chopped cooked chicken (10 ounces)

1. In a large skillet or Dutch oven combine water and broth. Bring to boiling. Stir in spinach, carrot, zucchini, tortellini, sweet pepper, onion, basil, oregano, and black pepper. Reduce heat. Simmer, covered, about 15 minutes or until tortellini and vegetables are nearly tender.

2. Stir in cooked chicken. Cook, covered, about 5 minutes more or until tortellini and vegetables are tender.

Nutrition Facts per serving: 210 cal., 6 g total fat (1 g sat. fat), 42 mg chol., 537 mg sodium, 19 g carbo., 3 g fiber, 20 g pro.
Exchanges: 1½ Vegetable, 1 Starch, 2 Very Lean Meat, ½ Fat

Chicken and Barley Bake

Prep: 20 minutes Cook: 10 minutes Bake: 30 minutes Oven: 350°F Makes: 4 servings

1 cup water

1 cup chopped onion (1 large)

³/₄ cup chopped carrot (2 small)

¹/₂ cup uncooked regular barley

1¹/₂ teaspoons instant chicken bouillon granules

1 teaspoon dried parsley flakes, crushed

1 clove garlic, minced

¹/₂ teaspoon poultry seasoning

1 to 1¹/₄ pounds chicken thighs, skinned

Salt

Black pepper

1. In a medium saucepan combine water, onion, carrot, barley, bouillon granules, parsley, garlic, and poultry seasoning. Bring to boiling; reduce heat. Cover and simmer for 10 minutes.

2. Transfer hot barley mixture to an ungreased 2-quart square baking dish. Place chicken on top of barley mixture. Sprinkle chicken with salt and pepper.

3. Bake, covered, in a 350° oven for 30 to 35 minutes or until barley is tender and chicken is tender and no longer pink (180°F).

Nutrition Facts per serving: 170 cal., 3 g total fat (1 g sat. fat), 54 mg chol., 539 mg sodium, 21 g carbo., 3 g fiber, 15 g pro.
Exchanges: ¹/₂ Vegetable, 1 Starch, 2 Lean Meat

Turkey and Vegetable Bake

Prep: 35 minutes Bake: 30 minutes Stand: 15 minutes Oven: 350°F Makes: 6 servings

2 cups sliced fresh mushrooms

¾ cup chopped red or yellow sweet pepper (1 medium)

½ cup chopped onion (1 medium)

2 cloves garlic, minced

2 tablespoons butter or margarine

¼ cup all-purpose flour

¾ teaspoon salt

½ teaspoon dried thyme, crushed

¼ teaspoon black pepper

2 cups fat-free milk

2 cups chopped cooked turkey or chicken (10 ounces)

2 cups cooked brown or white rice

1 10-ounce package frozen chopped spinach, thawed and well drained

½ cup finely shredded Parmesan cheese (2 ounces)

1. In a 12-inch skillet cook and stir mushrooms, sweet pepper, onion, and garlic in hot butter over medium heat until tender. Stir in flour, salt, thyme, and black pepper. Add milk all at once; cook and stir until thickened and bubbly.

2. Stir turkey, rice, spinach, and ¼ cup of the Parmesan cheese into the thickened mixture. Spoon mixture into a 2-quart rectangular baking dish. Sprinkle with remaining Parmesan cheese.

3. Bake, covered, in a 350° oven for 20 minutes. Uncover and bake about 10 minutes more or until heated through. Let stand 15 minutes before serving.

Nutrition Facts per serving: 297 cal., 10 g total fat (5 g sat. fat), 53 mg chol., 602 mg sodium, 28 g carbo., 3 g fiber, 24 g pro.
Exchanges: ½ Milk, 1 Vegetable, 1 Starch, 2 Lean Meat, ½ Fat

One-Dish Turkey and Biscuits

Prep: 30 minutes Bake: 20 minutes Oven: 425°F Makes: 4 servings

1 cup chicken broth

½ cup finely chopped onion (1 medium)

½ cup finely chopped celery (1 stalk)

1½ cups loose-pack frozen peas and carrots

1 cup reduced-fat or fat-free milk

3 tablespoons all-purpose flour

2 cups cubed cooked turkey breast (10 ounces)

½ teaspoon dried sage, crushed

⅛ teaspoon black pepper

1¼ cups packaged biscuit mix

½ cup reduced-fat or fat-free milk

2 teaspoons dried parsley flakes, crushed

1. In a medium saucepan combine broth, onion, and celery. Bring to boiling; reduce heat. Cover and simmer for 5 minutes. Add peas and carrots; return to boiling.

2. In a small bowl stir the 1 cup milk into flour until well mixed; stir into vegetable mixture in saucepan. Cook and stir until thickened and bubbly. Stir in turkey, sage, and pepper. Transfer to an ungreased 2-quart casserole.

3. In a small bowl combine biscuit mix, the ½ cup milk, and the parsley. Stir with a fork just until moistened. Spoon into 8 mounds on top of the hot turkey mixture in casserole. Bake, uncovered, in a 425° oven for 20 to 25 minutes or until biscuits are golden brown.

Nutrition Facts per serving: 356 cal., 8 g total fat (3 g sat. fat), 67 mg chol., 844 mg sodium, 41 g carbo., 3 g fiber, 30 g pro.
Exchanges: 2½ Starch, 3 Very Lean Meat, ½ Vegetable, 1 Fat

Pasta Pizza

Prep: 25 minutes Bake: 30 minutes Oven: 350°F Makes: 6 servings

Nonstick cooking spray

5 ounces packaged dried tricolored or plain corkscrew pasta (2 cups)

2 eggs, slightly beaten

½ cup milk

1 cup shredded 4-cheese pizza cheese or mozzarella cheese (4 ounces)

¾ cup chopped sweet pepper and/or chopped zucchini

1 14½-ounce can Italian-style stewed tomatoes, undrained

½ teaspoon dried Italian seasoning, crushed

1 4½-ounce jar sliced mushrooms, drained (optional)

½ of a 6-ounce package sliced turkey pepperoni

2 tablespoons grated Parmesan cheese

1. Lightly coat a 12-inch pizza pan (with sides) with cooking spray; set aside. Cook pasta according to package directions. Drain pasta; rinse with cold water. Drain again.

2. For pasta crust, in a large bowl combine eggs, milk, and ½ cup of the pizza cheese. Stir in pasta. Spread pasta mixture evenly in prepared pan. Bake in a 350° oven for 20 minutes.

3. Meanwhile, coat a large skillet with cooking spray. Heat over medium heat. Add sweet pepper and cook until crisp-tender. Add undrained tomatoes and Italian seasoning. Bring to boiling; reduce heat. Simmer, uncovered, for 10 minutes or until most of the liquid is evaporated, stirring occasionally. If desired, stir in mushrooms.

4. Arrange pepperoni over the pasta crust. Spoon tomato mixture over pepperoni. Sprinkle with remaining ½ cup pizza cheese and the Parmesan cheese. Bake for 10 to 12 minutes more or until heated through and cheese is melted. To serve, cut into wedges.

Nutrition Facts per serving: 242 cal., 6 g total fat (2 g sat. fat), 96 mg chol., 574 mg sodium, 31 g carbo., 2 g fiber, 14 g pro.
Exchanges: 1 Vegetable, 1½ Starch, 1½ Lean Meat

Oven-Baked Cassoulet

Prep: 20 minutes Bake: 40 minutes Oven: 325°F Makes: 5 servings

Nonstick cooking spray

12 ounces lean boneless pork, cut into 1/2-inch cubes

1 teaspoon cooking oil

1 cup chopped onion (1 large)

1 cup chopped carrot (2 medium)

2 cloves garlic, minced

2 15-ounce cans cannellini (white kidney) beans, rinsed and drained

4 roma tomatoes, chopped

2/3 cup reduced-sodium chicken broth

2/3 cup water

2 ounces smoked turkey sausage, halved lengthwise and cut into 1/4-inch slices

1 teaspoon dried thyme, crushed

1/4 teaspoon dried rosemary, crushed

1/4 teaspoon black pepper

2 tablespoons snipped fresh thyme or flat-leaf parsley (optional)

1. Coat an unheated ovenproof Dutch oven with cooking spray. Preheat over medium-high heat. Add pork to Dutch oven; cook and stir until pork is brown. Remove pork from Dutch oven. Reduce heat. Carefully add oil to the hot Dutch oven. Add onion, carrot, and garlic; cook until onion is tender. Stir pork, beans, tomato, broth, water, turkey sausage, thyme, rosemary, and pepper into Dutch oven.

2. Bake, covered, in a 325° oven for 40 to 45 minutes or until pork and carrot are tender. Serve in bowls. If desired, sprinkle with snipped fresh thyme.

Nutrition Facts per serving: 263 cal., 6 g total fat (2 g sat. fat), 48 mg chol., 500 mg sodium, 33 g carbo., 10 g fiber, 28 g pro.
Exchanges: 2 1/2 Vegetable, 1 1/2 Starch, 2 1/2 Medium-Fat Meat

Savory Ham and Rice Casserole

Prep: 20 minutes Cook: 30 minutes Oven: 350°F Makes: 4 servings

1 cup chopped carrot
    (2 medium)

½ cup chopped onion (1 medium)

½ cup chopped green or red
    sweet pepper (1 small)

½ cup water

1 10¾-ounce can reduced-fat
    and reduced-sodium con-
    densed cream of celery soup

¾ cup uncooked quick-cooking
    rice

8 ounces cooked reduced-sodium
    ham, cut into bite-size pieces
    (1½ cups)

¼ teaspoon ground sage

⅛ teaspoon black pepper

    Paprika (optional)

1. In a medium saucepan combine carrot, onion, sweet pepper, and water. Bring to boiling; reduce heat. Simmer, covered, for 4 to 5 minutes or until crisp-tender. Do not drain.

2. Stir in soup, rice, ham, sage, and black pepper. Transfer to an ungreased 1-quart casserole. If desired, sprinkle with paprika.

3. Bake, covered, in a 350° oven for 30 to 35 minutes or until rice is tender and mixture is heated through.

Nutrition Facts per serving: 191 cal., 3 g total fat (1 g sat. fat), 26 mg chol., 908 mg sodium, 28 g carbo., 1 g fiber, 13 g pro.
Exchanges: ½ Vegetable, 1½ Starch, 1 Lean Meat

Spinach and Ham Lasagna

Prep: 40 minutes Bake: 30 minutes Stand: 10 minutes Oven: 375°F Makes: 6 servings

6 packaged dried lasagna noodles (4 ounces)

1 10-ounce package frozen chopped spinach

2 cups fat-free milk

¼ cup chopped onion

3 tablespoons cornstarch

1½ cups diced low-fat, reduced-sodium cooked ham (8 ounces)

½ teaspoon dried Italian seasoning, crushed

1 cup low-fat cottage cheese

1 cup shredded reduced-fat mozzarella cheese (4 ounces)

1. Cook lasagna noodles according to package directions; drain. Rinse with cold water; drain again. Set aside.

2. Meanwhile, cook spinach according to package directions; drain well. Set aside.

3. For sauce, in a medium saucepan combine milk, onion, and cornstarch. Cook and stir until thickened and bubbly. Cook and stir for 2 minutes more.

4. Spread 2 tablespoons of the sauce evenly on the bottom of a 2-quart rectangular baking dish. Stir ham and Italian seasoning into remaining sauce.

5. Arrange 3 lasagna noodles in the dish. Spread with one-third of the remaining sauce. Layer the spinach on top. Layer another one-third of the sauce, the cottage cheese, and half of the mozzarella cheese over the spinach. Place remaining noodles on top. Top with remaining sauce and mozzarella cheese.

6. Bake in a 375° oven for 30 to 35 minutes or until heated through. Let stand 10 minutes before serving.

Nutrition Facts per serving: 239 cal., 5 g total fat (3 g sat. fat), 31 mg chol., 777 mg sodium, 26 g carbo., 2 g fiber, 21 g pro.
Exchanges: ½ Vegetable, 1½ Starch, 2½ Lean Meat

Spicy Skillet Pork Chops

Start to Finish: 40 minutes Makes: 4 servings

1½ cups loose-pack frozen whole kernel corn

1 10-ounce can chopped tomatoes and green chile peppers, undrained

½ teaspoon ground cumin

¼ teaspoon bottled hot pepper sauce

2 cloves garlic, minced

4 boneless pork loin chops, cut ¾ inch thick (about 1½ pounds)

½ teaspoon chili powder

2 teaspoons cooking oil

1 medium onion, cut into thin wedges

1 tablespoon snipped fresh cilantro

Fresh cilantro sprigs (optional)

1. In a medium bowl combine corn, undrained tomatoes, cumin, hot pepper sauce, and garlic; set aside.

2. Trim fat from chops. Sprinkle both sides of each chop with chili powder. In a 12-inch nonstick skillet heat oil over medium-high heat. Add chops; cook chops about 4 minutes or until brown, turning once. Remove chops from skillet, reserving drippings. Reduce heat to medium. Add onion to skillet. Cook and stir for 3 minutes. Stir corn mixture into onion mixture in skillet. Place chops on corn mixture. Bring to boiling; reduce heat. Simmer, covered, for 10 to 12 minutes or until pork juices run clear (160°F).

3. To serve, remove chops from skillet. Stir snipped cilantro into corn mixture in skillet; serve corn mixture with chops. If desired, garnish with cilantro leaves.

Nutrition Facts per serving: 330 cal., 11 g total fat (3 g sat. fat), 93 mg chol., 360 mg sodium, 18 g carbo., 2 g fiber, 40 g pro.
Exchanges: 1 Vegetable, 1 Starch, 5 Medium-Fat Meat

Pork Chops with Winter Squash

Prep: 20 minutes   Cook: 5 to 6 hours (low) or 2½ to 3 hours (high)   Makes: 6 servings

2 small or medium acorn squash
   (1½ to 2 pounds)

1 large onion, halved and sliced

6 pork chops (with bone), cut
   ¾ inch thick

½ cup reduced-sodium chicken
   broth

⅓ cup reduced-sugar orange marmalade

1 tablespoon Dijon-style mustard

1 teaspoon dried marjoram or
   thyme, crushed

¼ teaspoon black pepper

2 tablespoons cornstarch

2 tablespoons cold water

1. Cut squash in half lengthwise. Remove and discard seeds and membranes. Cut each squash half into 3 wedges. In a 5- to 6-quart slow cooker place squash and onion. Trim fat from chops. Place chops in cooker. In a small bowl combine chicken broth, marmalade, mustard, marjoram, and pepper. Pour over mixture in cooker.

2. Cover and cook on low-heat setting for 5 to 6 hours or on high-heat setting for 2½ to 3 hours.

3. Transfer chops and vegetables to a serving platter, reserving cooking liquid. Cover chops and vegetables with foil to keep warm.

4. For sauce, strain cooking liquid into a glass measuring cup. Skim off fat. Measure 1¾ cups liquid (add water, if necessary, to make 1¾ cups). Pour liquid into a medium saucepan. In a small bowl combine cornstarch and water. Stir into liquid in saucepan. Cook and stir over medium heat until thickened and bubbly. Cook and stir 2 minutes more. Serve chops and vegetables with sauce.

Nutrition Facts per serving: 283 cal., 8 g total fat (3 g sat. fat), 78 mg chol., 176 mg sodium, 18 g carbo., 2 g fiber, 33 g pro.
Exchanges: 1 Starch, 4 Lean Meat

Tortilla Bean and Rice Bake

Prep: 30 minutes Bake: 35 minutes Oven: 350°F Makes: 6 servings

1½ cups water

⅔ cup uncooked long grain rice

¼ teaspoon salt

6 6-inch corn tortillas

1 14½-ounce can Mexican-style stewed tomatoes, undrained

1 cup bottled salsa

1 15-ounce can kidney beans or small red beans, rinsed and drained

1 cup shredded reduced-fat Monterey Jack cheese (4 ounces)

Light dairy sour cream (optional)

1. In a medium saucepan combine water, rice, and salt. Bring to boiling; reduce heat. Simmer, covered, about 20 minutes or until rice is tender and water is absorbed. Meanwhile, stack tortillas and wrap in foil. Heat in a 350° oven for 10 minutes to soften.

2. In a medium bowl combine the undrained tomatoes and salsa. Stir beans into cooked rice. Cut softened tortillas into quarters and arrange half of them in the bottom of a lightly greased 2-quart square baking dish. Layer half of the rice mixture over tortillas. Top with half of the tomato mixture and ½ cup of the cheese. Repeat layers.

3. Bake, covered, in a 350° oven for 35 to 40 minutes or until heated through. If desired, serve with sour cream.

Nutrition Facts per serving: 280 cal., 5 g total fat (2 g sat. fat), 13 mg chol., 739 mg sodium, 49 g carbo., 6 g fiber, 14 g pro.
Exchanges: ½ Vegetable, 3 Starch, ½ Very Lean Meat, ½ Lean Meat

Vegetable Curry

Start to Finish: 35 minutes Makes: 6 servings

1 large red onion, halved and cut into thin wedges

1 tablespoon olive oil

2 teaspoons curry powder

1 teaspoon ground cumin

¼ teaspoon garam masala

⅛ teaspoon cayenne pepper

3 cups cauliflower florets

1 14½-ounce can diced tomatoes, undrained

2 medium potatoes, peeled and cut into 1-inch cubes (about 1½ cups)

2 medium sweet potatoes, peeled and cut into 1-inch cubes (about 1½ cups)

1½ cups vegetable broth or water

¼ teaspoon salt

¼ teaspoon freshly ground black pepper

1 cup loose-pack frozen peas

4½ cups hot cooked couscous or brown rice

1. In a large saucepan cook onion in hot oil over medium heat about 5 minutes or until tender. Add curry powder, cumin, garam masala, and cayenne pepper. Cook and stir for 1 minute.

2. Stir in cauliflower, tomatoes, potato, sweet potato, broth, salt, and black pepper. Bring to boiling; reduce heat. Simmer, covered, for 10 to 12 minutes or until potatoes are tender. Stir in peas; heat through. Serve over hot cooked couscous.

Nutrition Facts per serving: 284 cal., 3 g total fat (0 g sat. fat), 0 mg chol., 516 mg sodium, 55 g carbo., 7 g fiber, 9 g pro. **Exchanges:** 2 Vegetable, 3 Starch

Vegetable Primavera Casserole

Prep: 30 minutes Bake: 30 minutes Stand: 5 minutes Oven: 375°F Makes: 8 servings

1½ cups dried elbow macaroni
    (6 ounces)

1 16-ounce package loose-pack
    frozen vegetable blend

2 medium zucchini, halved
    lengthwise and sliced

½ cup chopped red sweet pepper

2 12-ounce cans (3 cups)
    evaporated milk

1 cup vegetable or chicken broth

⅓ cup all-purpose flour

1 teaspoon dried oregano,
    crushed

½ teaspoon garlic powder

½ teaspoon salt

½ teaspoon black pepper

¾ cup grated Parmesan cheese or
    Romano cheese

1 medium tomato, halved and
    sliced

1. In a 4- to 5-quart Dutch oven cook macaroni in lightly salted boiling water for 8 minutes, adding the frozen vegetables, zucchini, and sweet pepper for the last 3 minutes of cooking; drain. Return macaroni mixture to Dutch oven.

2. Meanwhile, in a medium saucepan whisk together evaporated milk, broth, flour, oregano, garlic powder, salt, and black pepper. Cook and stir over medium heat until thickened and bubbly. Add to macaroni mixture; toss to coat. Stir in ½ cup of the Parmesan cheese. Transfer macaroni mixture to a lightly greased 3-quart rectangular baking dish.

3. Bake, uncovered, in a 375° oven for 25 minutes. Top with tomato slices and remaining ¼ cup Parmesan cheese. Bake about 5 minutes more or until heated through. Let stand for 5 minutes before serving.

Nutrition Facts per serving: 277 cal., 9 g total fat (5 g sat. fat), 31 mg chol., 493 mg sodium, 35 g carbo., 3 g fiber, 13 g pro.
Exchanges: 1 Milk, 2 Vegetable, 1 Starch

Roasted Vegetables and Spinach with Pasta

Prep: 30 minutes Bake: 40 minutes Oven: 400°F Makes: 6 servings

1 eggplant (about 1 pound), peeled and cut into 1-inch cubes (about 6 cups)

1 large red onion, cut into thin wedges

1½ cups coarsely chopped yellow and/or green sweet pepper (2 medium)

1 tablespoon olive oil

½ teaspoon salt

1 teaspoon olive oil

2 cloves garlic, minced

½ teaspoon dried thyme, crushed

¼ teaspoon crushed red pepper

¼ teaspoon fennel seeds, crushed

¼ teaspoon black pepper

1 18.7-ounce can ready-to-serve tomato soup

12 ounces dried ziti or rotini pasta (4 cups)

1 6-ounce bag prewashed baby spinach (about 8 cups)

1 cup shredded mozzarella cheese (4 ounces)

1. In a shallow roasting pan combine eggplant, onion, sweet peppers, and the 1 tablespoon oil. Sprinkle with salt. Bake in a 400° oven for 30 to 35 minutes or until vegetables begin to brown, stirring twice.

2. Meanwhile, in a small saucepan heat the 1 teaspoon oil over medium heat. Add garlic, thyme, crushed red pepper, fennel seeds, and black pepper. Cook and stir for 2 minutes. Stir in soup. Bring to boiling; reduce heat. Simmer, uncovered, for 5 minutes, stirring occasionally.

3. Meanwhile, cook pasta according to package directions; drain. Transfer to a very large bowl. Add soup mixture and roasted vegetables; toss to coat. Stir in spinach.

4. Spoon pasta mixture into a greased 3-quart rectangular baking dish. Sprinkle with cheese. Bake, uncovered, in the 400° oven for 10 to 15 minutes or until heated through and cheese is melted.

Nutrition Facts per serving: 378 cal., 8 g total fat (3 g sat. fat), 16 mg chol., 636 mg sodium, 63 g carbo., 6 g fiber, 15 g pro. **Exchanges:** 3 Vegetable, 3 Starch, ½ Lean Meat, ½ Fat

make-ahead meals

The recipes in this section are designed to help you stock your freezer in the 3rd trimester so you'll have heat-and-eat meals for those first few weeks home with baby. Make a few or prepare a whole month's worth. It's up to you. Make-ahead meals are great for any time life gets super busy, and with a new baby on the way, there's no better time to give them a try than now.

Allspice Meatball Stew

Prep: 15 minutes Cook: 15 minutes Reheat: 30 minutes Freeze: up to 3 months
Makes: 2 (4-serving) portions

1 16-ounce package frozen prepared Italian-style meatballs

3 cups green beans, cut into 1-inch pieces, or frozen cut green beans

2 cups packaged peeled baby carrots

1 14-ounce can reduced-sodium beef broth

2 teaspoons Worcestershire sauce

½ to ¾ teaspoon ground allspice

½ teaspoon ground cinnamon

2 14½-ounce cans stewed tomatoes, undrained

1. In a Dutch oven combine the meatballs, green beans, carrots, broth, Worcestershire sauce, allspice, and cinnamon. Bring to boiling; reduce heat. Simmer, covered, for 10 minutes.

2. Stir in the undrained tomatoes. Return to boiling; reduce heat. Simmer, covered, about 5 minutes more or until vegetables are crisp-tender.

3. Divide soup between two 1½-quart freezer containers. Cool for 30 minutes. Seal, label, and freeze for up to 3 months.

4. To serve, place 1 portion of the frozen stew in a large saucepan. Heat, covered, over medium heat about 30 minutes or until heated through, stirring occasionally. Ladle into bowls.

Nutrition Facts per serving: 238 cal., 14 g total fat (6 g sat. fat), 37 mg chol., 729 mg sodium, 17 g carbo., 5 g fiber, 12 g pro.
Exchanges: 3 Vegetable, 2 Medium-Fat Meat

Barbecue Beef Sandwiches

Prep: 30 minutes Cook: 1½ hours Reheat: 8 minutes Freeze: up to 3 months Makes: 8 servings

1 2-pound beef round steak, cut ¾ inch thick

Nonstick cooking spray

1 14½-ounce can diced tomatoes, undrained

1 cup chopped onion (1 large)

¾ cup chopped carrot (1 large)

1 clove garlic, minced

2 tablespoons Worcestershire sauce

2 tablespoons vinegar

2 teaspoons chili powder

1 teaspoon dried oregano, crushed

¼ teaspoon salt

Salt

Black pepper

8 whole wheat hamburger buns

1. Trim fat from meat. Cut meat into 4 to 6 pieces. Coat a Dutch oven with cooking spray. Brown meat, half at a time, in Dutch oven over medium heat, turning to brown both sides. Return all meat to Dutch oven.

2. Add undrained tomatoes, onion, carrot, garlic, Worcestershire sauce, vinegar, chili powder, oregano, and the ¼ teaspoon salt. Bring to boiling; reduce heat. Simmer, covered, for 1½ to 2 hours or until meat is very tender.

3. Remove meat from sauce. Use 2 forks to shred meat. Return shredded meat to sauce; heat through. Season to taste with additional salt and pepper.

4. Transfer meat and sauce to 1-, 2-, or 4-serving-size freezer containers. Cover, label, and freeze for up to 3 months. To reheat, transfer mixture to a saucepan; add 1 tablespoon water. Cook over low heat until heated through, stirring occasionally. Allow 8 to 10 minutes for 1 or 2 servings; 25 to 30 minutes for 4 servings. Serve on buns.

Nutrition Facts per serving: 294 cal., 6 g total fat (1 g sat. fat), 65 mg chol., 515 mg sodium, 28 g carbo., 3 g fiber, 29 g pro.
Exchanges: ½ Vegetable, 2 Starch, 3 Lean Meat

Penne with Meat Sauce

Prep: 25 minutes Reheat: 20 minutes Bake: 25 minutes Freeze: up to 3 months Oven: 350°F
Makes: 4 to 6 servings

1 14½-ounce can whole Italian-style tomatoes, undrained

1 8-ounce can tomato sauce

¼ cup reduced-sodium beef broth

1 tablespoon snipped fresh oregano or 1 teaspoon dried oregano, crushed

½ teaspoon sugar

¼ teaspoon black pepper

1 pound lean ground beef

½ cup chopped onion (1 medium)

2 tablespoons water

8 ounces dried penne pasta

¼ cup sliced pitted ripe olives

1 cup shredded reduced-fat mozzarella cheese (4 ounces)

1. For sauce, in a blender or food processor combine undrained tomatoes, tomato sauce, broth, dried oregano (if using), sugar, and pepper. Cover and blend or process until smooth. Set aside. In a large skillet cook ground beef and onion until meat is brown. Drain off fat. Stir in tomato mixture. Bring to boiling; reduce heat. Simmer, covered, for 10 minutes. Cool. Transfer sauce to a freezer container. Seal, label, and freeze for up to 3 months.

2. To serve, transfer frozen sauce to a large saucepan. Add the water. Cook, covered, over medium heat about 20 to 25 minutes or until heated through, stirring occasionally.

3. Meanwhile, cook pasta according to package directions. Drain. Toss sauce with cooked pasta, fresh oregano (if using), and olives.

4. Spoon all of the pasta mixture into a 2-quart casserole or divide pasta mixture among four to six 12- to 16-ounce individual casseroles. Bake the 2-quart casserole, covered, in a 350° oven, for 20 minutes (bake individual casseroles, covered, for 15 minutes). Sprinkle with mozzarella cheese. Bake, uncovered, about 5 minutes more or until cheese is melted and pasta mixture is heated through.

Nutrition Facts per serving: 528 cal., 18 g total fat (8 g sat. fat), 92 mg chol., 759 mg sodium, 53 g carbo., 3 g fiber, 35 g pro.
Exchanges: 1 Vegetable, 2 Starch, 1 Other Carbo., 1 Lean Meat, 3 Medium-Fat Meat

Sloppy Beef Burgers

Prep: 25 minutes Reheat: 20 minutes Freeze: up to 3 months Makes: 8 servings

1½ pounds lean ground beef

½ cup chopped onion (1 medium)

⅓ cup chopped green sweet pepper

1 10¾-ounce can reduced-fat and reduced-sodium condensed tomato soup

1 tablespoon Worcestershire sauce

1 tablespoon yellow mustard

8 whole wheat or white hamburger buns, split and toasted

Dill pickle slices (optional)

1. In a large skillet cook ground beef, onion, and sweet pepper until beef is brown. Drain off fat. Stir in the soup, Worcestershire sauce, and mustard. Bring to boiling; reduce heat. Simmer, covered, for 5 minutes.

2. Divide beef mixture between 2 freezer containers; cool. Cover, label, and freeze for up to 3 months.

3. To serve, transfer meat mixture from 1 of the containers to a large saucepan. Cook, covered, over medium heat until heated through, stirring occasionally. If necessary, stir in 1 to 2 tablespoons water. Serve on toasted hamburger buns. If desired, top with pickles.

Nutrition Facts per serving: 289 cal., 11 g total fat (4 g sat. fat), 54 mg chol., 417 mg sodium, 27 g carbo., 2 g fiber, 20 g pro.
Exchanges: 2 Starch, 2 Medium-Fat Meat

Mozzarella-Stuffed Meat Loaves

Prep: 20 minutes Bake: 1¼ hours Stand: 5 minutes Freeze: up to 3 months Oven: 325°F
Makes: 6 servings

1 egg, beaten

1 cup soft bread crumbs (about 1½ slices)

½ cup bottled pasta sauce

1 or 2 cloves garlic, minced

½ teaspoon dried rosemary, crushed

1½ pounds lean ground beef

6 2½×½×½-inch sticks reduced-fat mozzarella cheese

½ cup bottled pasta sauce

6 tablespoons shredded reduced-fat mozzarella cheese (about 2 ounces)

1. In a large bowl combine egg, bread crumbs, the ½ cup pasta sauce, garlic, and rosemary. Add ground beef; mix well.

2. Divide meat mixture into 6 equal portions; form each into a loaf. Press a stick of cheese lengthwise into the center of each loaf, shaping so that meat completely covers the cheese. Place loaves in a 13×9×2-inch baking pan. Cover and freeze until firm. Wrap meat loaves in moistureproof, vaporproof freezer wrap or heavy foil. Label and freeze for up to 3 months.

3. To serve, unwrap the desired number of meat loaves and place in a shallow baking pan. Bake in a 325° oven, covered loosely with foil, for 1 hour. Uncover and bake for 10 minutes more. Spoon the remaining ½ cup pasta sauce over the loaves and sprinkle each with 1 tablespoon of the shredded cheese. Bake about 5 minutes more or until a thermometer inserted in the thickest part of the loaf registers 160°F. Let stand for 5 minutes. Transfer meat loaves to a platter.

Nutrition Facts per serving: 304 cal., 16 g total fat (7 g sat. fat), 124 mg chol., 486 mg sodium, 10 g carbo., 1 g fiber, 28 g pro.
Exchanges: ½ Other Carbo., 3 Lean Meat, 1 Medium-Fat Meat

Taco Spaghetti

Prep: 40 minutes Bake: 1¾ hour Freeze: up to 3 months Oven: 375°F
Makes: 2 (6 servings each) casseroles

10 ounces packaged dried spaghetti, linguine, or fettuccine, broken

2 pounds ground lean beef or ground uncooked turkey

2 cups chopped onion (2 large)

1½ cups water

1 1¼-ounce envelope (2 tablespoons) taco seasoning mix

2 11-ounce cans whole kernel corn with sweet peppers, drained

1 cup sliced, pitted ripe olives

2 cups shredded reduced-fat Colby and Monterey Jack or cheddar cheese (8 ounces)

1 cup salsa

2 4-ounce cans diced green chile peppers, drained

4 cups shredded lettuce

1 medium tomato, chopped

1 cup broken tortilla chips (optional)

   Dairy sour cream (optional)

1. Cook pasta according to package directions; drain.

2. In a 4-quart Dutch oven cook ground meat and onion until meat is brown. Drain off fat. Stir in water and taco seasoning; bring to boiling. Reduce heat and simmer, uncovered, for 2 minutes, stirring occasionally. Stir in cooked pasta, corn, olives, 1 cup of the shredded cheese, salsa, and chile peppers.

3. Divide mixture evenly between 2 lightly greased 2-quart casseroles. Wrap, label, and freeze casseroles for up to 3 months.

4. To serve, bake 1 of the frozen casseroles, covered, in a 375° oven for 1¾ to 2 hours or until heated through. Stir casserole after 1¼ hours. (Or thaw frozen casserole in refrigerator overnight. Bake, covered, in a 375° oven for 1 hour or until heated through, stirring once about halfway through baking time.) Sprinkle with ½ cup of the remaining shredded cheese.

5. Serve with lettuce, chopped tomato, and, if desired, tortilla chips and sour cream.

Nutrition Facts per serving: 334 cal., 12 g total fat (5 g sat. fat), 61 mg chol., 742 mg sodium, 33 g carbo., 3 g fiber, 25 g pro.
Exchanges: 1 Vegetable, 2 Starch, 1 Lean Meat, 1 Medium-Fat Meat, 1 Fat

Beef Goulash Soup

Prep: 30 minutes   Reheat: 20 minutes   Freeze: up to 3 months   Makes: 4 servings

6 ounces boneless beef top sirloin steak

1 teaspoon olive oil

½ cup chopped onion (1 medium)

2 cups water

1 14-ounce can beef broth

1 14½-ounce can no-salt-added diced tomatoes, undrained

½ cup thinly sliced carrot (1 medium)

1 teaspoon unsweetened cocoa powder

1 clove garlic, minced

1 cup thinly sliced cabbage

1 ounce dried wide noodles (about ½ cup)

2 teaspoons paprika

¼ cup light dairy sour cream

Snipped fresh parsley (optional)

Paprika (optional)

1. Trim fat from meat. Cut meat into ½-inch cubes. In a large saucepan cook and stir meat cubes in hot oil over medium-high heat about 6 minutes or until meat is brown. Add onion; cook and stir about 3 minutes more or until tender.

2. Stir in the water, broth, undrained tomatoes, carrot, cocoa powder, and garlic. Bring to boiling; reduce heat. Simmer, uncovered, about 15 minutes or until meat is tender.

3. Transfer soup to a freezer container; cool. Seal, label, and freeze for up to 3 months.

4. To serve, thaw soup overnight in the refrigerator. Transfer soup to a large saucepan. Cover and cook over medium heat until heated through, stirring occasionally to break up any remaining frozen chunks. Bring soup to boiling. Stir in the cabbage, uncooked noodles, and the 2 teaspoons paprika. Simmer, uncovered, for 5 to 7 minutes more or until noodles are tender but still firm. Remove from heat. Top each serving with some of the sour cream. If desired, sprinkle with parsley and additional paprika.

Nutrition Facts per serving: 188 cal., 7 g total fat (3 g sat. fat), 36 mg chol., 397 mg sodium, 16 g carbo., 3 g fiber, 14 g pro.
Exchanges: 2 Vegetable, ½ Starch, 1½ Medium-Fat Meat

Cincinnati Chili
Prep: 25 minutes Cook: 45 minutes Reheat: 20 minutes Freeze: up to 3 months Makes: 8 servings

5 bay leaves

1 teaspoon whole allspice

2 pounds lean ground beef

2 cups chopped onion (2 large)

1 clove garlic, minced

2 tablespoons chili powder

1 teaspoon ground cinnamon

½ teaspoon cayenne pepper

4 cups water

1 15-ounce can red kidney beans, rinsed and drained

1 8-ounce can tomato sauce

1 tablespoon vinegar

1 teaspoon Worcestershire sauce

½ teaspoon salt

¼ teaspoon black pepper

Hot cooked spaghetti (optional)

Shredded reduced-fat cheddar cheese (optional)

1. Wrap bay leaves and allspice in a double thickness of 100-percent-cotton cheesecloth. Tie closed with 100-percent-cotton string; set aside.

2. In a 4-quart Dutch oven cook ground beef, onion, and garlic until the meat is brown. Drain off fat. Stir in chili powder, cinnamon, and cayenne pepper. Cook and stir for 1 minute.

3. Stir in water, beans, tomato sauce, vinegar, Worcestershire sauce, salt, and black pepper. Add spice bag. Bring to boiling; reduce heat. Simmer, covered, for 30 minutes. Uncover; simmer for 15 to 20 minutes more or until desired consistency. Remove and discard spice bag.

4. Divide chili between 2 freezer containers; cool. Seal, label, and freeze for up to 3 months.

5. To serve, thaw 1 container of chili overnight in refrigerator. Transfer chili to a large saucepan. Cook, covered, over medium heat until heated through, stirring occasionally to break up any remaining frozen chunks. If desired, serve chili over hot cooked spaghetti and sprinkle with cheese.

Nutrition Facts per serving: 257 cal., 11 g total fat (4 g sat. fat), 71 mg chol., 435 mg sodium, 16 g carbo., 5 g fiber, 25 g pro.
Exchanges: 1 Starch, 1 Very Lean Meat, 2½ Lean Meat

Feisty Italian Meatballs

Prep: 20 minutes   Bake: 20 minutes   Reheat: 20 minutes   Freeze: up to 3 months   Oven: 350°F
Makes: 6 servings

Nonstick cooking spray

1 tablespoon finely chopped, drained canned whole cherry pepper (1 pepper) or pepperoncini salad peppers

¼ cup chili sauce

¼ cup seasoned fine dry bread crumbs

2 tablespoons finely chopped onion

1 tablespoon grated Parmesan cheese or Romano cheese

1½ teaspoons fennel seeds, crushed

1 pound very lean ground pork

1 26- or 27-ounce jar chunky-style pasta sauce

¼ cup chopped, drained canned whole cherry peppers (4 peppers) or pepperoncini salad peppers

3 cups hot cooked wide noodles

1. Lightly coat a 15×10×1-inch baking pan with cooking spray; set aside. In a large bowl combine the 1 tablespoon finely chopped pepper, the chili sauce, bread crumbs, onion, Parmesan cheese, and fennel seeds. Add pork. Mix well. Shape into 36 meatballs. Place in prepared pan.

2. Bake, uncovered, in a 350° oven for 20 to 25 minutes or until brown and cooked through. Remove from oven; drain off fat. Freeze meatballs in pan until firm. Transfer meatballs to a large resealable freezer bag. Seal, label, and freeze for up to 3 months.

3. To serve, thaw meatballs in refrigerator for 24 hours. In a medium saucepan heat the pasta sauce until bubbly. Add thawed meatballs and the ¼ cup chopped peppers; heat through. Serve over hot cooked noodles.

Nutrition Facts per serving: 294 cal., 9 g total fat (3 g sat. fat), 62 mg chol., 993 mg sodium, 38 g carbo., 2 g fiber, 16 g pro.
Exchanges: 1 Vegetable, 2 Starch, 2 Medium-Fat Meat

Baked Cavatelli

Prep: 35 minutes Reheat: 15 minutes Bake: 5 minutes Freeze: up to 2 months Oven: 375°F
Makes: 6 servings

12 ounces uncooked Italian sausage links, cut into 1/2-inch slices

1/2 cup chopped onion (1 medium)

2 cloves garlic, minced

1 26- to 28-ounce can or jar pasta sauce

1/8 to 1/4 teaspoon black pepper

2 1/2 cups dried cavatelli (12 ounces) or wagon wheel pasta (7 ounces)

1 cup shredded reduced-fat mozzarella cheese (4 ounces)

1. For sauce, in a large skillet cook sausage until no pink remains. Remove sausage from skillet, reserving 1 tablespoon drippings in skillet. Drain sausage on paper towels. Cook onion and garlic in the reserved drippings until tender; drain. In a large bowl combine sausage, onion mixture, pasta sauce, and pepper.

2. Pack sauce in an airtight freezer container. Seal, label, and freeze for up to 2 months.

3. To serve, thaw sauce in the container in the refrigerator overnight (it will still be icy). Place sauce in a medium saucepan. Heat, covered, for 15 to 20 minutes over medium-low heat until bubbly, stirring occasionally.

4. Meanwhile, cook pasta according to package directions. Drain in a colander; return to pot. Stir the sausage-sauce mixture and 1/2 cup mozzarella cheese into the pasta. Turn into a 2-quart casserole; sprinkle with another 1/2 cup mozzarella cheese. Bake, uncovered, in a 375° oven for 5 to 10 minutes or until cheese is melted.

Nutrition Facts per serving: 338 cal., 13 g total fat (6 g sat. fat), 39 mg chol., 915 mg sodium, 39 g carbo., 4 g fiber, 15 g pro.
Exchanges: 1 Starch, 1 Other Carbo., 1 High-Fat Meat, 1 Fat

Make-Ahead Pizzas

Prep: 30 minutes Stand: 10 minutes Bake: 25 minutes Freeze: up to 1 month Oven: 375°F
Makes: 2 pizzas (4 servings each)

2¾ to 3¼ cups all-purpose flour

1 package active dry yeast

¼ teaspoon salt

1 cup warm water (120°F to 130°F)

2 tablespoons cooking oil

Cornmeal (optional)

1 15-ounce can pizza sauce

1 pound lean ground beef, cooked and well drained

½ cup sliced green onion (4) or sliced pitted ripe olives

1 cup sliced fresh mushrooms or chopped green sweet pepper

2 cups shredded reduced-fat mozzarella cheese (8 ounces)

1. For crust, in a large mixing bowl combine 1¼ cups of the flour, the yeast, and salt. Add water and oil. Beat with an electric mixer on low speed for 30 seconds, scraping bowl. Beat on high speed for 3 minutes. Stir in as much of the remaining flour as you can. Turn out onto a lightly floured surface. Knead in enough remaining flour to make a moderately stiff dough that is smooth and elastic (6 to 8 minutes total). Divide dough in half. Cover dough and let rest for 10 minutes.

2. Grease two 12-inch pizza pans or baking sheets. If desired, sprinkle with cornmeal. On a lightly floured surface roll each dough portion into a 13-inch circle. Transfer to prepared pans. Build up edges slightly. Bake in a 425° oven about 12 minutes or until brown.

3. Spread pizza sauce onto hot crusts. Top with meat, green onion, mushrooms, and cheese.

4. Cover assembled pizzas with plastic wrap and freeze until firm. Wrap each frozen pizza in moistureproof and vaporproof wrap. Wrap in heavy foil or place in a resealable freezer bag. Seal, label, and freeze for up to 1 month.

5. To serve, bake 1 of the assembled frozen pizzas in a 375° oven about 25 minutes or until cheese is bubbly.

Nutrition Facts per serving: 575 cal., 30 g total fat (12 g sat. fat), 78 mg chol., 1110 mg sodium, 41 g carbo., 2 g fiber, 26 g pro.
Exchanges: 2 Starch, 1 Other Carbo., 1 Lean Meat, 2 High-Fat Meat, 2 Fat

Minestrone

Prep: 50 minutes Reheat: 25 minutes Freeze: up to 3 months Makes: 2 (4-serving) portions

6 cups water

1 28-ounce can diced tomatoes, undrained

1 8-ounce can tomato sauce

1 cup chopped onion (1 large)

1 cup chopped cabbage

1/2 cup chopped carrot (1 medium)

1/2 cup chopped celery (1 stalk)

4 teaspoons instant beef bouillon granules

1 tablespoon dried Italian seasoning, crushed

1 teaspoon bottled minced garlic or 2 cloves garlic, minced

1/4 teaspoon black pepper

1 15-ounce can cannellini (white kidney) or Great Northern beans, undrained

1 10-ounce package frozen lima beans or one 9-ounce package frozen Italian-style green beans

4 ounces broken dried linguine or spaghetti

1 small zucchini, halved lengthwise and sliced

1/2 cup grated Parmesan cheese

2 to 3 tablespoons purchased pesto (optional)

1. In a 5- to 6-quart Dutch oven combine water, undrained tomatoes, tomato sauce, onion, cabbage, carrot, celery, bouillon granules, Italian seasoning, garlic, and pepper. Bring to boiling; reduce heat. Simmer, covered, for 10 minutes.

2. Stir in undrained cannellini beans, lima beans, linguine, and zucchini. Return to boiling; reduce heat. Simmer, uncovered, for 15 minutes. Remove from heat. Cool.

3. Divide soup between two 2-quart freezer containers. Seal, label, and freeze for up to 3 months.

4. To serve, transfer frozen soup from 1 of the containers to a large saucepan. Cover and cook over medium heat for 25 to 30 minutes or until heated through, stirring occasionally to break up mixture. Ladle soup into bowls. Top each serving with 1 tablespoon Parmesan cheese and, if desired, 1 teaspoon pesto.

Nutrition Facts per serving: 195 cal., 2 g total fat (1 g sat. fat), 4 mg chol., 871 mg sodium, 36 g carbo., 6 g fiber, 10 g pro.
Exchanges: 2 Vegetable, 1 1/2 Starch, 1 Very Lean Meat

Vegetable Soup with Cornmeal Croutons

Prep: 40 minutes Cook: 15 minutes Bake: 12 minutes Reheat: 10 minutes Freeze: up to 1 month
Oven: 350°F Makes: 6 to 8 servings (about 10 cups)

2 medium leeks, sliced, or
   1 medium onion, chopped
   (½ cup)

1 tablespoon olive oil or cooking
   oil

1 8-ounce package fresh
   mushrooms, quartered

1 large yellow or red sweet
   pepper, coarsely chopped

4 cloves garlic, minced

3 cups water

1 28-ounce can Italian-style
   tomatoes, undrained and
   cut up

1 15- to 19-ounce can cannellini
   (white kidney) beans, rinsed
   and drained

½ teaspoon salt

¼ teaspoon black pepper

1 recipe Cornmeal Croutons

4 cups baby spinach leaves

1. In a 4-quart Dutch oven cook leek in hot oil over medium heat until tender, stirring occasionally. Add mushrooms, sweet pepper, and garlic; cook 5 minutes more, stirring occasionally. Transfer vegetables to a 3-quart freezer container.

2. Add water, undrained cut-up tomatoes, cannellini beans, salt, and black pepper. Cover and freeze up to 1 month.

3. To serve, thaw soup and Cornmeal Croutons in refrigerator about 48 hours. Transfer soup to a 4-quart Dutch oven. Bring soup just to boiling; reduce heat. Simmer, uncovered, for 5 minutes or until heated through. Stir in spinach. Serve with Cornmeal Croutons.

Cornmeal Croutons: Grease a very large baking sheet or 2 large baking sheets; set aside. In a medium bowl lightly beat 1 egg. Add one 8½-ounce package corn muffin mix, ⅔ cup finely shredded Romano or Parmesan cheese, and 2 tablespoons milk. Drop into small mounds by scant teaspoonfuls onto prepared baking sheet(s). Lightly sprinkle with freshly ground black pepper and, if desired, coarse sea salt. Bake in a 350°F oven for 12 to 14 minutes or until golden. Remove from baking sheet; cool completely on a wire rack. Place Cornmeal Croutons in a freezer container. Freeze for up to 1 month. Makes about 24 croutons.

Nutrition Facts per serving: 333 cal., 11 g total fat (2 g sat. fat), 42 mg chol., 928 mg sodium, 50 g carbo., 6 g fiber, 15 g pro.
Exchanges: 2½ Vegetable, 2½ Starch, 1½ Fat

Turkey Sausage and Sweet Pepper Stew

Prep: 25 minutes Cook: 15 minutes Reheat: 20 minutes Freeze: up to 3 months Makes: 6 servings

1 pound cooked smoked turkey sausage or cooked turkey kielbasa, halved lengthwise and cut into $1/2$-inch pieces

4 medium red, yellow, and/or green sweet peppers, cut into 1-inch pieces

2 stalks celery, cut into $1/2$-inch pieces

1 cup chopped onion (1 large)

1 15-ounce can Great Northern or navy beans, rinsed and drained

1 $14^{1}/_{2}$-ounce can diced tomatoes, undrained

1 $10^{3}/_{4}$-ounce can reduced-fat and reduced-sodium condensed tomato soup

1 cup water

1. In a 4-quart Dutch oven combine sausage, sweet pepper, celery, and onion. Add beans, undrained tomatoes, tomato soup, and water. Bring to boiling; reduce heat. Simmer, covered, for 15 to 20 minutes or until vegetables are tender.

2. Transfer soup to a freezer container; cool. Seal, label, and freeze for up to 3 months.

3. To serve, transfer soup to 4-quart Dutch oven. Cook, covered, over medium heat until heated through, stirring occasionally to break up frozen chunks.

Nutrition Facts per serving: 253 cal., 8 g total fat (2 g sat. fat), 51 mg chol., 1,233 mg sodium, 30 g carbo., 5 g fiber, 17 g pro.
Exchanges: 2 Vegetable, 1 Starch, 2 Lean Meat

Chicken Tacos

Prep: 30 minutes   Reheat: 20 minutes   Freeze: up to 3 months   Makes: 6 servings

Nonstick cooking spray

1 cup chopped onion (1 large)

1 clove garlic, minced

2 cups chopped cooked chicken

1 8-ounce can tomato sauce

1 4-ounce can diced green chile peppers, drained

½ teaspoon chili powder (optional)

¼ teaspoon ground cumin (optional)

12 taco shells or twelve 6- to 8-inch corn or flour tortillas, warmed*

2 cups shredded lettuce

1 medium tomato, seeded and chopped

½ cup finely shredded reduced-fat cheddar cheese and/or Monterey Jack cheese (2 ounces)

1. Coat a large skillet with cooking spray. Heat over medium heat. Add onion and garlic; cook about 5 minutes or until onion is tender, stirring occasionally.

2. Stir in chicken, tomato sauce, chile peppers, and, if desired, chili powder and cumin. Cook and stir until heated through.

3. Transfer chicken mixture to a freezer container; cool. Seal, label, and freeze for up to 3 months.

4. To serve, transfer chicken mixture to a large saucepan. Cook over medium heat until heated through, stirring occasionally. Divide chicken mixture among taco shells or tortillas. Top with lettuce, tomato, and cheese. Roll up tortillas, if using.

*Note: To warm tortillas, wrap tortillas tightly in foil. Heat in a 350°F oven about 10 minutes or until heated through.

Nutrition Facts per serving: 275 cal., 12 g total fat (3 g sat. fat), 48 mg chol., 434 mg sodium, 24 g carbo., 3 g fiber, 19 g pro.
Exchanges: ½ Vegetable, 1 Starch, 2 Lean Meat, 1 Fat

Chicken Chowder

Prep: 40 minutes Cook: 15 minutes Freeze: up to 1 month Makes: 6 servings (8 cups)

1 pound skinless, boneless chicken breast halves

1 tablespoon olive oil or cooking oil

³/₄ cup coarsely chopped green, yellow, or red sweet pepper (1 medium)

¹/₂ cup chopped onion (1 medium)

3 cloves garlic, minced

1¹/₄ cups coarsely chopped zucchini and/or yellow summer squash (1 medium)

2 14-ounce cans reduced-sodium chicken broth

1 10-ounce package frozen baby lima beans

2 teaspoons ground cumin

2 teaspoons ground coriander

¹/₄ teaspoon salt

¹/₄ teaspoon black pepper

1 8-ounce carton light dairy sour cream

2 tablespoons all-purpose flour

Snipped fresh cilantro (optional)

Shredded reduced-fat Monterey Jack cheese (optional)

1. Cut chicken into cubes. In a 4-quart Dutch oven heat oil over medium heat. Add chicken, sweet pepper, onion, and garlic; cook and stir until chicken is brown and vegetables are tender. Add zucchini; cook 2 minutes more. Add broth, lima beans, cumin, coriander, salt, and black pepper. Bring to boiling; reduce heat. Simmer, uncovered, for 5 minutes.

2. Transfer chowder to a freezer container; cool. Seal, label, and freeze up to 1 month.

3. To serve, thaw chowder in refrigerator 24 hours. Transfer chowder to a 4-quart Dutch oven. Bring to boiling, stirring frequently. In a small bowl stir together the sour cream and flour. Whisk into soup mixture. Cook and stir until thickened and bubbly; cook and stir for 1 minute more. To serve, ladle into bowls. If desired, sprinkle with cilantro and cheese.

Nutrition Facts per serving: 258 cal., 7 g total fat (3 g sat. fat), 56 mg chol., 508 mg sodium, 21 g carbo., 4 g fiber, 27 g pro.
Exchanges: ¹/₂ Vegetable, 1 Starch, 3¹/₂ Very Lean Meat, 1 Fat

Creamy Chicken Enchiladas

Prep: 35 minutes Bake: 40 minutes Cook: 12 minutes Stand: 5 minutes Freeze: up to 3 months
Oven: 350°F Makes: 2 (6-servings) casseroles

1 pound skinless, boneless chicken breast halves

1 14-ounce can chicken broth

½ teaspoon black pepper

1 10-ounce package frozen chopped spinach, thawed and well drained

¼ cup thinly sliced green onion (2)

2 8-ounce cartons light dairy sour cream

½ cup plain low-fat yogurt

¼ cup all-purpose flour

½ teaspoon salt

½ teaspoon ground cumin

1 cup reduced-fat or fat-free milk

2 4-ounce cans diced green chile peppers, drained

12 7- to 8-inch flour tortillas

1 cup shredded reduced-fat cheddar or Monterey Jack cheese (4 ounces)

Chopped tomato or salsa (optional)

Thinly sliced green onion (optional)

1. In a large skillet place chicken, broth, and ½ teaspoon black pepper. Bring to boiling; reduce heat. Simmer, covered, for 12 to 14 minutes or until chicken is no longer pink. Drain well. When cool enough to handle, using 2 forks, pull meat apart into shreds. (You should have about 3 cups). Set aside.

2. In a large bowl combine the shredded chicken, spinach, and the ¼ cup green onion; set aside.

3. In a bowl whisk together sour cream, yogurt, flour, salt, and cumin until smooth. Stir in milk and chile peppers. Divide sauce in half. Set 1 portion aside.

4. For filling, combine 1 portion of the sauce and the chicken mixture. Divide filling among tortillas. Roll up tortillas. Place, seam sides down, in 2 ungreased 2-quart rectangular baking dishes. Divide remaining sauce evenly between the two baking dishes. Wrap, label, and freeze casseroles for up to 3 months.

5. To serve, thaw 1 of the casseroles in the refrigerator overnight. Bake casserole, covered, in a 350° oven for 20 minutes. Uncover and bake 20 minutes more or until heated through. Sprinkle with ½ cup cheese; let stand for 5 minutes before serving. If desired, garnish with chopped tomato and additional green onion.

Nutrition Facts per serving: 245 cal., 9 g total fat (4 g sat. fat), 43 mg chol., 555 mg sodium, 22 g carbo., 1 g fiber, 18 g pro.
Exchanges: ½ Vegetable, 1½ Starch, 1 Very Lean Meat, ½ Lean Meat, 1 Fat

Old-Fashioned Chicken Noodle Soup

Prep: 20 minutes Cook: 2¼ hours Reheat: 20 minutes Freeze: up to 3 months
Makes: 2 (4-serving) portions (10½ cups total)

1 4- to 5-pound stewing chicken, cut up

6 cups water

½ cup chopped onion (1 medium)

2 teaspoons salt

¼ teaspoon black pepper

1 bay leaf

1½ cups dried medium noodles

1 cup chopped carrot (2 medium)

1 cup chopped celery (2 stalks)

2 tablespoons snipped fresh parsley

1. In a 6- to 8-quart Dutch oven combine chicken, water, onion, salt, pepper, and bay leaf. Bring to boiling; reduce heat. Simmer, covered, about 2 hours or until chicken is tender.

2. Remove chicken from Dutch oven. When cool enough to handle, remove meat from bones. Discard bones. Cut meat into bite-size pieces; set aside. Remove and discard bay leaf. Skim fat from broth.

3. Bring broth to boiling. Stir in noodles, carrot, and celery. Simmer, covered, about 8 minutes or until noodles are tender but still firm. Stir in chicken and parsley; heat through.

4. Divide soup between 2 freezer containers; cool. Seal, label, and freeze for up to 3 months.

5. To serve, thaw 1 container of soup overnight in the refrigerator. Transfer soup to a large saucepan or 4-quart Dutch oven. Cook, covered, over medium heat until heated through, stirring occasionally to break up any remaining frozen chunks. Ladle soup into bowls.

Nutrition Facts per serving: 210 cal., 6 g total fat (2 g sat. fat), 84 mg chol., 665 mg sodium, 10 g carbo., 1 g fiber, 26 g pro.
Exchanges: ½ Vegetable, ½ Starch, 3½ Very Lean Meat, 1 Fat

Pizza Lover's Pasta Sauce

Prep: 25 minutes   Cook: 10 minutes   Reheat: 25 minutes   Freeze: up to 3 months
Makes: 6 to 8 servings

Nonstick cooking spray

1 cup chopped onion (1 large)

¾ cup chopped green, red, or yellow sweet pepper (1 medium)

2 cloves garlic, minced

1 14½-ounce can diced tomatoes, undrained

1 8-ounce can tomato sauce

½ cup thinly sliced cooked turkey pepperoni, chopped

1 4-ounce can sliced mushrooms, drained (optional)

1 tablespoon snipped fresh oregano or basil or 1 teaspoon dried oregano or basil, crushed

⅛ to ¼ teaspoon crushed red pepper (optional)

8 to 10 ounces dried pasta

⅓ cup shredded Parmesan cheese

1. Coat a large saucepan with cooking spray. Heat over medium heat. Add onion, sweet pepper, and garlic; cook until tender, stirring occasionally. Stir in undrained tomatoes, tomato sauce, pepperoni, mushrooms (if desired), dried oregano (if using), and, if desired, crushed red pepper. Bring to boiling; reduce heat. Simmer, uncovered, about 10 minutes or until mixture is desired consistency, stirring occasionally.

2. Transfer sauce to a freezer container; cool. Seal, label, and freeze for up to 3 months.

3. To serve, transfer sauce to a large saucepan. Cook, covered, over medium heat about 25 minutes or until heated through, stirring occasionally. If necessary, stir in 1 to 2 tablespoons water to reach desired consistency.

4. Meanwhile, cook pasta according to package directions; drain. Just before serving, stir fresh oregano, if using, into sauce. Serve sauce over hot cooked pasta. Sprinkle with cheese.

Nutrition Facts per serving: 233 cal., 3 g total fat (1 g sat. fat), 19 mg chol., 580 mg sodium, 38 g carbo., 2 g fiber, 11 g pro.
Exchanges: 1 Vegetable, 2 Starch, ½ Lean Meat, ½ Fat

Parmesan Chicken and Broccoli

Prep: 25 minutes Bake: 80 minutes Freeze: up to 3 months Oven: 350°F Makes: 6 servings

1 cup uncooked converted rice

1/2 cup sliced green onion (4)

1¼ pounds skinless, boneless chicken breast halves, cut into strips

1 tablespoon cooking oil

1 teaspoon dried Italian seasoning, crushed

1 teaspoon bottled minced garlic or 2 cloves garlic, minced

4 teaspoons cornstarch

2¾ cups reduced-fat or fat-free milk

1/2 of an 8-ounce package reduced-fat cream cheese (Neufchâtel), cut up

1½ cups loose-pack frozen cut broccoli

1/2 cup grated Parmesan cheese

1/3 cup diced reduced-sodium cooked ham

2 tablespoons sliced almonds, toasted

1. Cook rice according to package directions; remove from heat and stir in half the green onion. Spread rice mixture in a greased 2-quart rectangular baking dish; set aside.

2. In a large skillet cook half the chicken strips in hot oil over medium heat for 6 minutes or until chicken is no longer pink. Remove from skillet. Add remaining chicken strips, the Italian seasoning, and garlic to the skillet. Cook 6 minutes or until chicken is no longer pink. Remove from skillet; reserve drippings.

3. For sauce, cook the remaining green onion in reserved skillet drippings until tender, adding more oil as necessary. Stir in cornstarch; add milk all at once. Cook and stir over medium heat until slightly thickened and bubbly. Reduce heat; stir in cream cheese until nearly smooth. Remove sauce from heat; stir in cooked chicken strips, broccoli, Parmesan cheese, and ham.

4. Spoon chicken mixture over rice in baking dish; season with salt and pepper. Cover with heavy foil. Label and freeze for up to 3 months.

5. To serve, thaw covered frozen casserole in the refrigerator overnight (casserole may still be icy). Bake casserole, covered with foil, in a 350° oven for 1 hour. Uncover and bake for 20 to 25 minutes more or until heated through. Sprinkle with almonds.

Nutrition Facts per serving: 421 cal., 14 g total fat (6 g sat. fat), 88 mg chol., 389 mg sodium, 37 g carbo., 2 g fiber, 36 g pro.
Exchanges: 1/2 Milk, 1 Vegetable, 1½ Starch, 2 Very Lean Meat, 1½ Medium-Fat Meat, 1 Fat

Picadillo Chicken Loaves

Prep: 15 minutes Bake: 35 minutes Freeze: up to 3 months Oven: 350°F Makes: 8 loaves

2 eggs, slightly beaten

½ cup fine dry bread crumbs

½ cup raisins

¼ cup thinly sliced pimiento-
stuffed green olives

¼ cup apple juice or milk

1 teaspoon onion salt

1 teaspoon ground cinnamon

1 teaspoon ground cumin

2 pounds ground uncooked
chicken or turkey

½ cup toasted chopped almonds
or pecans

¼ cup shredded reduced-fat
cheddar or Monterey Jack
cheese

1. In a large bowl stir together the eggs, bread crumbs, raisins, olives, apple juice, onion salt, cinnamon, and cumin. Add ground chicken and nuts; mix well.

2. Shape the chicken mixture into eight 4×2½×1-inch loaves. Place loaves in a freezer container or in self-sealing freezer bags. Seal, label, and freeze for up to 3 months.

3. To serve, bake the desired number of frozen loaves, uncovered, in a 350° oven for 35 to 40 minutes or until temperature reaches 165°F. Sprinkle each loaf with 1 tablespoon shredded cheese. Bake about 3 minutes more or until cheese melts.

Nutrition Facts per loaf: 362 cal., 22 g total fat (1 g sat. fat), 55 mg chol., 561 mg sodium, 15 g carbo., 2 g fiber, 25 g pro.
Exchanges: 1 Other Carbo., 3 Lean Meat, ½ Medium-Fat Meat, 2 Fat

Make-Ahead Burritos

Prep: 30 minutes Bake: 60 minutes Freeze: up to 3 months Oven: 350°F
Makes: 8 (2-burrito) servings

1 pound cooked chicken, beef, or pork

1 16-ounce jar salsa

1 16-ounce can refried beans

1 4½-ounce can diced green chile peppers, undrained

1 1½-ounce envelope burrito or taco seasoning mix

¼ cup cooking oil

16 8-inch flour tortillas

16 ounces reduced-fat Monterey Jack or cheddar cheese, cut into sixteen 5×½-inch sticks

Salsa (optional)

Dairy sour cream (optional)

1. For filling, using 2 forks, shred cooked chicken or meat (should have about 3 cups). In a large skillet combine shredded chicken or meat, the 16 ounces salsa, refried beans, undrained chile peppers, and seasoning mix. Cook and stir over medium heat until heated through.

2. In another skillet heat 1 tablespoon of the cooking oil. Heat tortillas, 1 at a time, in the oil over medium-low heat about 30 seconds per side or until brown, adding more oil if necessary. Set aside to cool.

3. To assemble, place ⅓ cup filling onto each tortilla near 1 edge. Top each with a cheese stick. Fold in the sides; roll up, starting from edge with the cheese. Secure with wooden toothpicks. Place the burritos in a freezer container. Seal, label, and freeze for up to 3 months.

4. To serve, remove desired number of burritos from the freezer. Wrap each frozen burrito individually in foil. Place on baking sheet. Bake in a 350° oven for 50 minutes. (Or thaw frozen burritos in the refrigerator overnight. Wrap each burrito in foil. Bake in a 350° oven for 30 minutes.)

5. Remove foil. Bake about 10 minutes more or until tortillas are crisp and brown. If desired, serve with additional salsa and sour cream.

Nutrition Facts per serving: 292 cal., 13 g total fat (5 g sat. fat), 45 mg chol., 830 mg sodium, 22 g carbo., 2 g fiber, 20 g pro.
Exchanges: 2 Starch, 1 Very Lean Meat, 1 Lean Meat, 1 Fat

Roasted Turkey Calzones

Prep: 30 minutes Bake: 12 minutes Freeze: up to 3 months Oven: 350°F Makes: 8 calzones

1 pound boneless cooked turkey breast, chopped (about 3 cups)

2½ cups chopped fresh spinach

1½ cups shredded 4-cheese pizza cheese (6 ounces)

1 14- or 15-ounce jar pizza sauce

2 13.8-ounce packages refrigerated pizza dough

Milk

Grated Parmesan or Romano cheese (optional)

1. In a large bowl combine turkey, spinach, pizza cheese, and ½ cup of the pizza sauce. On a lightly floured surface, roll out 1 package of pizza dough to a 12×12-inch square. Cut into four 6×6-inch squares.

2. Place about ⅔ cup of the turkey mixture onto half of each square to within about ½ inch of edge. Moisten edges of dough with water and fold over, forming a triangle or rectangle. Pinch or press with a fork to seal edges. Prick tops of calzones with a fork; brush with milk and place on an ungreased baking sheet. Repeat with remaining dough and turkey mixture.

3. Freeze calzones until firm. Transfer to a resealable freezer bag or freezer container. Seal, label and freeze for up to 3 months. Transfer remaining pizza sauce to an airtight freezer container. Seal, label, and freeze for up to 3 months.

4. Thaw frozen calzones and frozen pizza sauce in the refrigerator overnight. Unwrap calzones and place on a lightly greased baking sheet. If desired, sprinkle with Parmesan cheese. Bake calzones, uncovered, in a 350° oven for 12 to 15 minutes or until heated through. Heat pizza sauce and serve with calzones.

Nutrition Facts per calzone: 390 cal., 11 g total fat (4 g sat. fat), 54 mg chol.., 708 mg sodium, 40 g carbo., 2 g fiber, 29 g pro.
Exchanges: 1 Vegetable, 3 Starch, 2 Very Lean Meat, 1 Medium-Fat Meat

Turkey Soup with Barley

Prep: 35 minutes Cook: 10 minutes Reheat: 25 minutes Freeze: up to 3 months Makes: 4 servings

12 ounces turkey breast tenderloin or skinless, boneless chicken breasts or thighs

1 tablespoon cooking oil

½ cup chopped onion (1 medium)

½ cup chopped red or green sweet pepper

1 clove garlic, minced

2 14-ounce cans reduced-sodium chicken broth

1½ cups loose-pack frozen cut green beans

1 cup loose-pack frozen whole kernel corn or one 8-ounce can whole kernel corn, drained

⅓ cup quick-cooking barley

2 tablespoons snipped fresh basil or 1½ teaspoons dried basil, crushed

¼ teaspoon salt

¼ teaspoon black pepper

1. Cut turkey into bite-size pieces or cubes. In a Dutch oven cook and stir turkey in hot oil for 5 minutes. Using a slotted spoon, remove turkey from pan. In pan drippings cook onion, sweet pepper, and garlic for 3 minutes, stirring occasionally. Drain off fat.

2. Return turkey to Dutch oven. Add broth, green beans, corn, barley, dried basil (if using), salt, and black pepper. Bring to boiling; reduce heat. Simmer, covered, for 10 to 15 minutes or until barley is cooked. Stir in fresh basil (if using).

3. Transfer soup to a freezer container; cool. Cover, label, and freeze for up to 3 months.

4. To serve, transfer soup to Dutch oven. Cover and cook over medium heat for 25 to 30 minutes or until heated through, stirring occasionally to break up mixture. Ladle soup into bowls.

Nutrition Facts per serving: 247 cal., 5 g total fat (1 g sat. fat), 51 mg chol., 703 mg sodium, 25 g carbo., 4 g fiber, 26 g pro.
Exchanges: 1 Vegetable, 1 Starch, 2 Medium-Fat Meat

Mediterranean-Style Fish Rolls

Prep: 25 minutes Bake: 63 minutes Freeze: up to 3 months Makes: 4 (2-roll) servings

8 4-ounce fresh or frozen flounder, sole, or other fish fillets

1½ pounds asparagus spears or
   two 10-ounce packages frozen
   asparagus spears

½ cup finely chopped onion
   (1 medium)

4 teaspoons olive oil or
   cooking oil

4 teaspoons cornstarch

1 teaspoon dried basil, crushed

½ teaspoon dried oregano,
   crushed

2 8-ounce cans tomato sauce

2 4-ounce cans diced green chile
   peppers, drained

2 tablespoons lemon juice

½ cup shredded Monterey Jack
   cheese (2 ounces)

Lemon slices (optional)

Sliced, pitted ripe olives
   (optional)

1. Thaw fish, if frozen. Cut the fresh asparagus, if using, into 6-inch spears; discard woody stems. Cook the fresh asparagus, covered, in a small amount of boiling water for 8 to 10 minutes or until crisp-tender. Or, if using frozen asparagus, cook according to package directions. Drain well.

2. Place 4 or 5 asparagus spears crosswise on each fillet. Roll into a spiral, starting from a narrow end. Place 4 fish rolls, seam sides down, in a 2-quart baking dish. Place remaining fish rolls, seam sides down, in another 2-quart baking dish.

3. For sauce, in a small saucepan cook the onion in oil until tender. Stir in the cornstarch, basil, and oregano. Add the tomato sauce, chile peppers, and lemon juice. Cook and stir until thickened and bubbly. Cook and stir for 2 minutes more. Spoon the sauce over fish rolls.

4. Wrap fish rolls in moistureproof and vaporproof freezer wrap. Label and freeze for up to 3 months.

5. To serve, bake 1 dish of frozen fish rolls, covered, in a 350° oven for 60 to 70 minutes or until fish is nearly done. Sprinkle each fish roll with 1 tablespoon shredded Monterey Jack cheese. Bake, uncovered, for 3 to 5 minutes more or just until fish begins to flake easily and cheese is melted. If desired, garnish with lemon slices and sliced, pitted ripe olives.

Nutrition Facts per serving: 166 cal., 4 g total fat (1 g sat. fat), 54 mg chol., 439 mg sodium, 7 g carbo., 1 g fiber, 24 g pro.
Exchanges: 3 Lean Meat

good-for-you
sweets

Your pregnancy may be giving you constant cravings for the taste of something sweet, but most sweet treats are not very nutritious. Here are the best of both worlds—desserts that can satisfy your cravings for sweets but aren't over the top on calories, fat, and sugar. Make a few extra and share them with friends and family. Anyone can enjoy a good-for-you sweet!

Berry Dessert Nachos

Prep: 20 minutes Bake: 5 minutes Cool: 15 minutes Oven: 400°F Makes: 6 servings

½ cup light dairy sour cream

½ cup frozen light whipped dessert topping, thawed

2 tablespoons sugar

⅛ teaspoon ground cinnamon

6 7- to 8-inch flour tortillas

Butter-flavor nonstick cooking spray

1 tablespoon sugar

⅛ teaspoon ground cinnamon

3 cups raspberries and/or blackberries

2 tablespoons sliced almonds, toasted

1½ teaspoons grated semisweet chocolate

1. In a small bowl stir together sour cream, dessert topping, the 2 tablespoons sugar, and ⅛ teaspoon cinnamon; cover and refrigerate until serving time.

2. Cut each tortilla into 8 wedges. Arrange wedges on 2 baking sheets. Lightly coat wedges with cooking spray. In a small bowl stir together the 1 tablespoon sugar and ⅛ teaspoon cinnamon; sprinkle over tortilla wedges.

3. Bake in a 400° oven about 5 minutes or until crisp. Cool completely on a wire rack.

4. To serve, place 8 tortilla wedges on each of 6 dessert plates. Top with berries and sour cream mixture. Sprinkle with almonds and grated chocolate.

Nutrition Facts per serving: 205 cal., 7 g total fat (3 g sat. fat), 7 mg chol., 133 mg sodium, 32 g carbo., 5 g fiber, 5 g pro. **Exchanges:** 1 Fruit, 1 Starch, 1½ Fat

Fruit and Granola Bake

Prep: 25 minutes Bake: 40 minutes Oven: 350°F Makes: 6 servings

3 medium apples, peeled and cut into bite-size pieces

3 medium pears, peeled and cut into bite-size pieces

⅓ cup dried tart cherries

⅓ cup apple butter

¼ cup apple juice

½ teaspoon ground cinnamon

1 cup low-fat granola cereal

1. In an ungreased 2-quart rectangular baking dish combine apple, pear, and dried cherries. In a small bowl whisk together apple butter, apple juice, and cinnamon. Pour mixture over fruit in dish and toss to combine.

2. Bake, covered, in a 350° oven for 30 minutes. Uncover; stir fruit mixture. Sprinkle with granola and bake, uncovered, for 10 to 15 minutes more or until top is golden and fruit is tender. Serve warm.

Nutrition Facts per serving: 258 cal., 1 g total fat (0 g sat. fat), 0 mg chol., 51 mg sodium, 63 g carbo., 6 g fiber, 2 g pro. **Exchanges:** 1 Fruit, 2 Starch, 1 Other Carbo.

Baked Red Pears

Prep: 15 minutes Bake: 40 minutes Oven: 350°F Makes: 4 servings

1¼ cups apricot nectar

⅓ cup snipped dried apricots

2 tablespoons dried tart red cherries or dried cranberries

4 firm medium red pears

2 tablespoons sugar

¼ teaspoon ground nutmeg

½ teaspoon vanilla

⅛ teaspoon ground cardamom

1. In a small saucepan combine apricot nectar, apricots, and dried cherries. Bring to boiling. Remove from heat; let stand for 5 minutes. Drain fruit, reserving liquid.

2. Meanwhile, cut off tops of pears; set aside. Core pears almost through to bottom. Place pears and pear tops in a 2-quart square baking dish. In a small bowl combine drained fruit mixture, sugar, and nutmeg. Spoon into centers of pears.

3. In another small bowl combine reserved liquid, vanilla, and cardamom; pour over and around pears.

4. Bake, covered, in a 350° oven for 20 minutes. Uncover; bake for 20 to 25 minutes more or until pears are tender, basting occasionally with cooking liquid.

5. To serve, place tops on pears; spoon liquid over pears. Serve warm.

Nutrition Facts per serving: 206 cal., 1 g total fat (0 g sat. fat), 0 mg chol., 4 mg sodium, 52 g carbo., 6 g fiber, 1 g pro.
Exchanges: 3½ Fruit

Fun-Day Sundae Parfait

Start to Finish: 15 minutes Makes: 2 servings

1½ cups frozen vanilla or fruit-flavored yogurt or light ice cream

½ cup coarsely crushed vanilla wafers or honey or cinnamon graham crackers

1 cup fresh fruit, such as sliced bananas or strawberries; peeled, sliced kiwifruit, peaches, or mangoes; cut-up pineapple; raspberries; and/or blueberries

6 tablespoons strawberry ice cream topping

¼ cup frozen light whipped dessert topping, thawed (optional)

2 maraschino cherries with stems (optional)

1. Chill 2 tall parfait glasses.

2. Place ¼ cup frozen yogurt in the bottom of each chilled glass. Top each with 2 tablespoons of the crushed wafers, ¼ cup fruit, and 1 tablespoon strawberry topping. Repeat layers. Top each with ¼ cup frozen yogurt. Drizzle each with remaining strawberry topping. If desired, top with whipped topping and garnish with maraschino cherries. Serve with long-handled spoons.

Nutrition Facts per serving: 375 cal., 9 g total fat (4 g sat. fat), 15 mg chol., 138 mg sodium, 70 g carbo., 2 g fiber, 4 g pro.
Exchanges: 1 Fruit, 3½ Other Carbo., 1½ Fat

Mango Parfaits

Start to Finish: 15 minutes Makes: 2 servings

1 6-ounce carton vanilla low-fat yogurt

¼ of an 8-ounce container frozen light whipped dessert topping, thawed

1½ cups chopped seeded and peeled mango, papaya, peaches, or apricots

Frozen light whipped dessert topping, thawed (optional)

Fresh fruit (such as sliced kiwifruit or raspberries) (optional)

1. Spoon yogurt into a small bowl. Fold in the ¼ of an 8-ounce carton whipped topping. Spoon one-fourth of the yogurt mixture into each of 2 parfait glasses. Top with half of the mango. Repeat layers with remaining yogurt mixture and mango. If desired, top with additional whipped topping and fresh fruit.

Nutrition Facts per serving: 216 cal., 5 g total fat (4 g sat. fat), 4 mg chol., 59 mg sodium, 39 g carbo., 2 g fiber, 5 g pro.
Exchanges: ½ Milk, 2 Fruit, 1 Fat

Baked Apples

Prep: 25 minutes Bake: 50 minutes Oven: 350°F Makes: 4 servings

2 medium cooking apples, such as Rome Beauty, Granny Smith, or Jonathan

¼ cup raisins, dried cranberries, or mixed dried fruit bits

2 tablespoons red cinnamon candies

1 tablespoon packed brown sugar

⅓ cup apple juice or water

⅓ cup caramel ice cream topping

1 tablespoon maple-flavored syrup

1 cup frozen vanilla yogurt

Chopped toasted walnuts or pecans (optional)

1. Core apples; peel a strip from the top of each. Place apples in a 2-quart square baking dish. In a small bowl combine raisins, cinnamon candies, and brown sugar; spoon into center of apples. Pour apple juice into baking dish.

2. Bake, uncovered, in a 350° oven for 50 to 55 minutes or until the apples are tender, basting occasionally during baking.

3. Meanwhile, for topping, in a small bowl combine caramel topping and maple syrup; set aside.

4. To serve, halve warm apples lengthwise. Transfer apple halves to dessert dishes. Top each serving with a scoop of frozen yogurt. Drizzle with topping. If desired, sprinkle with nuts. Serve immediately.

Nutrition Facts per serving: 256 cal., 2 g total fat (1 g sat. fat), 5 mg chol., 81 mg sodium, 60 g carbo., 2 g fiber, 3 g pro.
Exchanges: 1½ Fruit, 2½ Other Carbo.

Granola-Topped Nectarine Gratin

Prep: 35 minutes Bake: 37 minutes Oven: 325°F/450°F Makes: 4 servings

1 cup Almond-Fruit Granola

4 medium nectarines, pitted and sliced

½ cup fresh blueberries

2 tablespoons orange juice

2 tablespoons packed brown sugar

1. Prepare Almond-Fruit Granola; set aside.

2. For gratin, in a medium bowl combine nectarine, blueberries, and orange juice; toss to coat. Spoon fruit into 4 gratin dishes or casseroles (12 to 16 ounces each). Sprinkle with brown sugar.

3. Bake in a 450° oven for 7 to 8 minutes or until fruit is warm and most of sugar is melted. Sprinkle ¼ cup Almond-Fruit Granola over each gratin. Serve immediately.

Almond-Fruit Granola: Lightly coat a 13×9×2-inch baking pan with nonstick cooking spray; set aside. In a medium bowl stir together 1¼ cups rolled oats, ½ cup bran cereal, ¼ cup toasted wheat germ, and 2 tablespoons sliced almonds. In a small bowl stir together ¼ cup raspberry, mixed berry, or plain applesauce (do not use "lite" applesauce); 3 tablespoons honey; and ⅛ teaspoon ground cinnamon. Pour applesauce mixture over cereal mixture. Use a wooden spoon to mix well. Spread granola evenly in prepared pan. Bake in a 325° oven about 25 minutes or until golden, stirring occasionally. Carefully stir in ¼ cup dried berries and cherries. Bake for 5 minutes more. Spread on foil; cool completely. Store in an airtight container for up to 2 weeks. Makes 3 cups.

Nutrition Facts per serving: 222 cal., 2 g total fat (0 g sat. fat), 0 mg chol., 12 mg sodium, 46 g carbo., 5 g fiber, 4 g pro.
Exchanges: 1 Fruit, ½ Starch

Peach-Filled Phyllo Bundles

Prep: 25 minutes Bake: 20 minutes Stand: 5 minutes Oven: 375°F Makes: 4 bundles

3 medium peaches, peeled, pitted, and coarsely chopped, or 2¼ cups frozen unsweetened peach slices, thawed and coarsely chopped*

2 tablespoons granulated sugar

4 teaspoons miniature semisweet chocolate pieces

1 tablespoon all-purpose flour

1 teaspoon lemon juice

Nonstick cooking spray

8 sheets frozen phyllo dough (9×14-inch rectangles), thawed

2 teaspoons powdered sugar

1. For filling, in a medium bowl combine peaches, granulated sugar, chocolate pieces, flour, and lemon juice. Toss to combine; set aside.

2. Lightly coat four 6-ounce custard cups with cooking spray; set aside. Lightly coat 1 phyllo sheet with cooking spray. (Keep remaining phyllo sheets covered with a damp cloth to keep them from drying out.) Place another sheet of phyllo on top of the first sheet; lightly coat with nonstick spray. Repeat twice. Cut stack in half lengthwise, forming 2 rectangles. Repeat with remaining phyllo.

3. Gently ease 1 stack of phyllo into bottom and up the sides of 1 custard cup (phyllo will hang over edge). Spoon about ½ cup of the peach filling into center. Bring phyllo up over filling, pinching together to form a ruffled edge. Lightly coat again with nonstick spray. Repeat with remaining cups, phyllo, and filling. Place custard cups in a 15×10×1-inch baking pan.

4. Bake in a 375° oven for 20 minutes. Cool 5 minutes in custard cups; remove from cups. Serve warm or cool. Sift powdered sugar over pastry tops before serving.

*Note: If using frozen peaches, blot them well with paper towels after thawing to remove excess moisture.

Nutrition Facts per bundle: 173 cal., 2 g total fat (1 g sat. fat), 0 mg chol., 107 mg sodium, 37 g carbo., 3 g fiber, 3 g pro
Exchanges: 1 Fruit, 1½ Starch

Spicy Roasted Plums

Prep: 15 minutes Bake: 20 minutes Oven: 450°F Makes: 6 servings

Nonstick cooking spray

6 medium plums

½ cup unsweetened pineapple juice

¼ cup packed brown sugar

½ teaspoon ground cinnamon

¼ teaspoon ground cardamom

⅛ teaspoon ground cumin

⅓ cup light dairy sour cream

1 tablespoon packed brown sugar

2 tablespoons sliced almonds, toasted

1. Coat a 2-quart rectangular baking dish with cooking spray. Halve and pit plums. Place plums, cut sides up, in prepared baking dish. Stir together pineapple juice, the ¼ cup brown sugar, the cinnamon, cardamom, and cumin. Drizzle over plums.

2. Bake in a 450° oven about 20 minutes or until plums are tender. In a small bowl stir together sour cream and the 1 tablespoon brown sugar. To serve, arrange plums in dessert dishes; top with sour cream mixture and almonds.

Nutrition Facts per serving: 129 cal., 3 g total fat (1 g sat. fat), 4 mg chol., 14 mg sodium, 25 g carbo., 2 g fiber, 2 g pro. **Exchanges:** 2 Fruit

Strudel Triangles with Apples

Prep: 35 minutes Bake: 6 minutes Oven: 375°F Makes: 6 servings

¼ cup low-fat cinnamon graham cracker crumbs

1 tablespoon granulated sugar

4 sheets frozen phyllo dough (9×14-inch rectangles), thawed

Nonstick cooking spray

1 tablespoon butter or margarine

1 tablespoon packed brown sugar

3 medium apples, peeled, cored, and thinly sliced

¼ cup raisins or dried cherries

1 tablespoon water

¼ teaspoon ground cinnamon

⅛ teaspoon ground nutmeg

⅓ cup fat-free caramel ice cream topping

Ground cinnamon (optional)

1. In a small bowl combine graham cracker crumbs and sugar; set aside.

2. For strudel triangles, lightly coat phyllo sheets with cooking spray. Sprinkle one-fourth of the crumb mixture on 1 phyllo half. Top with a phyllo sheet and one-fourth of the crumb mixture; repeat with remaining phyllo and crumb mixture. Cut the 4-layer stack into nine 2¾×4-inch rectangles. Cut each rectangle diagonally in half to form 2 triangles (18 triangles total). Lightly coat a large baking sheet with cooking spray. Carefully place triangles on baking sheet. Bake in a 375° oven for 6 to 8 minutes or until golden brown.

3. Meanwhile, in a large skillet melt butter; stir in brown sugar. Stir in apple slices, raisins, water, cinnamon, nutmeg, and 3 tablespoons of the ice cream topping. Cook, uncovered, about 5 minutes or until apples are tender, stirring occasionally.

4. To serve, place a strudel triangle on each of 6 dessert plates. Spoon one-third of apple mixture over each of the 6 triangles. Add a second strudel triangle. Top with half of the remaining apple mixture. Repeat with remaining triangles and apple mixture. Drizzle with remaining ice cream topping. If desired, sprinkle with cinnamon. Serve immediately.

Nutrition Facts per serving: 173 cal., 3 g total fat (1 g sat. fat), 5 mg chol., 136 mg sodium, 36 g carbo., 1 g fiber, 1 g pro.
Exchanges: ½ Fruit, 1½ Starch, ½ Fat

Strawberry Gelato

Prep: 25 minutes Chill: 6 to 24 hours Freeze: per manufacturer's directions
Makes: 14 servings (about 7 cups)

2 cups low-fat milk

1 cup refrigerated or frozen egg product, thawed

½ cup sugar

4 cups strawberries

1 teaspoon lemon juice

Fresh strawberries (optional)

1. In a medium saucepan combine milk, egg product, and sugar. Cook and stir over medium heat about 10 minutes or until mixture is thickened. Do not boil. Remove saucepan from heat.

2. Place saucepan in a sink or bowl of ice water for 1 to 2 minutes, stirring constantly. Pour custard mixture into a bowl; set aside.

3. Place strawberries in a blender or food processor. Cover and blend or process until nearly smooth. Stir the strawberries and lemon juice into custard mixture. Cover the surface of custard with plastic wrap. Refrigerate for several hours or overnight until completely chilled. (Or, to chill quickly, place bowl in a sink of ice water.)

4. Freeze mixture in a 2- or 3-quart ice cream freezer according to the manufacturer's directions. If desired, serve with additional fresh strawberries.

Nutrition Facts per serving: 65 cal., 1 g total fat (0 g sat. fat), 3 mg chol., 41 mg sodium, 12 g carbo., 1 g fiber, 3 g pro.
Exchanges: ½ Milk, ½ Fruit

Peach Gelato: Prepare as above, except substitute 4 cups cut-up pitted and peeled peaches (5 to 6 peaches) for the strawberries.

Peach Freeze

Prep: 20 minutes Stand: 15 minutes Freeze: 4 to 24 hours Makes: 6 servings

4 cups sliced, peeled fresh peaches or one 16-ounce package frozen unsweetened peach slices, thawed

⅓ cup sugar

2 teaspoons finely shredded lemon peel

3 tablespoons lemon juice

½ of an 8-ounce container frozen fat-free whipped dessert topping, thawed

½ cup light dairy sour cream

Fresh raspberries (optional)

1. In a food processor combine peaches, sugar, lemon peel, and lemon juice. Cover and process until smooth. Transfer to a large bowl. Fold in whipped topping and sour cream.

2. Transfer to a freezer container. Cover and freeze for 4 to 24 hours. Before serving, let stand at room temperature for 15 to 20 minutes to soften slightly. If desired, garnish with raspberries.

Nutrition Facts per serving: 200 cal., 2 g total fat (1 g sat. fat), 7 mg chol., 24 mg sodium, 44 g carbo., 5 g fiber, 3 g pro.
Exchanges: 3 Fruit, ½ Fat

Fruited Yogurt Brûlée

Prep: 20 minutes Bake: 7 minutes Oven: 450°F Makes: 4 servings

6 cups fresh fruit (such as blueberries; raspberries; sliced
   strawberries, nectarines,
   peaches, pears, apricots, or
   bananas; and/or mango,
   papaya, or pineapple chunks)

1 cup vanilla low-fat yogurt

½ cup part-skim ricotta cheese

¼ cup packed brown sugar

1. Divide fruit among four 10- to 12-ounce gratin dishes. Place dishes in a 15×10×1-inch baking pan. In a small bowl stir together yogurt and ricotta cheese. Spoon the yogurt mixture over fruit. Sprinkle with brown sugar.

2. Bake, uncovered, in a 450° oven for 7 to 8 minutes or until brown sugar melts. Serve immediately.

Nutrition Facts per serving: 211 cal., 4 g total fat (2 g sat. fat), 13 mg chol., 86 mg sodium, 39 g carbo., 5 g fiber, 7 g pro.
Exchanges: ½ Milk, 2 Fruit

Orange-Cranberry Cake

Prep: 25 minutes Bake: 40 minutes Cool: 1 hour Oven: 350°F Makes: 12 servings

Nonstick cooking spray

2 cups all-purpose flour

1¼ teaspoons baking powder

½ teaspoon baking soda

3 tablespoons butter, softened

1 cup granulated sugar

2 eggs

⅔ cup plain fat-free yogurt

2 cups fresh or frozen cranberries, chopped

1 teaspoon finely shredded orange peel

Powdered sugar (optional)

1. Coat a 10-inch fluted tube pan with cooking spray; set aside. In a medium bowl combine flour, baking powder, and baking soda; set aside.

2. In a large mixing bowl beat butter with an electric mixer on medium speed for 30 seconds. Add granulated sugar and beat until fluffy. Add eggs, 1 at a time, beating well after each addition. Alternately add flour mixture and yogurt to egg mixture, beating after each addition just until combined. Fold in cranberries and orange peel.

3. Spoon batter into the prepared pan, spreading evenly. Bake in a 350° oven about 40 minutes or until a toothpick inserted near the center comes out clean. Cool in pan on a wire rack for 10 minutes. Remove from pan. Cool completely on a wire rack. If desired, sift powdered sugar over cake.

Nutrition Facts per serving: 186 cal., 4 g total fat (2 g sat. fat), 43 mg chol., 121 mg sodium, 34 g carbo., 1 g fiber, 4 g pro.
Exchanges: 1 Starch, 1 Other Carbo., 1 Fat

Citrus Pumpkin Flan

Bake: 40 minutes Chill: 4 to 24 hours Oven: 325°F Makes: 4 servings

⅔ cup sugar

¾ cup refrigerated or frozen egg product, thawed

¾ cup canned pumpkin

1 5-ounce can (⅔ cup) evaporated fat-free milk

¼ cup sugar

1 teaspoon pumpkin pie spice*

1 teaspoon finely shredded orange peel

1 teaspoon vanilla

1. To caramelize sugar, in a heavy medium skillet heat the ⅔ cup sugar over medium-high heat until sugar begins to melt, shaking skillet occasionally to heat evenly (do not stir). Reduce heat to low; cook sugar until melted and golden brown, stirring as necessary with a wooden spoon. Quickly divide caramelized sugar among four 6-ounce custard cups; tilt cups to coat bottoms evenly.

2. Place custard cups in a 3-quart rectangular baking dish. In a medium bowl stir together egg product, pumpkin, evaporated milk, the ¼ cup sugar, pumpkin pie spice, orange peel, and vanilla. Pour pumpkin mixture over caramelized sugar in cups. Place dish on oven rack. Pour boiling water into dish around cups to a depth of 1 inch.

3. Bake in a 325° oven for 40 to 45 minutes or until a knife inserted near the centers comes out clean. Remove cups from pan. Cool slightly. Cover; refrigerate for 4 to 24 hours.

4. To serve, loosen edges of flans with a knife, slipping the point down the sides to let air in. Invert flans onto four dessert plates, spooning caramelized sugar onto flans.

*Note: To make your own pumpkin pie spice, stir together ½ teaspoon ground cinnamon, ¼ teaspoon ground ginger, ⅛ teaspoon ground nutmeg, and ⅛ teaspoon ground allspice.

Nutrition Facts per serving: 287 cal., 4 g total fat (1 g sat. fat), 161 mg chol., 100 mg sodium, 55 g carbo., 1 g fiber, 8 g pro.
Exchanges: ½ Milk, ½ Lean Meat, ½ Fat

Lunch Box Oatmeal Cookies

Prep: 25 minutes Bake: 7 minutes per batch Oven: 375°F Makes: about 40 cookies

½ cup butter or margarine, softened

½ cup reduced-fat peanut butter

⅓ cup granulated sugar

⅓ cup packed brown sugar

½ teaspoon baking soda

2 egg whites

½ teaspoon vanilla

1 cup all-purpose flour

1 cup quick-cooking rolled oats

1. In a large mixing bowl beat butter and peanut butter with an electric mixer on medium to high speed about 30 seconds or until combined.

2. Add granulated sugar, brown sugar, and baking soda. Beat until combined, scraping side of bowl occasionally. Beat in egg whites and vanilla until combined. Beat in as much flour as you can with the mixer. Stir in any remaining flour. Stir in oats.

3. Drop dough by rounded teaspoons 2 inches apart on ungreased cookie sheets. Bake in a 375° oven for 7 to 8 minutes or until edges are golden. Cool on cookie sheet for 1 minute. Transfer to a wire rack and let cool.

Nutrition Facts per cookie: 76 cal., 4 g total fat (2 g sat. fat), 7 mg chol., 69 mg sodium, 9 g carbo., 1 g fiber, 2 g pro.
Exchanges: ½ Other Carbo., ½ Fat

Chocolate Soufflés

Prep: 30 minutes Bake: 25 minutes Oven: 350°F Makes: 8 soufflés

⅔ cup granulated sugar

⅓ cup unsweetened cocoa
   powder

1 tablespoon all-purpose flour

⅛ teaspoon salt

½ cup fat-free milk

2 egg yolks

4 egg whites

1 teaspoon vanilla

⅛ teaspoon cream of tartar

   Sifted powdered sugar (optional)

1. Place eight 6-ounce ramekins in a shallow baking pan; set aside.

2. In a small saucepan stir together ⅓ cup of the granulated sugar, the cocoa powder, flour, and salt. Gradually stir in milk. Cook and stir over medium-high heat until thickened and bubbly. Reduce heat; cook and stir for 1 minute more. Remove from heat. Slightly beat egg yolks. Slowly add chocolate mixture to egg yolks, stirring constantly.

3. In a large mixing bowl combine egg whites, vanilla, and cream of tartar. Beat with an electric mixer on high speed until soft peaks form (tips curl). Gradually add the remaining ⅓ cup granulated sugar, beating on high speed until stiff peaks form (tips stand straight). Stir about one-fourth of the egg whites into chocolate mixture to lighten. Gently fold chocolate mixture into egg white mixture. Spoon into ramekins.

4. Bake in a 350° oven about 25 minutes or until knife inserted near centers comes out clean. If desired, sprinkle with powdered sugar. Serve immediately.

Nutrition facts per soufflé: 109 cal., 2 g total fat (0 g sat. fat), 52 mg chol., 73 mg sodium, 19 g carbo., 0 g fiber, 4 g pro.
Exchanges: 1 Other Carbo., 1 Medium-Fat Meat

Mini Cheesecakes

Prep: 20 minutes Bake: 18 minutes Stand: 5 minutes Chill: 4 hours Oven: 325°F
Makes: 10 mini cheesecakes

Nonstick cooking spray

$^1/_3$ cup crushed vanilla wafers (about 8 wafers)

$1^1/_2$ 8-ounce tubs fat-free cream cheese, softened (12 ounces total)

$^1/_2$ cup sugar

1 tablespoon all-purpose flour

1 teaspoon vanilla

$^1/_4$ cup refrigerated or frozen egg product, thawed

$^3/_4$ cup fresh fruit (such as halved grapes, cut-up pineapple, cut-up peeled kiwifruit or papaya, red raspberries, blueberries, sliced strawberries, sliced plums, and/or orange and grapefruit sections)

1. Coat ten $2^1/_2$-inch muffin cups with cooking spray. Sprinkle the bottom and side of each cup with a rounded teaspoon of the crushed vanilla wafers. Set aside.

2. In a medium mixing bowl beat the cream cheese with an electric mixer on medium speed until smooth. Add sugar, flour, and vanilla. Beat on medium speed until smooth. Add egg product; beat on low speed just until combined. Divide evenly among the prepared muffin cups.

3. Bake in a 325° oven for 18 to 20 minutes or until set. Cool in muffin cups on a wire rack for 5 minutes. Cover and refrigerate for 4 to 24 hours.

4. Remove the cheesecakes from muffin cups. Just before serving, top the cheesecakes with fresh fruit.

Nutrition Facts per mini cheesecake: 97 cal., 1 g total fat (0 g sat. fat), 5 mg chol., 24 mg sodium, 17 g carbo., 0 g fiber, 6 g pro.
Exchanges: 1 Milk, $^1/_2$ Other Carbo.

Warm Chocolate Bread Pudding

Prep: 25 minutes Bake: 15 minutes Oven: 350°F Makes: 2 servings

Nonstick cooking spray

1 cup firm-textured white bread cubes (about 1¼ slices of Italian or sourdough bread)

⅓ cup fat-free milk

2 tablespoons granulated sugar

2 tablespoons miniature semisweet chocolate pieces

3 tablespoons refrigerated or frozen egg product, thawed, or 1 egg

½ teaspoon finely shredded orange or tangerine peel

¼ teaspoon vanilla

Powdered sugar or fat-free pressurized whipped dessert topping (optional)

1. Coat two 6-ounce individual soufflé dishes or custard cups with cooking spray. Divide the bread cubes between the prepared dishes.

2. In a small saucepan combine the milk, granulated sugar, and chocolate pieces. Cook and stir over low heat until chocolate is melted. Remove from heat. If necessary, use a wire whisk to beat until smooth.

3. In a small bowl combine the egg product, orange peel, and vanilla. Gradually stir in the chocolate mixture. Pour over the bread cubes in dishes. Press lightly with the back of a spoon to thoroughly moisten bread. If desired, cover and refrigerate for up to 2 hours before baking.

4. Bake, uncovered, in a 350° oven for 15 to 20 minutes until the tops appear firm and a knife inserted near centers comes out clean. Cool slightly on a wire rack. If desired, sift powdered sugar over the warm puddings.

Nutrition Facts per serving: 163 cal., 4 g total fat (0 g sat. fat), 0 mg chol., 125 mg sodium, 29 g carbo., 0 g fiber, 5 g pro.
Exchanges: 2½ Fat

Cinnamon Raisin Apple Indian Pudding

Prep: 20 minutes Bake: 30 minutes Cool: 20 minutes Oven: 350°F Makes: 6 servings

Nonstick cooking spray

2 cups fat-free milk

⅓ cup yellow cornmeal

2 tablespoons packed brown sugar

½ teaspoon ground cinnamon

¼ teaspoon salt

1 egg

2 medium cooking apples, chopped

¼ cup raisins

1. Lightly coat six 6-ounce custard cups with cooking spray; place in a shallow baking pan and set aside.

2. In a medium saucepan heat 1½ cups of the milk over medium heat just until boiling. In a small bowl combine cornmeal with the remaining ½ cup milk; slowly whisk into hot milk. Cook and stir until mixture returns to boiling. Reduce heat to low. Cook and stir for 5 to 7 minutes or until thick. Remove from heat. Stir in brown sugar, cinnamon, and salt.

3. In a small bowl beat egg with a fork; gradually stir the hot mixture into egg. Stir in apples and raisins. Divide mixture among prepared custard cups.

4. Bake in a 350° oven about 30 minutes or until a knife inserted in centers comes out clean. Cool on a wire rack for 20 minutes; serve warm.

Nutrition Facts per serving: 129 cal., 1 g total fat (0 g sat. fat), 37 mg chol., 146 mg sodium, 26 g carbo., 2 g fiber, 5 g pro.
Daily Values: 5% vit. A, 4% vit. C, 12% calcium, 3% iron
Exchanges: ½ Milk, ½ Fruit, 1 Other Carbo.

Peachy Rice Pudding

Start to Finish: 30 minutes Makes: 5 servings

1⅓ cups water

⅔ cup uncooked long grain rice

½ of a 12-ounce can (¾ cup)
   evaporated fat-free milk

⅓ cup mixed dried fruit bits

2 teaspoons honey

¼ teaspoon pumpkin pie spice or
   ground cinnamon

⅛ teaspoon salt

1 cup sliced peeled peaches or
   frozen sliced peaches, thawed

¼ cup fat-free vanilla yogurt

   Pumpkin pie spice or ground
   cinnamon (optional)

1. In a medium saucepan stir together the
water and uncooked rice. Bring to boiling;
reduce heat. Simmer, covered, for 15 to
20 minutes or until rice is tender.

2. Stir evaporated milk, fruit bits, honey, the
¼ teaspoon pumpkin pie spice, and the salt
into cooked rice. Bring just to boiling; reduce
heat to medium-low. Cook, uncovered, about
5 minutes or until mixture is thick and
creamy, stirring frequently. Serve pudding
warm, topped with peaches and yogurt. If
desired, sprinkle with additional pumpkin
pie spice.

Nutrition Facts per serving: 175 cal., 0 g total fat (0 g sat. fat), 2 mg
chol., 120 mg sodium, 47 g carbo., 1 g fiber, 6 g pro.
Exchanges: 1½ Fruit, 1½ Starch

healthy eating
meal plans

The following Healthy Eating Meal Plan checklists are a smart tool that can help you get your diet on track. Use them to get an idea of healthy portion sizes and types of foods to have at each meal.

Tips for using the meal plans:

- Check off your daily water/fluid intake in the appropriate place under Snack "B."
- When you take your vitamin each day, you can check that off next to the reminder under each plan.
- If you are still hungry and you have used all of your exchanges for the day, fill up on vegetables and lean protein.
- Some foods are considered "combination foods," and they will count under more than one food group/exchange: 1 medium egg is both 1 lean protein source and 1 fat, as are 10–15 nuts and 1 tablespoon peanut butter. When eating a combination food, take your best guess as to how to count it. One slice of cheese pizza is approximately 1 starch, 1 ounce of lean meat/meat substitute, and 1–2 fats.
- Copy the checklists and take them with you when you grocery shop to help increase your variety!
- Use these meal plans as a tool. They are not meant to be a strict diet but to provide a sense of what a calorie-controlled and nutritionally balanced day can look like.

1,600 calories: Postpartum, Not Breastfeeding

BREAKFAST

Fruit/Fruit juices (choose 1)	Starches (choose 2)	Milk/Yogurt (choose 1)	Fats (choose 2)
☐ 3–4 oz juice	☐ ½ small bagel	☐ 1 c fat-free milk	☐ 1 tsp butter
☐ 1 small banana	☐ 1 slice bread/toast	☐ 1 c low-fat milk	☐ 1 tsp margarine
☐ 1 apple/orange/pear	☐ ½ English muffin	☐ 1 c soymilk	☐ 1 tsp oil
☐ ¾ c pineapple	☐ ¾ c dry cereal	☐ ¾ c fortified rice milk	☐ 1 Tbsp low-fat margarine
☐ ½ grapefruit	☐ ½ c hot cereal	☐ 1 c evap milk (low-fat)	☐ 2 Tbsp sour cream
☐ 1 c cut-up melon or berries	☐ 3–4 graham crackers	☐ 8 oz low-fat yogurt	☐ 1 Tbsp cream cheese
☐ ½ c fruit salad	☐ 1 small pancake	**Lean Meat/Meat Substitutes** (Choose 1)	☐ 2 Tbsp half-and-half
☐ 12–15 cherries/grapes	☐ 1 small waffle	☐ 1 slice cheese	☐ 1 slice bacon
☐ 2 plums/kiwifruits		☐ ¼ c cottage cheese	☐ 2 Tbsp flaxseed
☐ 3 prunes		☐ 1 medium egg (+1 fat)	
☐ 2 Tbsp raisins		☐ ¼ c egg substitute	
☐ ½ c canned fruit in juice or water		☐ 10–15 nuts (+1 fat)	
		☐ 1 Tbsp peanut butter (+1 fat)	

LUNCH

Starches (choose 2)	Lean Meat/ Meat Substitutes (choose 2)	Vegetables (choose 1 minimum)	Fats (choose 2)	Fruit/Fruit juices (choose 1)
☐ ½ bagel	☐ 1 oz turkey/ chicken	☐ ½ c cooked vegetables	☐ 1 tsp butter	☐ 3–4 oz juice
☐ ½ 6" pita	☐ 1 oz fish	- carrots	☐ 1 tsp margarine	☐ 1 small banana
☐ 1 slice bread/ toast	☐ 1 oz beef	- beets	☐ 1 tsp oil	☐ 1 apple/orange/ pear
☐ 1 flour/corn tortilla	☐ 1 medium egg (+1 fat)	- broccoli	☐ 1 Tbsp low-fat marg	☐ ¾ c pineapple
☐ ⅓ c pasta/ noodles	☐ 1 oz lean ham/ pork	- cauliflower	☐ 2 Tbsp sour cream	☐ ½ grapefruit
☐ ½ English muffin	☐ ½ c beans or ¼ c hummus	- spinach	☐ 1 Tbsp cream cheese	☐ 1 c cut-up melon/ berries
☐ ¾ c cereal	☐ 1 oz feta cheese	- greens	☐ 2 Tbsp half-and- half	☐ ½ c fruit salad
☐ 1 small baked potato	☐ ¼ c egg substitute	- cabbage	☐ ⅛ avocado	☐ 12–15 cherries/ grapes
☐ ½ c mashed potato	☐ 1 Tbsp peanut butter (+1 fat)	- asparagus	☐ 1 tsp mayo	☐ 2 plums/ kiwifruits
☐ 6 crackers	☐ 1 oz low-fat cheese	- green beans	☐ 1 Tbsp salad dressing	☐ 3 prunes
☐ ½ c peas or corn	☐ 1–2 oz tuna in water	- other	☐ 2 Tbsp light dressing	☐ 2 Tbsp raisins
☐ ½ c beans or legumes (may count as protein)	☐ 1 oz seafood	☐ 1 c raw vegetables	☐ 2 tsp Miracle Whip salad dressing	☐ ½ cup canned fruit in juice or water
☐ ⅓ c rice	☐ 1–2 oz veggie burger	- lettuce		☐ ¼ c dried fruit
☐ ⅔ c lentils	☐ 1–2 oz salmon, canned	- tomato		
☐ 1 c soup	☐ 2 oz tofu	- cucumber		☐ **+1 c milk/ yogurt**
☐ ½ hamburger/ hot dog bun		- celery		
☐ 1 c winter squash		- peppers		
		- onions		
		- other		
		☐ ½ c chunky veggie tomato sauce		
		☐ 4–6 oz tomato/ V8 juice		

DINNER

Starches (choose 2)	Lean Meat/Meat Substitutes (choose 3)	Vegetables (choose 2 minimum)	Fats (choose 2–3)	Fruit/Fruit juices (choose 1)
☐ ½ 6" pita	☐ 1 oz turkey/ chicken	☐ ½ c cooked vegetables	☐ 1 tsp butter	☐ 3–4 oz juice
☐ 1 slice bread	☐ 1 oz fish	- carrots	☐ 1 tsp margarine	☐ 1 small banana
☐ 1 flour/corn tortilla	☐ 1 oz beef	- beets	☐ 1 tsp oil	☐ 1 apple/orange/ pear
☐ ⅓ c pasta/ noodles	☐ 1 medium egg (+1 fat)	- broccoli	☐ 1 Tbsp low-fat margarine	☐ ¾ c pineapple
☐ ½ English muffin	☐ 1 oz lean ham/ pork	- cauliflower	☐ 2 Tbsp sour cream	☐ ½ grapefruit
☐ ¾ c cereal	☐ ½ c beans	- spinach	☐ 1 Tbsp cream cheese	☐ 1 c cut-up melon/berries
☐ 1 small baked potato	☐ 1 oz feta cheese	- greens	☐ 2 Tbsp half-and-half	☐ ½ c fruit salad
☐ ½ c mashed potato	☐ ¼ c egg substitute	- cabbage	☐ ⅛ avocado	☐ 12–15 cherries/ grapes
☐ 6 crackers	☐ 1 Tbsp peanut butter (+1 Fat)	- asparagus	☐ 1 tsp mayo	☐ 2 plums/ kiwifruits
☐ ½ c peas or corn	☐ 1 oz low-fat cheese	- green beans	☐ 1 Tbsp salad dressing	☐ 3 prunes
☐ ½ c beans or legumes	☐ 1–2 oz tuna in water	- other	☐ 2 Tbsp light dressing	☐ 2 Tbsp raisins
☐ ⅓ c rice	☐ 1 oz seafood	☐ 1 c raw vegetables	☐ 2 tsp Miracle Whip salad dressing	☐ ½ c canned fruit in juice or water
☐ ⅔ c lentils	☐ 1–2 oz veggie burger	- lettuce		☐ ¼ c dried fruit
☐ 1 c soup	☐ 1–2 oz salmon, canned	- tomato		☐ 1 small mango
☐ ½ hamburger/ hot dog bun/ dinner roll	☐ 2 oz tofu	- cucumber		
☐ 1 c winter squash		- celery		
		- peppers		
		- onions		
		- other		
		☐ ½ c chunky veggie tomato sauce		
		☐ 4 oz tomato/ V8 juice		

SNACK A (choose 1)

- ☐ 1 slice low-fat cheese + 3 small crackers
- ☐ Small snack bar such as Pria or Luna
- ☐ ¼ c hummus or bean dip w/veggies
- ☐ 1 hard-cooked egg + 3 whole grain crackers such as Triscuits
- ☐ 1 oz bag soy crisps such as Glenny's or Stacy's
- ☐ 2 c air-popped popcorn + 1 low-fat string cheese
- ☐ 1 small fruit + 10 nuts
- ☐ ¾ c high-protein, high-fiber cereal such as Kashi GOLEAN
- ☐ 1 Tbsp peanut butter w/celery

SNACK B (choose 1)

- ☐ 1 c yogurt
- ☐ 1 c fat-free/low-fat milk
- ☐ 1 c soymilk
- ☐ ¾ c fortified rice milk
- ☐ ½ c low-fat frozen yogurt

- ☐ 1–2 oz lean meat/ meat substitutes + vegs if still hungry

Extras

☐☐☐☐☐☐☐☐
8 cups water/day

Activity

Vitamin supplement?
This plan provides 7 starch servings, 6–7oz protein, 3 servings vegetables minimum, 3 fruit servings, 3 milk servings, and 7 added-fat servings/day.

1,800 calories: Postpartum, Breastfeeding or Overweight Pregnancy

BREAKFAST

Fruit/Fruit juices (choose 1)	Starches (choose 2)	Milk/Yogurt (choose 1)	Fats (choose 1-2)
☐ 3–4 oz juice ☐ 1 small banana ☐ 1 apple/orange/pear ☐ ¾ c pineapple ☐ ½ grapefruit ☐ 1 c cut-up melon or berries ☐ ½ c fruit salad ☐ 12–15 cherries/grapes ☐ 2 plums/kiwifruits ☐ 3 prunes ☐ 2 Tbsp raisins ☐ ½ c canned fruit in juice or water	☐ ½ small bagel ☐ 1 slice bread/toast ☐ ½ English muffin ☐ ¾ c dry cereal ☐ ½ c hot cereal ☐ 3–4 graham crackers ☐ 1 small pancake ☐ 1 small waffle	☐ 1 c fat-free milk ☐ 1 c low-fat milk ☐ 1 c soymilk ☐ ¾ c fortified rice milk ☐ 1 c evaporated milk (low-fat) ☐ 8 oz low-fat yogurt **Lean Meat/Meat Substitutes (choose 1)** ☐ 1 slice cheese ☐ ¼ c cottage cheese ☐ 1 medium egg (+1 fat) ☐ ¼ c egg substitute ☐ 10–15 nuts (+1 fat) ☐ 1 Tbsp peanut butter (+1 fat)	☐ 1 tsp butter ☐ 1 tsp marg. ☐ 1 tsp oil ☐ 1 Tbsp low-fat margarine ☐ 2 Tbsp sour cream ☐ 1 Tbsp cream cheese ☐ 2 Tbsp half-and-half ☐ 1 slice bacon

LUNCH

Starches (choose 2)	Lean Meat/ Meat Substitutes (choose 2)	Vegetables (choose 1 minimum)	Fats (choose 2–3)	Fruit/Fruit juices (choose 1)
☐ ½ bagel ☐ ½ 6" pita ☐ 1 slice bread/ toast ☐ 1 flour/corn tortilla ☐ ⅓ c pasta/ noodles ☐ ½ English muffin ☐ ¾ c cereal ☐ 1 small baked potato ☐ ½ c mashed potato ☐ 6 saltine crackers ☐ ½ c peas or corn ☐ ½ c beans or legumes (may count as protein) ☐ ⅓ c rice ☐ ⅔ c lentils ☐ 1 c soup ☐ ½ hamburger/ hot dog bun ☐ 1 c winter squash	☐ 1 oz turkey/ chicken ☐ 1 oz fish ☐ 1 oz beef ☐ 1 medium egg (+1 fat) ☐ 1 oz lean ham/ pork ☐ ½ c beans or ¼ c hummus ☐ 1 oz feta cheese ☐ ¼ c egg substitute ☐ 1 Tbsp peanut butter (+1 fat) ☐ 1 oz low-fat cheese ☐ 1–2 oz tuna in water ☐ 1 oz seafood ☐ 1–2 oz veggie burger ☐ 1–2 oz salmon, canned ☐ 2 oz tofu	☐ ½ c cooked vegetables - carrots - beets - broccoli - cauliflower - spinach - greens - cabbage - asparagus - green beans - other ☐ 1 c raw vegetables - lettuce - tomato - cucumber - celery - peppers - onions - other ☐ ½ c chunky veggie tomato sauce ☐ 4–6 oz tomato/ V8 juice	☐ 1 tsp butter ☐ 1 tsp marg. ☐ 1 tsp oil ☐ 1 Tbsp low-fat margarine ☐ 2 Tbsp sour cream ☐ 1 Tbsp cream cheese ☐ 2 Tbsp half-and-half ☐ ⅛ avocado ☐ 1 tsp mayo ☐ 1 Tbsp salad dressing ☐ 2 Tbsp light dressing ☐ 2 tsp Miracle Whip salad dressing	☐ 3–4 oz juice ☐ 1 small banana ☐ 1 apple/orange/ pear ☐ ¾ c pineapple ☐ ½ grapefruit ☐ 1 c cut-up melon/berries ☐ ½ c fruit salad ☐ 12–15 cherries/ grapes ☐ 2 plums/ kiwifruits ☐ 3 prunes ☐ 2 Tbsp raisins ☐ ½ c canned fruit in juice or water ☐ ¼ c dried fruit **☐ +1 cup milk/ yogurt**

DINNER

Starches (choose 2)	Lean Meat/Meat Substitutes (choose 4)	Vegetables (choose 2 minimum)	Fats (choose 2-3)	Fruit/Fruit juices (choose 1)
□ ½ bagel	□ 1 oz turkey/	□ ½ c cooked	□ 1 tsp butter	□ 3-4 oz juice
□ ½ 6" pita	chicken	vegetables	□ 1 tsp margarine	□ 1 small banana
□ 1 slice bread	□ 1 oz fish	- carrots	□ 1 tsp oil	□ 1 apple/orange/
□ 1 flour/corn	□ 1 oz beef	- beets	□ 1 Tbsp low-fat	pear
tortilla	□ 1 medium egg	- broccoli	margarine	□ ¾ c pineapple
□ ⅓ c pasta/	(+1 fat)	- cauliflower	□ 2 Tbsp sour	□ ½ grapefruit
noodles	□ 1 oz lean ham/	- spinach	cream	□ 1 c cut-up
□ ½ English	pork	- greens	□ 1 Tbsp cream	melon/berries
muffin	□ ½ c beans	- cabbage	cheese	□ ½ c fruit salad
□ ¾ c cereal	□ 1 oz feta cheese	- asparagus	□ 2 Tbsp half-and-	□ 12–15 cherries/
□ 1 small baked	□ ¼ c egg	- green beans	half	grapes
potato	substitute	- other	□ ⅛ avocado	□ 2 plums/
□ ½ c mashed	□ 1 Tbsp peanut	□ 1 c raw	□ 1 tsp mayo	kiwifruits
potato	butter (+1 fat)	vegetables	□ 1 Tbsp salad	□ 3 prunes
□ 6 saltine	□ 1 oz low-fat	- lettuce	dressing	□ 2 Tbsp raisins
crackers	cheese	- tomato	□ 2 Tbsp light	□ ½ c canned fruit
□ ½ c peas or corn	□ 1 oz tuna in	- cucumber	dressing	in juice or water
□ ½ c beans or	water	- celery	□ 2 tsp Miracle	□ ¼ c dried fruit
legumes	□ 1 oz seafood	- peppers	Whip salad	□ 1 small mango
□ ⅓ c rice	□ 1–2 oz veggie	- onions	dressing	
□ ⅔ c lentils	burger	- other		
□ 1 c soup	□ 1 oz salmon,	□ ½ c chunky		
□ ½ hamburger/	canned	veggie tomato		
hot dog bun/	□ 2 oz tofu	sauce		
dinner roll		□ 4 oz tomato/V8		
□ 1 c winter		juice		
squash				

SNACK A (choose 1-2) | SNACK B (choose 1) | Extras | Activity

SNACK A (choose 1-2)	SNACK B (choose 1)	Extras	Activity
□ 1 slice low-fat cheese + 3 small crackers	□ 1 c yogurt		
	□ 1 c 1% milk		
□ Small snack bar such as Luna or Pria	□ 1 c soymilk		
	□ ¾ c fortified rice milk		
□ ¼ c hummus or bean dip w/veggies	□ ½ c fat free frozen yogurt		
□ 1 hard-boiled egg + 3 whole grain crackers such as Triscuits	□ (1–2 oz lean meat/ meat substitutes + vegs if still hungry		
□ 1 oz bag soy crisps such as Glenny's or Stacy's	□□□□□□□□ **8 c water/day**		
□ 2 c air-popped popcorn + 1 low-fat string cheese			
□ 1 small fruit + 10 nuts			
□ ¾ c high-protein/ high-fiber cereal such as Kashi GOLEAN			
□ 1 Tbsp peanut butter w/celery			

Vitamin supplement?
This plan provides 7–8 starch servings, 7–8 oz protein, 3 servings vegetables minimum, 3 fruit servings, 3 milk servings, and 8 added-fat servings/day.

2,000–2,200 calories: Normal-weight pregnancy

BREAKFAST

Fruit/Fruit juices (choose 1)	Starches (choose 2)	Milk/Yogurt (choose 1)	Fats (choose 2-3)
☐ 3–4 oz juice	☐ ½ small bagel	☐ 1 c fat-free milk	☐ 1 tsp butter
☐ 1 small banana	☐ 1 slice bread/toast	☐ 1 c low-fat milk	☐ 1 tsp margarine
☐ 1 apple/orange/pear	☐ ½ English muffin	☐ 1 c soymilk	☐ 1 tsp oil
☐ ¾ c pineapple	☐ ¾ c dry cereal	☐ ¾ c fortified rice milk	☐ 1 Tbsp low-fat
☐ ½ grapefruit	☐ ½ c hot cereal	☐ 1 c evap. milk	margarine
☐ 1 c cut-up melon/	☐ 3–4 graham crackers	(reduced-fat)	☐ 2 Tbsp sour cream
berries	☐ 1 small pancake	☐ 8 oz low-fat yogurt	☐ 1 Tbsp cream cheese
☐ ½ c fruit salad	☐ 1 small waffle		☐ 2 Tbsp half-and-half
☐ 12–15 cherries/grapes		**Lean Meat/Meat**	☐ 1 slice bacon
☐ 2 plums/kiwifruits		**Substitutes** (choose 2)	
☐ 3 prunes		☐ 1 slice low-fat cheese	
☐ 2 Tbsp raisins		☐ ¼ c cottage cheese	
☐ ½ c canned fruit in		☐ 1 medium egg	
juice or water		(+1 fat)	
		☐ ¼ c egg substitute	
		☐ 10–15 nuts (+1 fat)	
		☐ 1 Tbsp peanut butter	
		(+1 fat)	

LUNCH

Starches (choose 3)	Lean Meat/ Meat Substitutes (choose 3)	Vegetables (choose 2 minimum)	Fats (choose 2–3)	Fruit/Fruit juices (choose 1–2)
☐ ½ bagel	☐ 1 oz turkey/	☐ ½ c cooked	☐ 1 tsp butter	☐ 3-4 oz juice
☐ ½ 6" pita	chicken	vegetables	☐ 1 tsp margarine	☐ 1 small banana
☐ 1 slice bread/	☐ 1 oz fish	- carrots	☐ 1 tsp oil	☐ 1 apple/orange/
toast	☐ 1 oz beef	- beets	☐ 1 Tbsp low-fat	pear
☐ 1 flour/corn	☐ 1 medium egg	- broccoli	margarine	☐ ¾ c pineapple
tortilla	(+1 fat)	- cauliflower	☐ 2 Tbsp sour	☐ ½ grapefruit
☐ ⅓ c pasta/	☐ 1 oz lean ham/	- spinach	cream	☐ 1 c cut-up
noodles	pork	- greens	☐ 1 Tbsp cream	melon/berries
☐ ½ English	☐ ½ c beans or	- cabbage	cheese	☐ ½ c fruit salad
muffin	¼ c hummus	- asparagus	☐ 2 Tbsp half-and-	☐ 12-15 cherries/
☐ ⅓ c cereal	☐ 1 oz feta cheese	- green beans	half	grapes
☐ 1 small baked	☐ ¼ c egg	- other	☐ ⅛ avocado	☐ 2 plums/
potato	substitute	☐ 1 c raw	☐ 1 tsp mayo	kiwifruits
☐ ½ c mashed	☐ 1 Tbsp peanut	vegetables	☐ 1 Tbsp salad	☐ 3 prunes
potato	butter (+ 1 fat)	- lettuce	dressing	☐ 2 Tbsp raisins
☐ 6 saltine	☐ 1 oz low-fat	- tomato	☐ 2 Tbsp light	☐ ½ c canned fruit
crackers	cheese	- cucumber	dressing	in juice or water
☐ ½ c baked	☐ 1-2 oz tuna in	- celery	☐ 2 tsp Miracle	☐ ¼ c dried fruit
plantains	water	- peppers	Whip salad	
☐ ½ c peas or corn	☐ 1 oz seafood	- onions	dressing	☐ +1–2 c milk/
☐ ½ c beans or	☐ 1-2 oz veggie	- other		**yogurt**
legumes (may	burger	☐ ½ c chunky		
count as	☐ 1-2 oz salmon,	veggie tomato		
protein)	canned	sauce		
☐ ⅓ c rice	☐ 2 oz tofu	☐ 4-6 oz tomato/		
☐ ⅔ c lentils		V8 juice		
☐ 1 c soup				
☐ ½ hamburger/				
hot dog bun				
☐ 1 c winter				
squash				

DINNER

Starches (choose 3)	Lean Meat/ Meat Substitutes (choose 3)	Vegetables (choose 2 minimum)	Fats (choose 3)	Fruit/Fruit juices (choose 1)
☐ ½ bagel ☐ ½ 6" pita ☐ 1 slice bread ☐ 1 flour/corn tortilla ☐ ⅓ c pasta/ noodles ☐ ½ English muffin ☐ ¾ c cereal ☐ 1 small baked potato ☐ ½ c mashed potato ☐ 6 saltine crackers ☐ ½ c peas or corn ☐ ½ c beans or legumes ☐ ⅓ c rice ☐ ⅔ c lentils ☐ 1 c soup ☐ ½ hamburger/ hot dog bun/ dinner roll ☐ 1 c winter squash	☐ 1 oz turkey/ chicken ☐ 1 oz fish ☐ 1 oz beef ☐ 1 medium egg (+1 fat) ☐ 1 oz lean ham/ pork ☐ ½ c beans ☐ 1 oz feta cheese ☐ ¼ c egg substitute ☐ 1 Tbsp peanut butter (+1 fat) ☐ 1 oz low-fat cheese ☐ 1–2 oz tuna in water ☐ 1 oz seafood ☐ 1–2 oz veggie burger ☐ 1–2 oz salmon, canned ☐ 2 oz tofu	☐ ½ c cooked vegetables - carrots - beets - broccoli - cauliflower - spinach - greens - cabbage - asparagus - green beans - other ☐ 1 c raw vegetables - lettuce - tomato - cucumber - celery - peppers - onions - other ☐ ½ c chunky veggie tomato sauce ☐ 4 oz tomato/V8 juice	☐ 1 tsp butter ☐ 1 tsp margarine ☐ 1 tsp oil ☐ 1 Tbsp low-fat margarine ☐ 2 Tbsp sour cream ☐ 1 Tbsp cream cheese ☐ 2 Tbsp half- and-half ☐ ⅛ avocado ☐ 1 tsp mayo ☐ 1 Tbsp salad dressing ☐ 2 Tbsp light dressing ☐ 2 tsp Miracle Whip salad dressing	☐ 3-4 oz juice ☐ 1 small banana ☐ 1 apple/orange/ pear ☐ ¾ c pineapple ☐ ½ grapefruit ☐ 1 c cut-up melon/ berries ☐ ½ c fruit salad ☐ 12–15 cherries/ grapes ☐ 2 plums/kiwifruits ☐ 3 prunes ☐ 2 Tbsp raisins ☐ ½ c canned fruit in juice or water ☐ ¼ c dried fruit ☐ 1 small mango

SNACK A (choose 1-2)	SNACK B (choose 1)	Extras	Activity
☐ 1 slice low-fat cheese + 3 small crackers ☐ Small snack bar such as Pria or Luna ☐ ¼ c hummus or bean dip w/veggies ☐ 1 hard-cooked egg + 3 whole grain crackers such as Triscuits ☐ 1 oz bag soy crisps such as Glenny's or Stacy's ☐ 2 c air-popped popcorn + 1 low-fat string cheese ☐ 1 small fruit + 10 nuts ☐ ¾ c high-protein/ high-fiber cereal such as Kashi GOLEAN ☐ 1 Tbsp peanut butter w/celery	☐ 1 c yogurt ☐ 1 c low-fat milk ☐ 1 c soymilk ☐ ¾ c rice milk ☐ ½ c fat free frozen yogurt ☐ (1–2 oz lean meat/meat substitutes + vegs if still hungry ☐☐☐☐☐☐☐☐☐ **8 c water/day**		

Vitamin supplement??
This plan provides 9–10 starch servings, 9–10 oz protein, 4 servings vegetables minimum, 4 fruit servings, 3–4 milk servings, and 9 added-fat servings/day.

2,400 calories: Underweight Pregnancy/Twins (minimum)

BREAKFAST

Fruit/Fruit juices (choose 1)	Starches (choose 2)	Milk/Yogurt (choose 1)	Fats (choose 2–3)
☐ 3–4 oz juice	☐ ½ small bagel	☐ 1 c fat-free milk	☐ 1 tsp butter
☐ 1 small banana	☐ 1 slice bread/toast	☐ 1 c low-fat milk	☐ 1 tsp margarine
☐ 1 apple/orange/pear	☐ ½ English muffin	☐ 1 c soymilk	☐ 1 tsp oil
☐ ¾ c pineapple	☐ ¾ c dry cereal	☐ ¾ c fortified rice milk	☐ 1 Tbsp low-fat margarine
☐ ½ grapefruit	☐ ½ c hot cereal	☐ 1 c evaporated milk (low-fat)	☐ 2 Tbsp sour cream
☐ 1 c cut-up melon/ berries	☐ 3–4 graham crackers	☐ 8 oz low-fat yogurt	☐ 1 Tbsp cream cheese
☐ ½ cup fruit salad	☐ 1 small pancake		☐ 2 Tbsp half-and-half
☐ 12–15 cherries/ grapes	☐ 1 small waffle	**Lean Meat/Meat Substitutes** (choose 2)	☐ 1 slice bacon
☐ 2 plums/kiwifruits		☐ 1 slice low-fat cheese	
☐ 3 prunes		☐ ¼ c cottage cheese	
☐ 2 Tbsp raisins		☐ 1 medium egg (+1 fat)	
☐ ½ c canned fruit in juice or water		☐ ¼ c egg substitute	
		☐ 10-15 nuts (+1 fat)	
		☐ 1 Tbsp peanut butter (+1 fat)	

LUNCH

Starches (choose 3)	Lean Meat/ Meat Substitutes (choose 3)	Vegetables (choose 3 minimum)	Fats (choose 3–4)	Fruit/Fruit juices (choose 2)
☐ ½ bagel	☐ 1 oz turkey/ chicken	☐ ½ c cooked vegetables	☐ 1 tsp butter	☐ 3–4 oz juice
☐ ½ 6" pita	☐ 1 oz fish	- carrots	☐ 1 tsp marg.	☐ 1 small banana
☐ 1 slice bread/ toast	☐ 1 oz beef	- beets	☐ 1 tsp oil	☐ 1 apple/orange/ pear
☐ 1 flour/corn tortilla	☐ 1 medium egg (+1 fat)	- broccoli	☐ 1 Tbsp low-fat marg	☐ ¾ c pineapple
☐ ⅓ c pasta/ noodles	☐ 1 oz lean ham/ pork	- cauliflower	☐ 2 Tbsp sour cream	☐ ½ grapefruit
☐ ½ English muffin	☐ ½ c beans or ¼ c hummus	- spinach	☐ 1 Tbsp cream cheese	☐ 1 c cut-up melon/berries
☐ ¾ c cereal	☐ 1 oz feta cheese	- greens	☐ 2 Tbsp half-and- half	☐ ½ c fruit salad
☐ 1 small baked potato	☐ ¼ c egg substitute	- cabbage	☐ ⅛ avocado	☐ 12–15 cherries/ grapes
☐ ½ c mashed potato	☐ 1 Tbsp peanut butter (+1 fat)	- asparagus	☐ 1 tsp mayo	☐ 2 plums/ kiwifruits
☐ 6 saltine crackers	☐ 1 oz low-fat cheese	- green beans	☐ 1 Tbsp salad dressing	☐ 3 prunes
☐ ½ c peas or corn	☐ 1–2 oz tuna in water	- other	☐ 2 Tbsp light dressing	☐ 2 Tbsp raisins
☐ ½ c beans or legumes (may count as protein)	☐ 1 oz seafood	☐ 1 c raw vegetables	☐ 2 tsp Miracle Whip salad dressing	☐ ½ c canned fruit in juice or water
☐ ⅓ c rice	☐ 1–2 oz veggie burger	- lettuce		☐ ¼ c dried fruit
☐ ⅔ c lentils	☐ 1–2 oz salmon canned	- tomato		
☐ 1 c soup	☐ 2 oz tofu	- cucumber		☐ **+2 c milk/ yogurt**
☐ ½ hamburger/ hot dog bun		- celery		
☐ 1 c winter squash		- peppers		
		- onions		
		- other		
		☐ ½ c chunky veggie tomato sauce		
		☐ 4-6 oz tomato/ V8 juice		

DINNER

Starches (choose 3)	Lean Meat/ Meat Substitutes (choose 3)	Vegetables (choose 2 minimum)	Fats (choose 3)	Fruit/Fruit juices (choose 1–2)
☐ ½ bagel ☐ ½ 6" pita ☐ 1 slice bread ☐ 1 flour/corn tortilla ☐ ⅓ c pasta/ noodles ☐ ½ English muffin ☐ ¾ c cereal ☐ 1 small baked potato ☐ ½ c mashed potato ☐ 6 saltine crackers ☐ ½ c peas or corn ☐ ½ c beans or legumes ☐ ⅓ c rice ☐ ⅔ c lentils ☐ 1 c soup ☐ ½ hamburger/ hot dog bun/ dinner roll ☐ 1 c winter squash	☐ 1 oz turkey/ chicken ☐ 1 oz fish ☐ 1 oz beef ☐ 1 medium egg (+1 fat) ☐ 1 oz lean ham/ pork ☐ ½ c beans ☐ 1 oz feta cheese ☐ ¼ c egg substitute ☐ 1 Tbsp peanut butter (+1 fat) ☐ 1 oz low-fat cheese ☐ 1–2 oz tuna in water ☐ 1 oz seafood ☐ 1–2 oz veggie burger ☐ 1–2 oz salmon canned ☐ 2 oz tofu	☐ ½ c cooked vegetables - carrots - beets - broccoli - cauliflower - spinach - greens - cabbage - asparagus - green beans - other ☐ 1 c raw vegetables - lettuce - tomato - cucumber - celery - peppers - onions - other ☐ ½ c chunky veggie tomato sauce ☐ 4 oz tomato/V8 juice	☐ 1 tsp butter ☐ 1 tsp margarine ☐ 1 tsp oil ☐ 1 Tbsp low-fat margarine ☐ 2 Tbsp sour cream ☐ 1 Tbsp cream cheese ☐ 2 Tbsp half-and-half ☐ ⅛ avocado ☐ 1 tsp mayo ☐ 1 Tbsp salad dressing ☐ 2 Tbsp light dressing ☐ 2 tsp Miracle Whip	☐ 3–4 oz juice ☐ 1 small banana ☐ 1 apple./ orange/pear ☐ ¾ c pineapple ☐ ½ grapefruit ☐ 1 c cut-up melon/berries ☐ ½ c fruit salad ☐ 12–15 cherries/ grapes ☐ 2 plums/ kiwifruits ☐ 3 prunes ☐ 2 tbsp raisins ☐ ½ c canned fruit in juice or water ☐ ¼ c dried fruit ☐ 1 small mango

SNACK A (choose 2)	SNACK B (choose 1)	Extras	Activity
☐ 1 slice low-fat cheese + 3 small crackers ☐ Small snack bar such as Pria or Luna ☐ ¼ c hummus or bean dip w/veggies ☐ 1 hard-cooked egg + 3 whole grain crackers such as Triscuits ☐ 1 oz bag Soy Crisps such as Glenny's or Stacy's ☐ 2 c air popped popcorn + 1 low-fat string cheese ☐ 1 small fruit + 10 nuts ☐ ¾ c high-protein, high-fiber cereal such as Kashi GOLEAN ☐ 1 Tbsp peanut butter w/celery	☐ 1 c yogurt ☐ 1 c low-fat milk ☐ 1 c soymilk ☐ ¾ c fortified rice milk ☐ ½ c fat-free frozen yogurt ☐ (1–2 oz lean meat/ meat substitutes + vegs if still hungry ☐☐☐☐☐☐☐☐ **8 c water/day**		

Vitamin supplement?
This plan provides 10 starch servings, 10 oz protein, 5 servings vegetables minimum, 5–6 fruit servings, 4 milk servings, and 10 added-fat servings/day.

Index

Recipe Index

You & Your BABY™

Essential Books

for Life's Most Amazing Journey

You & Your Baby: Pregnancy

This up-to-date, week-by-week pregnancy guide authored by Dr. Laura E. Riley, an OB/GYN who is a mother herself, answers everything expectant parents need to know in an easy-to-read and comforting manner. Eight full-color in-utero fetal photos deliver an unforgettable visual journey.

You & Your Baby: Pregnancy Organizer

This ideal companion helps mothers-to-be prepare for important events and track memorable milestones such as baby's first kick, prenatal appointments, diet plans and shopping lists, and more.

You & Your Baby: Healthy Eating During Pregnancy

With medically sound weight-management guidance and more than 200 great-tasting and healthy recipes, this is the ultimate guide on optimum nutrition and health for expectant mothers.

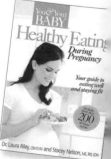

All-new *You & Your Baby*™ pregnancy book series authored by leading OB/GYN, Dr. Laura Riley.